NEUROANATOMY
A FUNCTIONAL ATLAS OF PARTS AND PATHWAYS

RAY PORITSKY, Ph.D.

Associate Professor
Department of Anatomy
Case Western University School of Medicine
Lecturer in Medical Illustration
Cleveland Institute of Art
Cleveland, Ohio

HANLEY & BELFUS, INC./Philadelphia
MOSBY — YEAR BOOK, INC./St. Louis • Baltimore • Boston • Chicago • London
Philadelphia • Toronto

Publisher: HANLEY & BELFUS, INC.
                  210 S. 13th Street
                  Philadelphia, PA 19107
                  (215) 546-7293

North American and worldwide sales and distribution:

                  MOSBY-YEAR BOOK, INC.
                  11830 Westline Industrial Drive
                  St. Louis, MO 63146

In Canada: THE C.V. MOSBY COMPANY, LTD.
                  5240 Finch Avenue East
                  Unit 1
                  Scarborough, Ontario M1S 5A2
                  Canada

NEUROANATOMY: A Functional Atlas of Parts and Pathways   ISBN   156053-008-1

Library of Congress catalog card number   91-77427

Last digit is the print number: 9   8   7   6   5   4   3   2

CONTENTS

PREFACE

This book presents the reader with a simple and direct method of learning the essentials of neuroanatomy. It illustrates the brain and spinal cord in easy-to-understand three-dimensional drawings. It allows the reader to learn the pathways and parts of the brain and spinal cord by reading about them and coloring and labeling them at the same time.

The author has lent heavy emphasis to explaining and understanding the basic terminology of the nervous system.

Carefully thought-out black and white illustrations explain and depict the basic structure of the brain and spinal cord and their major components. Recent discoveries about their functions and interrelationships are represented.

The illustrations of the structure of the eye and ear are comprehenisve and reveal their ultra-structure in exceptional detail.

Some of the long pathways involve tearing out successive pages, pasting them together, and tracing the tracts using different color pencils for each modality. This results in large colored "road maps" of the ascending sensory tracts and the descending motor tracts.

Instead of simply reading about these vital structures, the reader is able to learn and remember by becoming physically active and using his or her own muscles. Many individuals remember better if they combine passive reading with some kind of physical activity, thus employing a type of muscular memory.

The use of colors to enforce memory is obviously optional. The reader may choose to doodle with an ordinary lead pencil or the use of any colors or art materials; however, the traditional color scheme or color code of anatomy textbooks and atlases is red for arteries, blue for veins, yellow for nerves, pink to reddish brown for muscles, and light tan for bones, roughly representing natural colors. Color pencils or color markers can be used for this purpose. The reader will find that good quality, sharp, color pencils work quite well. One can employ many colors or just a few, depending on the time and effort one wishes to invest.

The author has included here and there etymological cartoons of neuroanatomical terms. Many of these cartoons are used in his lectures to medical students at the Case Western Reserve Medicine School. There are a few admittedly shameless puns to which the author pleads guilty on words such as *hippocampus*. The author is unable to explain why hippos seem to have assumed such a dominant role in his etymological cartoons.

RAY PORITSKY, Ph.D.
Cleveland, Ohio

1 CNS: Brain and spinal cord

The central nervous system (CNS) consists of the brain and spinal cord. They are both soft and delicate, with a consistency somewhat like gelatin. They are well protected by bones and ligaments.

Color and label

1   Brain
2   Spinal cord. Figure in lower right shows tapering lower end of spinal cord within its bony canal.
3   Cerebellum
4   Pons
5   Medulla oblongata
6   Flocculus (Latin, a small lock or pile of wool) of cerebellum
7   Olive (bump on side of medulla)
8   Central sulcus (of Rolando). Separates frontal lobe from parietal lobe.
9   Temporal lobe
10   Occipital lobe
11   Olfactory bulb

Parts of the Spinal Cord

12   Conus medullaris. Tapering inferior end of spinal cord. Note that the tip of the conus usually lies between lumbar vertebrae L1 and L2 in the adult.
13   Filum terminale. This is a thread-like extension of the pia mater and connective tissue that stretches from the tip of the conus to sacral level S2.
14   Anterior horn of spinal cord gray matter
15   Posterior horn of spinal cord gray matter. Note the butterfly or H shape of the gray matter. The gray matter contains the neuron cell bodies.
16   White matter of spinal cord. The white matter consists of longitudinally running myelinated axons.
17   Posterior root filaments (rootlets)
18   Anterior root filaments (rootlets)
19   Spinal nerve
20   Anterior ramus of spinal nerve. Most of the nerves of the body such as the median nerve, sciatic nerve, and intercostal nerves are derived from anterior rami.
21   Posterior ramus of spinal nerve
22   Dorsal root ganglion (spinal ganglion)

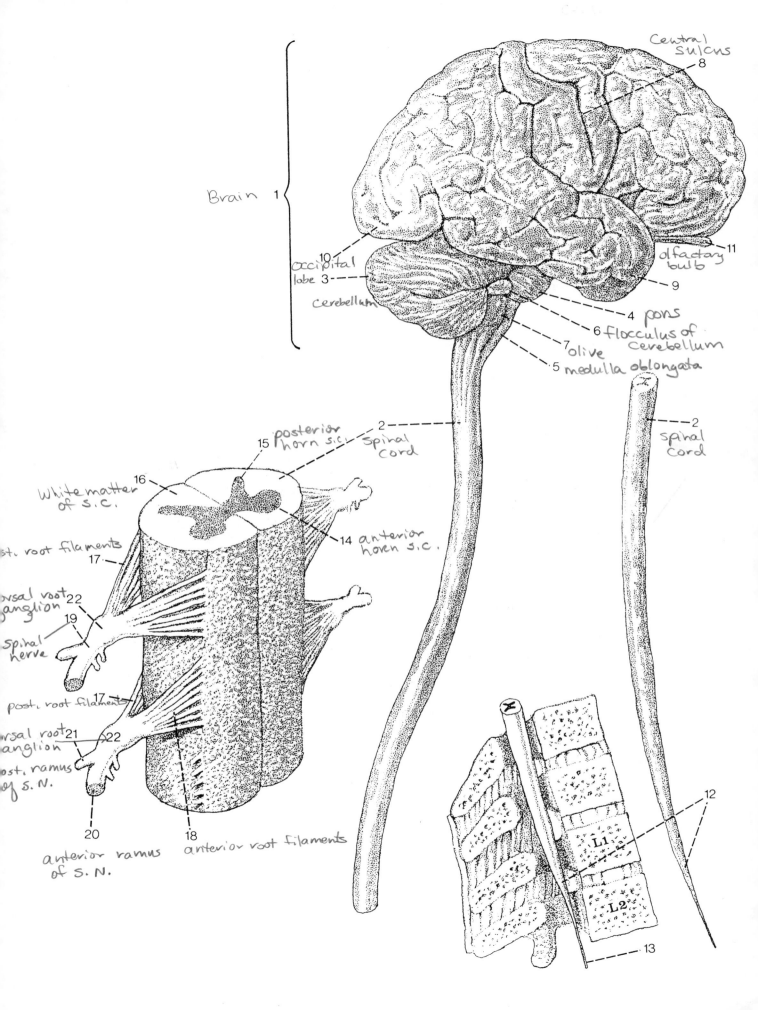

Central
sulcus
8

Brain 1

10
occipital
lobe 3
Cerebellum

olfactory
bulb
11

9

4 pons
6 flocculus of
cerebellum
7 olive
5 medulla oblongata

posterior
15 horn s.c.
2 spinal
cord

2
spinal
cord

White matter 16
of s.c.

14 anterior
horn s.c.

st. root filaments
17

rsal root 22
anglion
19
spinal
nerve

post. root filaments 17

rsal root 21 22
anglion

post. ramus
of s.N.

20

18 anterior root filaments

anterior ramus
of s.N.

12

L1

L2

13

2 Some basic terms

UPPER FIGURE

Color and label

1 **Ganglion.** A ganglion is a collection of nerve cell bodies outside the CNS. These cell bodies are connected to their fibers by a single process. Hence, these neurons are unipolar. These fibers travel through this ganglion with no break or synapse.

2 **Nucleus.** A nucleus in neuroanatomy is a collection of nerve cell bodies inside the brain or spinal cord. A nucleus may be so small that it consists of a few hundred neurons; or it may consist of millions of neurons and be so large that it is readily seen with the naked eye (the brain is estimated to be made up of a million million cells). Six neuronal cell bodies comprise the nucleus, here labelled 2. Nucleus is derived from the Latin, *nux* (nut or kernel), and originally meant a little kernel. Each neuron, or nerve cell, like any other cell, has its own nucleus within its cell body.

3 **Nerve.** A nerve is a collection of nerve fibers (or axons) connecting the CNS to other parts of the body. Larger nerves contain both outgoing and incoming fibers. They also consist of connective tissue sheaths, blood vessels, lymphatics, and some white blood cells.

4 **Tract or fasciculus.** This is a bundle of axons within the brain or spinal cord (within the CNS).

5 **Afferent fibers.** Afferent means incoming or travelling toward. Fibers labelled 5 are bringing information toward the CNS. Hence they are afferent fibers.

6 **Efferent fibers.** Efferent means outgoing, or in this case travelling away from the CNS. These fibers (6) arise from the cell bodies in the nucleus marked 2. Thus these neurons (2) are the **cells of origin** or the **parent cell bodies** of these efferent fibers (6).

7 **Second-order neurons.** These five neurons (7) comprise a nucleus and receive the endings of incoming or afferent fibers marked 5. Since these neurons comprise the second link in this particular neuronal pathway, they are called second-order neurons.

8 **Second-order fibers.** These fibers arise from second-order neuron cell bodies (7) and form a tract or fasciculus within the CNS.

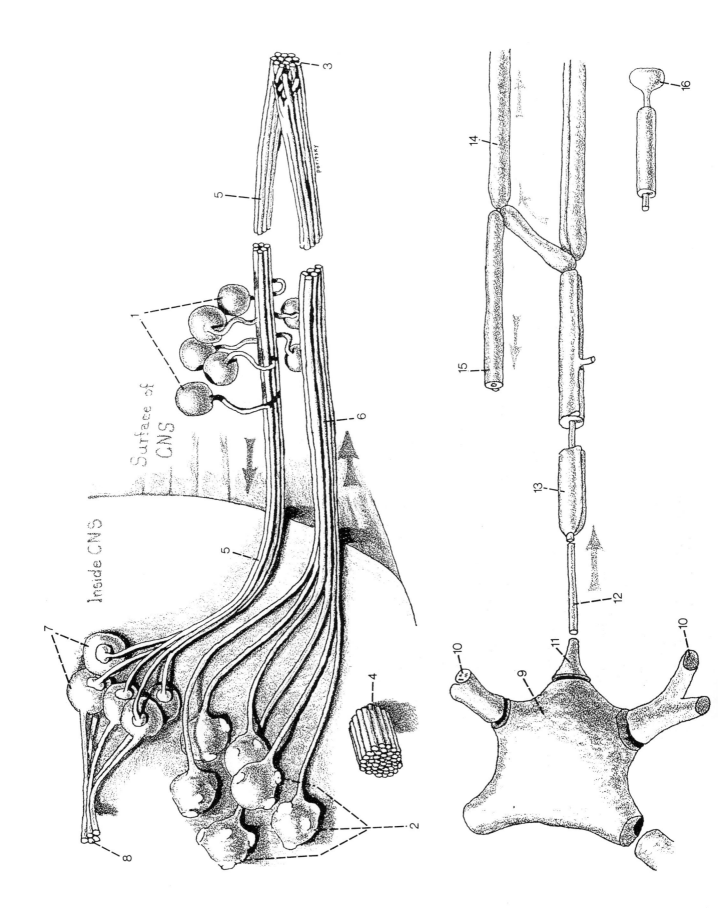

(Continued)

A disassembled neuron and its component parts

LOWER FIGURE

9   **Soma or perikaryon.** Both these terms mean neuron cell body (plurals: somata, perikarya).

10   **Dendrites.** Tree-like extensions of the cell body that greatly increase its receptive surface for synaptic contact with incoming fibers. Only the proximal truncated portions of the dendrites are shown here.

11   **Axon hillock.** This cone-like projection of the cell body is the site of origin of the axon. It is devoid of Nissl substance (basophilic material within the cytoplasm of active neurons).

12   **Initial unmyelinated segment of axon.** Experiments have shown that the nerve impulse begins here.

13   **Myelin.** A layer of insulation derived from Schwann cell membranes in the peripheral nervous system (PNS) and from oligodendrocyte membranes in the CNS.

14   **Collateral branch.** A side branch of an axon running more or less parallel to the main branch.

15   **Recurrent collateral.** A branch of an axon running back toward its cell of origin.

16   **Axon terminal.** Small bag-like swelling at the end of each axon branch. Each of these forms a synapse with other nerve cells. This is also called a *bouton* (French, button).

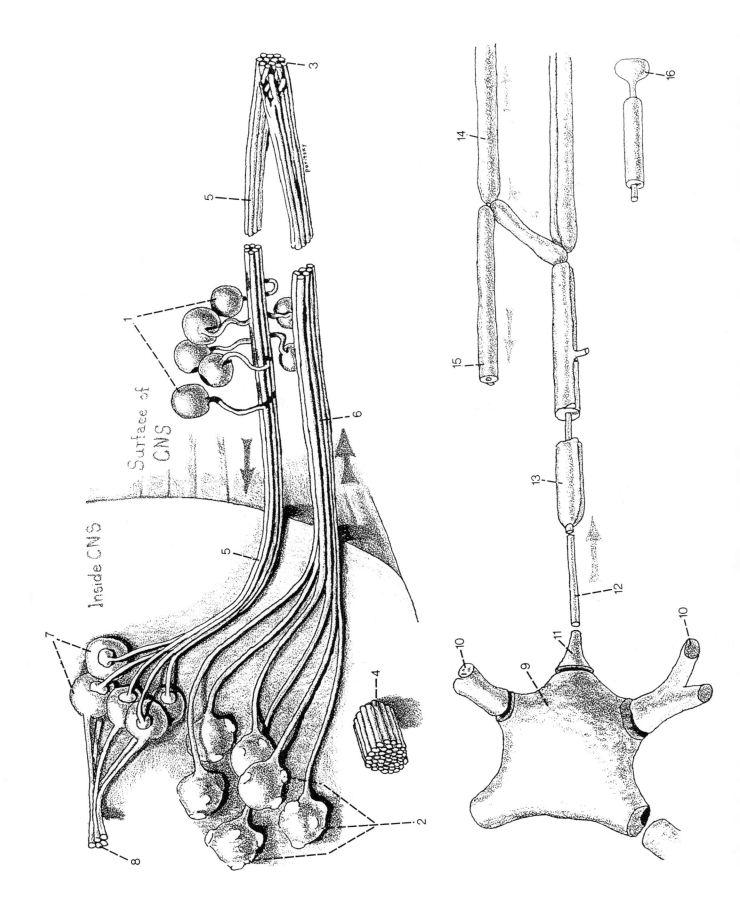

3 Ascending pathways

Color and label

1   **First-order sensory neuron** or **primary afferent.** This is the number-one neuron in a chain of neurons that carries sensory information up the neural axis (brain and spinal cord) to the cerebral cortex. This chain of neurons constitutes a neural pathway. Note its unipolar (one-process) cell body located in a dorsal root ganglion. Its peripheral process may extend to the big toe and be a meter in length. The central process enters the spinal cord and synapses upon a second-order neuron. Sensory modalities such as pain, touch, temperature, and proprioception (knowledge of body's position and movement), plus subconscious visceral information concerned with heart rate and breathing, are all brought to the CNS by neurons such as these. Some long ascending fibers belong to dorsal root ganglion cells and are primary afferent fibers.

2   **Second-order neurons.** This neuron relays this information to two third-order neurons.

3   **Third-order neurons.** One of these neurons sends its axon across the midline, where it ascends in a crossed (contralateral) tract. The other third-order neuron's axon ascends in an uncrossed (homolateral or ipsilateral) tract. Because these cells give rise to ascending fibers, they are tract cells or cells of origin or parent cell bodies.

4   **Fourth-order neurons.** These receive synapses from third-order neurons and project their axons to fifth-order neurons in the cerebral cortex.

5   **Fifth-order neurons** in the cerebral cortex.

The figure on the lower right shows how such fibers and their cell bodies are indicated in the usual "wiring" diagrams commonly used in neuroanatomy. One such neuron and its fiber may represent hundreds, thousands, or even millions of neurons. Note how the synapse is indicated by the Y shape at the fiber's end.

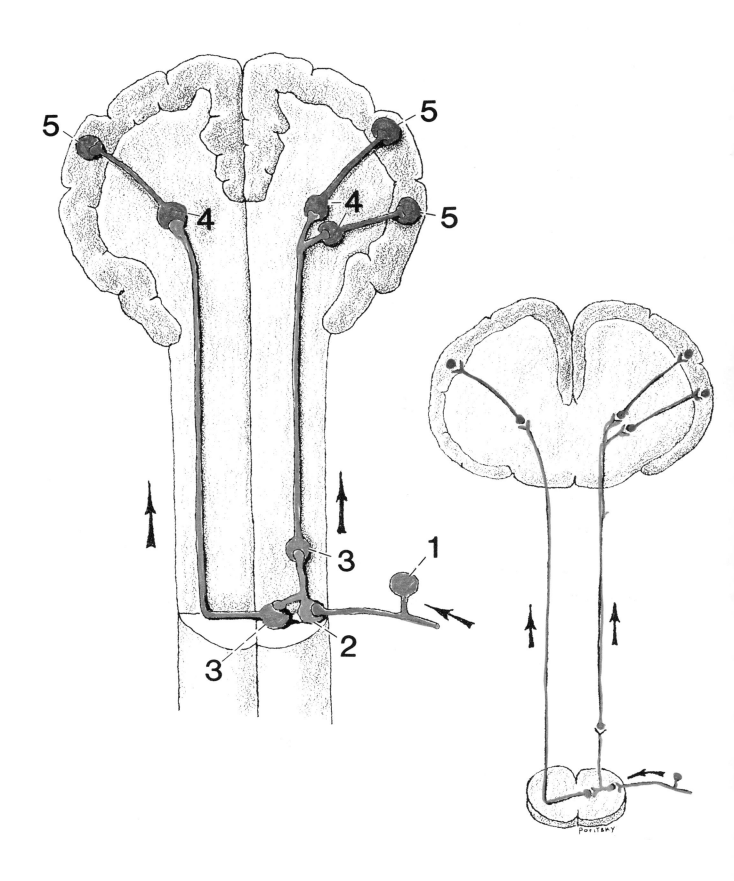

4 Descending pathways

Color and label

1   **Cortical neurons that project homolateral** (uncrossed) **fibers** down the spinal cord.

2   **Cortical neurons that project contralateral** (crossed) **fibers** down the spinal cord. Fibers such as these that arise from somata (cell bodies) in the cerebral cortex and end in the spinal cord are corticospinal fibers. The name conveys both their origin and destination. The largest descending tract in the human neural axis is the lateral corticospinal tract (also called the pyramidal tract). It arises in the cerebral cortex of one hemisphere, crosses the midline (decussates) in the lower medulla, and ends in the opposite side of the spinal cord.

3   **Commissural neuron and its fiber.** Commissures are bundles of axons that project from one side of the neural axis to the corresponding region on the other side. The largest commissure by far is the corpus callosum, which consists of approximately 300,000,000 fibers that link together the two cerebral hemispheres. The left cerebral hemisphere controls the right side of the body and the right cerebral hemisphere controls the left side of the body. Commissures provide a means of unifying the two halves of the brain. Possibly commissures arose by cortical neurons that had long descending fibers, such as pyramidal tract neurons, pulling adjacent cortical neurons or the fibers of adjacent cortical neurons to the opposite cerebral hemispheres when these neurons first crossed to the opposite side. The crossing of ascending and descending tracts and the resulting contralateral brain-to-body control may have facilitated the development of commissural fibers and the unification of the brain.

4   **Decussation of the crossing fibers.** As tracts from each side cross the midline and intersect, they form an X shape. Decussate comes from the Latin verb *decussare*, "to cut crosswise in the shape of the letter X."

5   **Alpha motor neurons.** These were formerly called **lower motor neurons**, and cortical neurons giving rise to corticospinal fibers were **upper motor neurons**. Alpha motor neurons innervate voluntary striated muscle and control all voluntary movement.

Note the wiring diagram in the lower right figure.

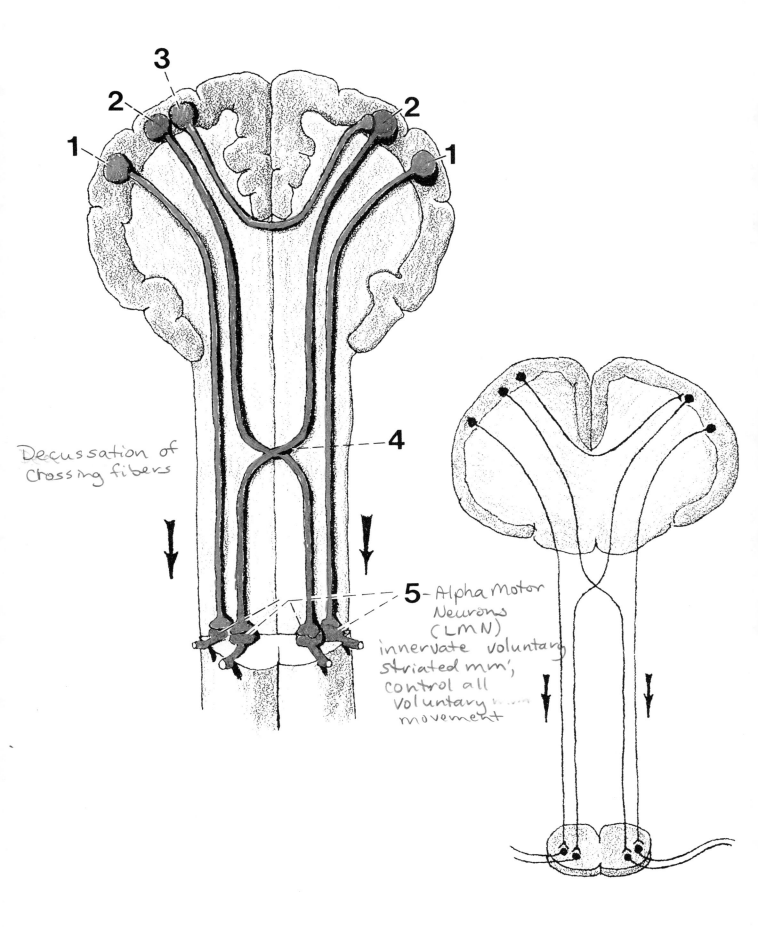

Decussation of Crossing fibers

5 - Alpha Motor Neurons (LMN) innervate voluntary striated mm', control all voluntary m..... movement

Color and label. Use boxes as color keys.

1 **Axodendritic synapse.** Axons end as small bag-like swellings called axon terminals (also called end bulbs, end feet, boutons terminaux, synaptic bulbs). Two afferent fibers ending upon dendrites are indicated at 1, thus forming axon-to-dendrite synapses or axodendritic synapses. The synapse is the site where the nerve impulse is transmitted from one neuron to the other.

2 **Axosomatic synapse.** Two axon-to-soma or axosomatic synapses are shown.

3 **Axoaxonic synapse.** An axon ending upon another axon—in this case the beginning of another axon—constitutes an axoaxonic synapse. One axon terminal synapsing upon another axon terminal is another type of axoaxonic synapse.

4 **Synapse in passing.** This type of synapse is formed by an axon contacting and synapsing upon the target cell at some site before it ends. Synapses formed in this manner are called synapses in passing (or *en passant*, French).

5 **Nissl substance.** This is the granular endoplasmic reticulum in nerve cells. It may be block-like, as shown, or take other forms. It consists of cisterns and ribosomes. The basophilia of the Nissl substance is due to the RNA within the ribosomes.

6 **Nucleus with nucleolus**

7 **Oligodendrocyte.** One of the neuroglial cells (neuroglia are, collectively, the non-neuronal cellular components of the CNS)

8 **Astrocyte.** Another type of neuroglia.

9 **Astrocytic processes.** These extend from the astrocyte cell body to the neuron. Astrocytes have exceedingly convoluted surfaces.

10 **Perivascular end feet.** These are formed by astrocyte processes that end upon capillaries in the CNS.

11 **Capillary.** Capillaries in the CNS are almost completely ensheathed by perivascular end feet from astrocytes.

12 **Axon.** The cytoplasm within the axon is called axoplasm. The cell membrane surrounding the axon is the **axolemma**.

13 **Oligodendrocytic cytoplasm.** Myelin within the CNS is made by the oligodendrocyte. After the myelin is formed, a thin "tongue" of oligodendrocyte cytoplasm remains both within the myelin sheath and on its external surface.

14 **Myelin sheath.** Synthesized by spirally wrapped oligodendrocyte plasma membrane. In nerves, that is, outside the CNS, myelin is formed by spirally wrapped Schwann cell membrane.

The study of neuroanatomy is mainly a study of the "wiring" or "circuitry" in the CNS. In a sense, one can think of nerve cells as tiny telephones and their fibers (or axons) as telephone wires grouped together into tracts. In addition to understanding the basic circuitry, the function of the tracts and their neurochemistry continue to be slowly unraveled. For example, it has been shown that certain neural tracts carry pain, and that by cutting these tracts, pain may be reduced. As more is learned about the neurotransmitter released at nerve endings, neuroscientists attempt to manage disorders such as epilepsy, depression, and schizophrenia with drugs rather than with more invasive approaches such as surgery.

The brain and spinal cord consist of billions of nerve cells and even more neuroglial cells that may outnumber the nerve cells by as much as ten to one. Memories appear to be stored in the brain in the form of networks of nerve cells. A stimulus reaching the brain jumps from nerve cell to nerve cell and activates a network of nerve cells in a matter of milliseconds. As this happens, it is believed that some kind of change occurs at each of the synapses between all neurons stimulated, thus linking them together as a network. This network of nerve cells is the neural substrate of the memory, and its activation evokes the memory. Exactly how this takes place is still largely unknown.

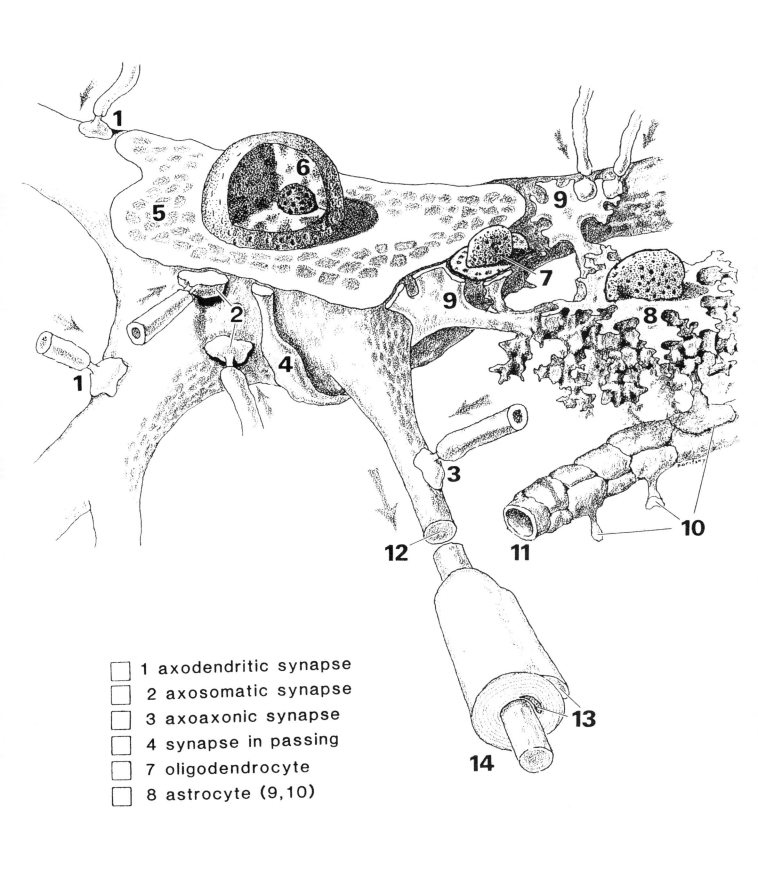

1 axodendritic synapse
2 axosomatic synapse
3 axoaxonic synapse
4 synapse in passing
7 oligodendrocyte
8 astrocyte (9,10)

6   Etymological cartoon: Tigroid bodies

Tigers have stripes and leopards have spots. Tigroid bodies are another name for Nissl substance, which is the granular endoplasmic reticulum of nerve cells. When stained with certain dyes, the Nissl substance appears as tiny particles in the nerve cell body and in the larger dendrites. This particulate pattern of the Nissl bodies certainly resembles leopard spots more than tiger stripes. The cartoon shows the unknown perpetrator of this egregious (Latin, "out of the herd," i.e., it's that bad) misnomer–a confused histologist who did not know the difference between tigers and leopards, and his class of confused students.

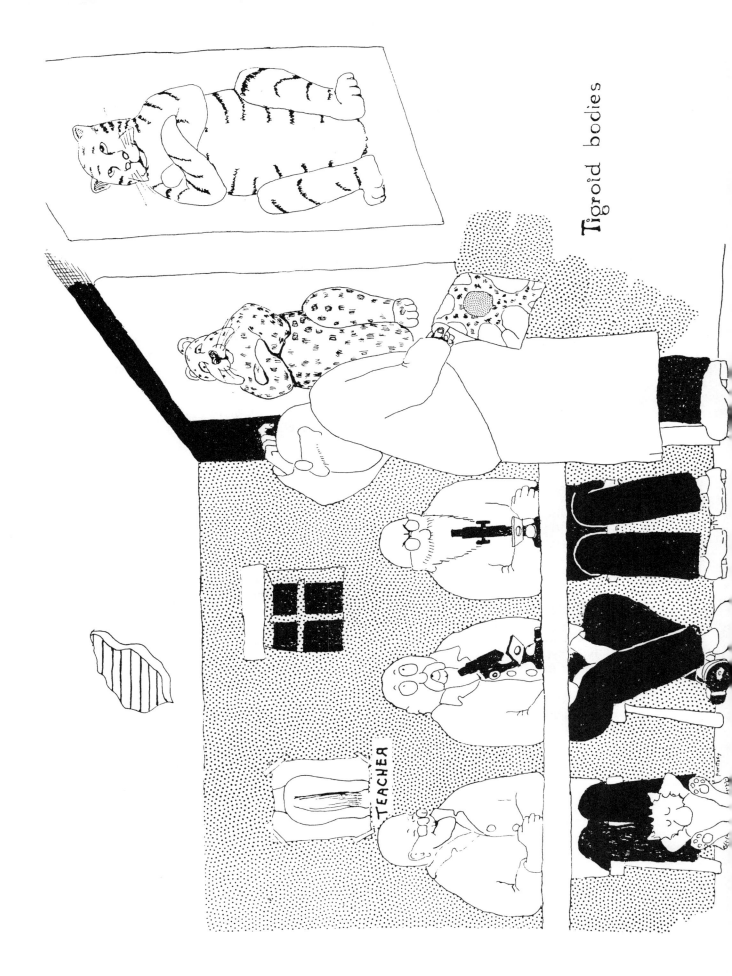

Tigroid bodies

7 Nerve* and its connective tissue sheaths

Color and label. Use boxes as color keys.

1   **Epineurium.** This is the outermost sheath surrounding a nerve. It consists mainly of collagen. It contains blood vessels and lymphatics that supply the nerve. Smaller nerves have no epineurium.

2   **Perineurium.** This is the connective tissue around each fascicle. It consists of several layers of flat perineural epithelial cells that are tightly bound to each other and appear to form a barrier to the surrounding tissue. The perineural epithelium forms several concentric layers that alternate with layers of collagen fibers.

3   **Endoneurium.** This is the innermost connective tissue sheath. It consists of longitudinally arrayed collagenous fibers that surround each axon.

4   **Fascicles.** These are bundles of nerve fibers (axons) surrounded by perineurium. Large nerves such as the ulnar and median each contain several fascicles.

5   **Axon.** Axons or nerve fibers are thin extensions of nerve cell bodies that carry the nerve impulse. The cytoplasm within the axon is **axoplasm** and the axon's membrane is the **axolemma.**

6   **Myelin.** Myelin is found on axons thicker than 0.5 μm. Myelin consists of tight spirally wound cell membranes. In the CNS, myelin is made by oligodendrocytes. In the peripheral nervous system (PNS), that is, in nerves, myelin is made by Schwann cells.

7   **Schwann cells.** These cells form a long tubular sheath around the myelin called the neurilemma or sheath of Schwann with one Schwann cell to each segment of myelin. Unmyelinated axons are also ensheathed by elongated Schwann cells, with one Schwann cell ensheathing up to 12 or more unmyelinated axons. Schwann cells are not present in the CNS.

8   **Capillaries**

9   **Arteries and veins.** Larger nerves contain arteries and veins, which, when temporarily blocked, cause the arm or leg to "fall asleep."

10 **Basal lamina.** A dense layer of fine filamentous material around the Schwann cell.

11 **Membrane-enclosed vesicles.** Believed to be derived from the smooth endoplasmic reticulum in the cell body from which they migrate down the axon.

12 **Microtubule.** These are found in the axon, dendrite, and perikaryon. About 240 ångströms (Å) (24 nm) in diameter.

13 **Neurofilaments.** Thinner than microtubule, about 80 Å (8 nm) in diameter, these are found in the axons, dendrites, and perikarya.

14 **Mitochondria.** These originate in the perikarya and move down the axon in a proximal-to-distal axoplasmic flow.

A nerve is a collection of axons outside the CNS. Larger nerves such as those shown here contain blood vessels, connective tissue sheaths, and cells such as fibroblasts, macrophages, and various white blood cells. Smaller nerves are too small to be seen with the unaided eye.

Microscopic units of length are:

   The millimeter (mm): (1000 mm = 1 meter)
   The micrometer (μm): (micron or μ is the old name); 1000 μm = 1 mm
   The nanometer (nm): 1000 nm = 1 μm
   The ångström (Å): 10 Å = 1 nm, or 10,000 Å = 1 μm

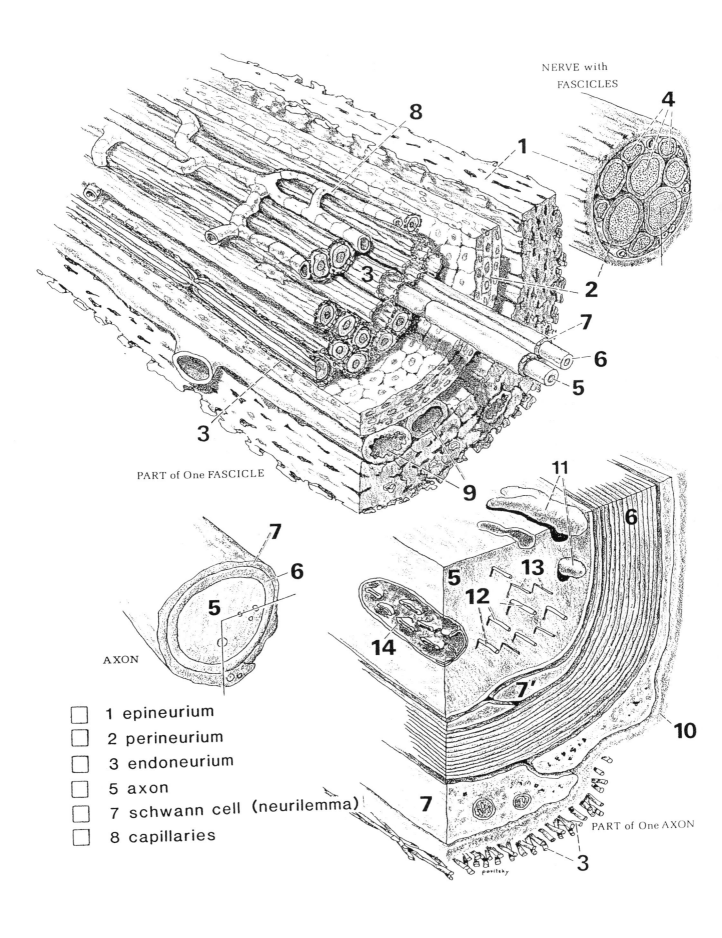

NERVE with FASCICLES

1

4

8

3

2

7

6

5

3

PART of One FASCICLE

9

11

6

5

13

12

14

7'

10

AXON

7

6

5

7

PART of One AXON

3

poritsky

1 epineurium
2 perineurium
3 endoneurium
5 axon
7 schwann cell (neurilemma)
8 capillaries

Color* and label

1	Olfactory bulb*
2	Olfactory tract*
3	Olfactory trigone*
4	Medial olfactory stria*
5	Lateral olfactory stria*
6	Anterior perforated substance
7	Optic nerve (II)*
8	Optic chiasma*
9	Optic tract*
10	Infundibulum
11	Tuber cinereum
12	Mamillary body
13	Cerebral peduncle
14	Uncus
15	Oculomotor nerve (III)*
16	Pons
17	Trigeminal nerve (V)*
18	Abducent nerve (VI)*
19	Facial nerve (VII)–motor*
20	Nervus intermedius (part of facial nerve, VII)*
21	Vestibulocochlear nerve (VIII)*
22	Glossopharyngeal nerve (IX)*
23	Vagus nerve (X)*
24	Accessory nerve (XI)*
25	Pyramids
26	Hypoglossal nerve (XII)*
27	Cerebellum (hemisphere)
28	Trochlear nerve (IV)

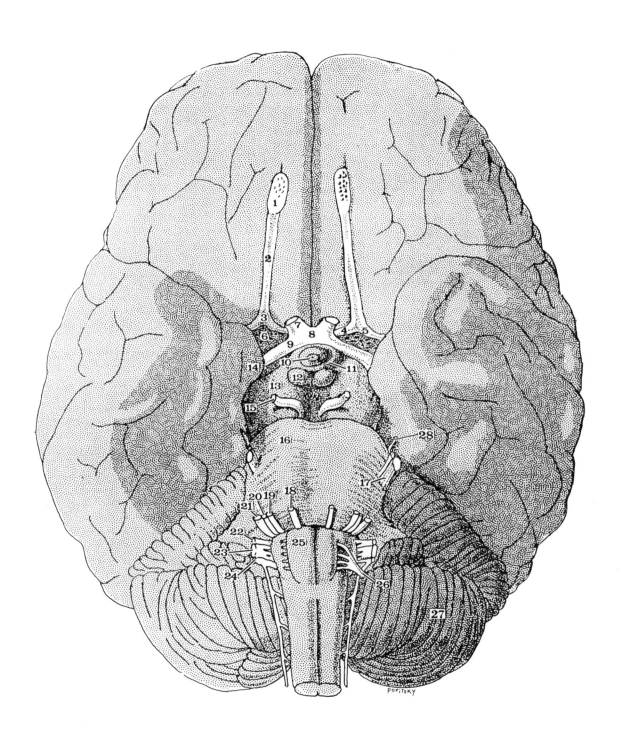

Medial view of right half of brain

Color* and label

1 Genu of corpus callosum*
2 Body of corpus callosum*
3 Splenium of corpus callosum*
4 Septum pellucidum*
5 Anterior commissure*
6 Fornix*
7 Thalamus*
8 Interthalamic adhesion*
9 Hypothalamus*
10 Lamina terminalis*
11 Optic chiasm*
12 Optic nerve*
13 Mamillary body*
14 Cerebral aqueduct
15 Decussation of the brachium conjunctivum*
16 Pineal body*
17 Mesencephalic tectum* (formerly lamina quadrigemina)
18 Pons

19 Medulla
20 Fourth ventricle
21 Infundibulum*
22 Oculomotor nerve*
23 Central canal of spinal cord
24 Olfactory bulb
25 Uncus on temporal lobe
26 Cingulate gyrus
27 Calcarine sulcus
28 Probe in interventricular foramen
29 Parieto-occipital sulcus
30 Occipital lobe
31 White matter of vermis
32 Anterior lobe of cerebellum
33 Posterior lobe of cerebellum
34 Nodulus of cerebellum
35 Common stem of parieto-occipital sulcus and calcarine sulcus
36 Cingulate sulcus
37 Marginal part of cingulate sulcus

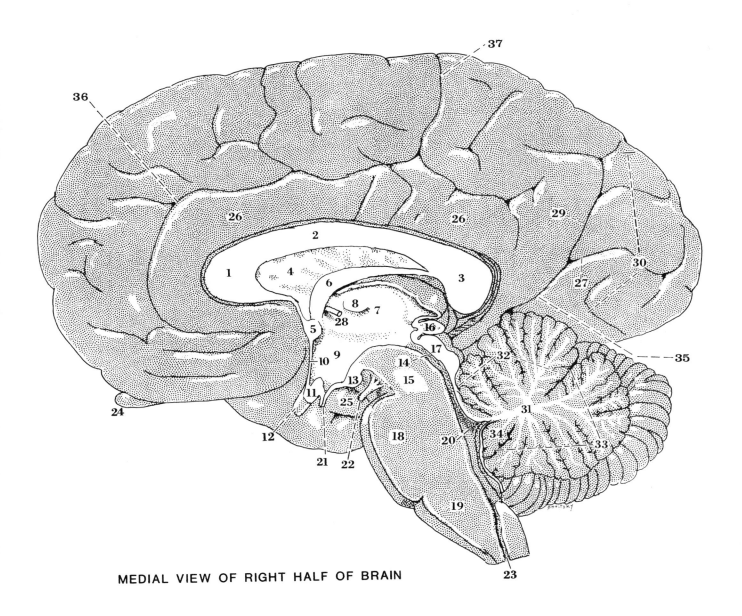

MEDIAL VIEW OF RIGHT HALF OF BRAIN

Color and label

1	Scalp
2	Calvaria of skull
3	Diploe (spongy marrow of cranial bones)
4	Superior sagittal sinus (cut open to show opening of superior cerebral veins)
5	Falx cerebri
6	Inferior sagittal sinus
7	Crista galli
8	Straight sinus
9	Great cerebral vein
10	Confluence of sinus
11	Opening of right transverse sinus
12	Occipital sinus
13	Falx cerebri
14	Frontal sinus
15	Corpus callosum
16	Anterior cerebral artery
17	Septum pellucidum
18	Fornix
19	Thalamus and interthalamic adhesion
20	Optic chiasm
21	Pituitary gland (hypophysis)
22	Sphenoidal sinus
23	Mamillary body
24	Midbrain (mesencephalon)
25	Mesencephalic tectum
26	Pineal gland
27	Cerebral aqueduct
28	Cerebellum
29	Fourth ventricle
30	Cisterna magna (cerebellomedullary cistern)
31	Basilar artery
32	Left vertebral artery
33	Pons
34	Medulla oblongata
35	Spinal cord
36	Anterior arch of atlas
37	Body and dens of atlas
38	Pharyngeal tonsil
39	Ostium (opening) of auditory tube (eustachian tube)
40	Nasal pharynx
41	Middle nasal concha
42	Inferior nasal concha
43	Hard palate
44	Soft palate and uvula
45	Mandible
46	Hyoid bone
47	Genioglossus muscle
48	Geniohyoid muscle
49	Mylohyoid muscle
50	Epiglottis
51	Thyroid cartilage
52	Cricoid cartilage
53	Trachea
54	Oral pharynx
55	Laryngeal pharynx
56	Esophagus

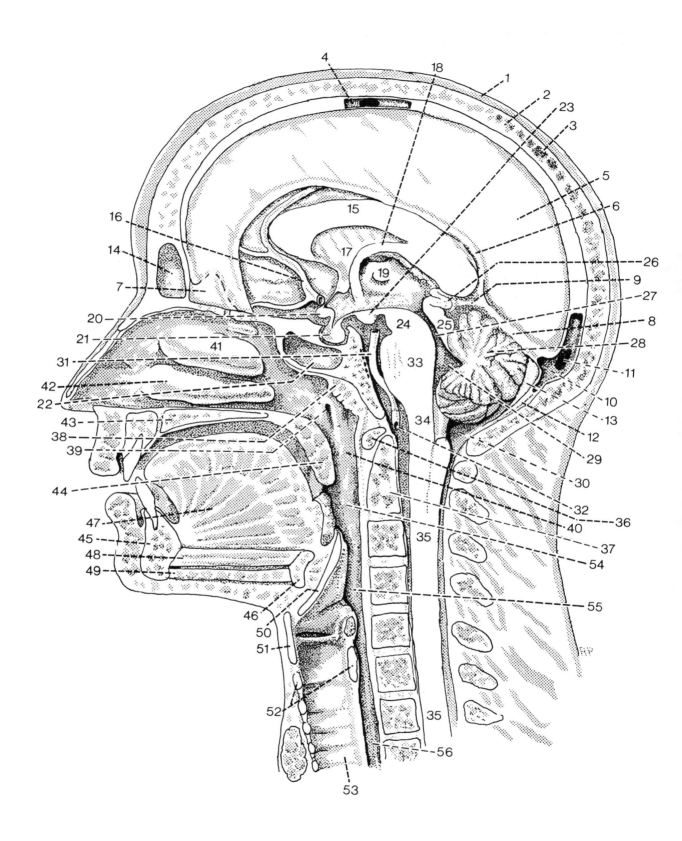

Color and label

1	Crista galli
2	Cribriform plate of ethmoid bone
3	Foramina for olfactory nerve fibers
4	Orbital part of frontal bone
5	Optic canal
6	Anterior clinoid process
7	Foramen rotundum
8	Foramen spinosum
9	Foramen ovale
10	Foramen lacerum
11	Dorsum sellae
12	Posterior clinoid process
13	Groove for middle meningeal artery
14	Groove for superior petrosal sinus
15	Internal auditory meatus
16	Jugular foramen
17	Sulcus for sigmoid sinus
18	Sulcus for transverse sinus
19	Hypoglossal canal
20	Foramen magnum
21	Sulcus for superior sagittal sinus

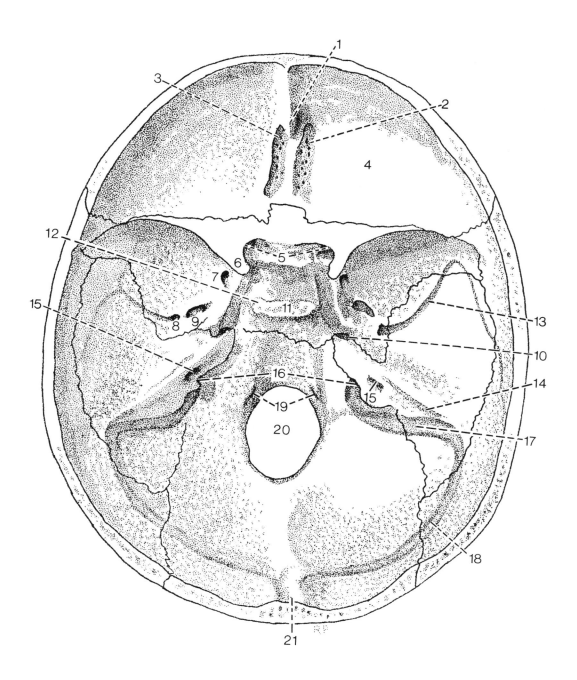

Cranial dural venous sinuses*

BENEATH THE BRAIN

Color and label

1   Superior sagittal sinus
     (cut open)
2   Straight sinus (cut open and pulled slightly to the right)
3   Right transverse sinus
     (cut open)
4   Sigmoid sinus (cut open)
5   Occipital sinus
6   Confluence of sinuses
7   Cavernous sinus (cut open on left)
8   Superior petrosal sinus
9   Inferior petrosal sinus
10   Basilar venous plexus
11   Middle meningeal vein
12   Sphenoparietal sinus
13   Anterior and posterior
     intercavernous sinuses
14   Superior ophthalmic vein
15   Tentorium cerebelli

* These are veins with walls of dura mater that carry blood from the brain and drain into veins in the neck.

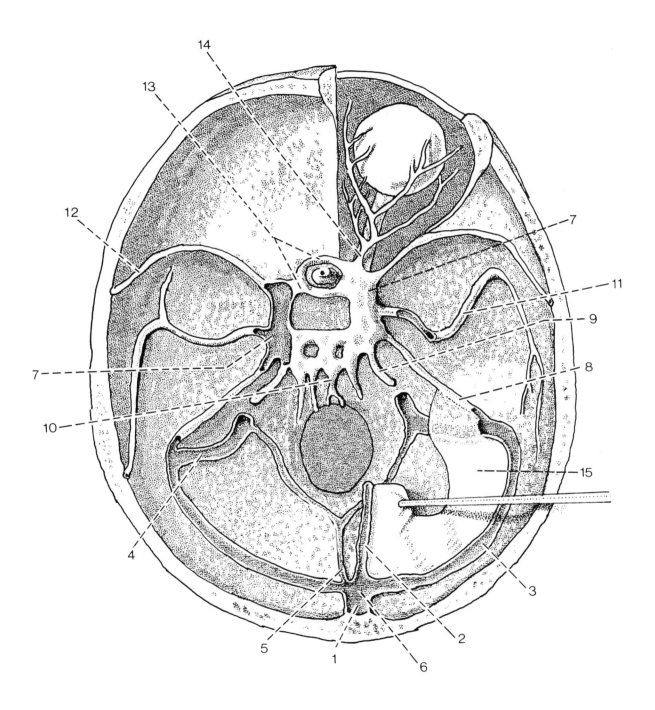

13 Superior sagittal sinus

Color and label

1   Bone of the skull
2   Dura mater (Latin, tough mother)
3   Arachnoid mater (Greek, spider-like or web-like)
4   Pia mater (Latin, tender or faithful mother)
5   Superior sagittal sinus (a large vein formed
     by walls of dura mater)
6   Inferior sagittal sinus
7   Arachnoid granulations (these allow the cerebrospinal
     fluid in the subarachnoid space to enter the superior
     sagittal sinus and mix with its venous blood)
8   Arachnoid trabeculae (a meshwork of small fibers that
     crisscross the subarachnoid space)
9   Lateral lacunae (outpouchings of the superior sagittal sinus)
10   Subarachnoid space containing cerebrospinal fluid
11   Superior cerebral vein emptying into the superior sagittal sinus
12   Cerebral cortex
13   Emissary veins (these pass completely through the skull)
14   Periosteum (in most areas the dura mater and the periosteum
     are fused together)
15   Falx cerebri
16   Pits on inner surface of skull caused by arachnoid granulations

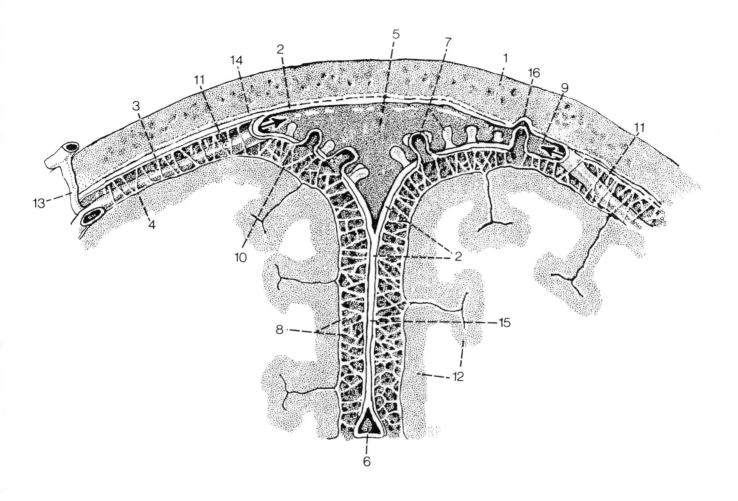

Ventral aspect of brain stem showing exit of cranial nerves.
There are twelve pairs of cranial nerves.

Color and label

Cranial nerve I is the olfactory nerve (Latin, *olfacia*, to smell). It is made up of the central processes or axons of bipolar olfactory receptors in the top of the nose. These axons group into about 20 bundles that penetrate the cribriform plate of the ethmoid bone and end in the olfactory bulb. The axons of the olfactory nerve are thin and unmyelinated and are easily broken when the **olfactory bulb** is raised.

Cranial nerve II is the **optic nerve**. It consists of about one million fibers that arise from ganglion cells in the retina. The optic nerve is the only nerve that is enclosed by the three meninges, the dura mater, arachnoid mater, and pia mater. By convention the optic nerve is "nerve" from eyeball to chiasm. From chiasm to its end in the lateral geniculate body it is called "optic tract."

Cranial nerve III is the **oculomotor nerve**. It supplies motor fibers and movement to four extrabulbar eye muscles and the raiser of the eyelid (levator palpebrae).

Cranial nerve IV is the **trochlear nerve** (Greek, *trochlea*, pulley). It supplies only one extrabulbar eye muscle, the superior oblique. It is the only cranial nerve that becomes completely crossed (it supplies the opposite superior oblique). It is also the only cranial nerve that exits from the dorsal aspect of the brain stem.

Cranial nerve V is the **trigeminal nerve** (Latin, *trigeminus*, three fold). It is mainly sensory and divides into three large branches–the ophthalmic, maxillary, and mandibular–that supply the face, eye, nose, mouth, teeth, and anterior two-thirds of the tongue with pain, touch, and temperature sensibilities. It has a small motor component that supplies the muscle of the jaw (and a few others).

Cranial nerve VI is the **abducent nerve** (Latin, *abducere*, to lead away). It supplies only one extrabulbar eye muscle, the lateral rectus muscle.

Cranial nerve VII is the **facial nerve**. It has two roots. Its larger motor root supplies the muscle of facial expression. Immediately lateral to the motor root is the smaller root of the facial nerve, the **nervus intermedius**. The nervus intermedius contains taste fibers from the anterior two-thirds of the tongue and parasympathetic fibers that supply the lacrimal gland, nasal glands, submandibular gland, and sublingual gland.

Cranial nerve VIII is the **vestibulocochlear nerve**. It carries two distinct sensory modalities from the inner ear. The older **vestibular** portion carries information about the position and movement of the head. The vestibular part of the inner ear responds to the head being turned, tilted, or accelerated in a straight line. The newer **cochlear** portion of the vestibulocochlear nerve carries hearing from the cochlea.

Cranial nerve IX is the **glossopharyngeal nerve** (Greek, literally "tongue-throat"). It is mainly sensory to the upper pharynx and soft palate. It supplies pain, touch, temperature, and taste to the posterior one-third of tongue. It supplies motor fibers that join with those of the vagus nerve to form the pharyngeal plexus, which innervates the soft palate and upper pharynx. Parasympathetic fibers in the glossopharyngeal nerve supply the parotid salivary gland.

Cranial nerve X is the **vagus nerve**. It contains five different kinds of fibers. These include preganglionic parasympathetic fibers that innervate the esophagus, heart, lungs, stomach, and intestines. Numerous visceral afferent fibers control cardiac and pulmonary reflexes. The vagus supplies motor control of the pharynx and larynx. Taste fibers from taste buds on the epiglottis travel within the vagus, as do a few afferent fibers from the skin of the ear.

Cranial nerve XI is the **accessory nerve** (old name, spinal accessory nerve). It arises by two roots, a cranial one in the medulla and a spinal one from the cervical spinal cord. The spinal root ascends through the foramen magnum and joins the cranial root as the latter emerges from the medulla. It supplies only two muscles, the trapezius and sternocleidomastoid.

Cranial nerve XII is the **hypoglossal nerve**. It supplies all the tongue muscles on the same side.

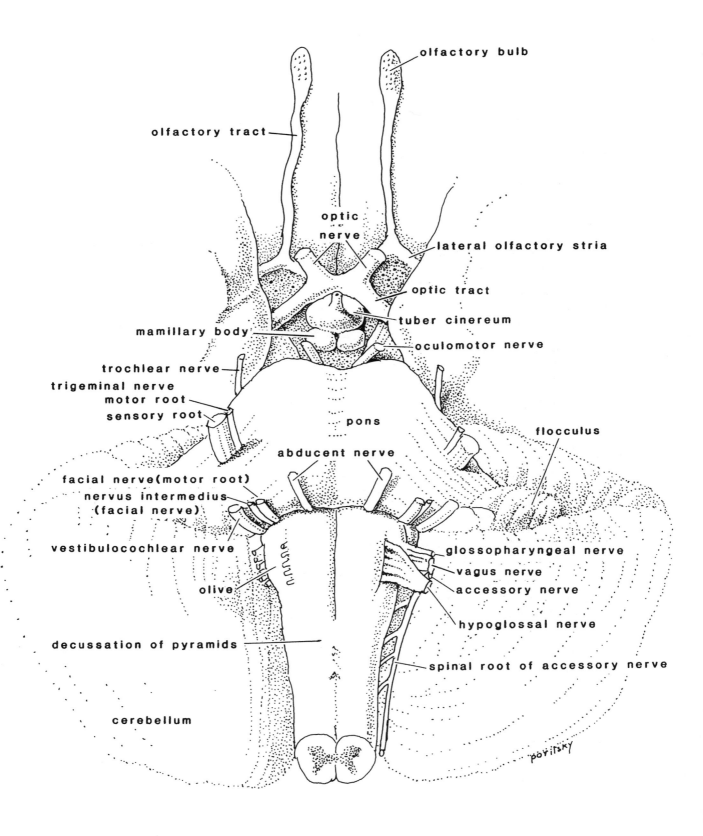

olfactory bulb

olfactory tract

optic nerve

lateral olfactory stria

optic tract

tuber cinereum

mamillary body

oculomotor nerve

trochlear nerve

trigeminal nerve
motor root
sensory root

pons

flocculus

abducent nerve

facial nerve(motor root)

nervus intermedius
(facial nerve)

vestibulocochlear nerve

glossopharyngeal nerve

vagus nerve

accessory nerve

olive

hypoglossal nerve

decussation of pyramids

spinal root of accessory nerve

cerebellum

povilsky

Color and label

1 Optic nerve (N II)
2 Internal carotid artery
3 Ophthalmic artery
4 Trigeminal ganglion
5 Sensory root of the trigeminal nerve (N V)
6 Motor root of trigeminal nerve
7 Oculomotor nerve (N III)
8 Trochlear nerve (N IV)
9 Abducent nerve (N VI)
10 Pituitary gland (hypophysis)
11 Cut edge of dura mater
12 Ophthalmic nerve
13 Frontal nerve
14 Nasociliary nerve
15 Lacrimal nerve
16 Supraorbital nerve
17 Supratrochlear nerve
18 Maxillary nerve
19 Mandibular nerve
20 Middle meningeal artery
21 Facial nerve motor root (N VII)
22 Nervus intermedius (N VII)
23 Vestibulocochlear nerve (N VIII)
24 Glossopharyngeal nerve (N IX)
25 Vagus nerve (N X)
26 Accessory nerve (N XI)
27 Hypoglossal nerve (N XII)
28 Vertebral artery
29 Internal auditory meatus
30 Jugular foramen
31 Hypoglossal canal
32 Roof of orbit removed
33 Roof of superior orbital fissure
removed

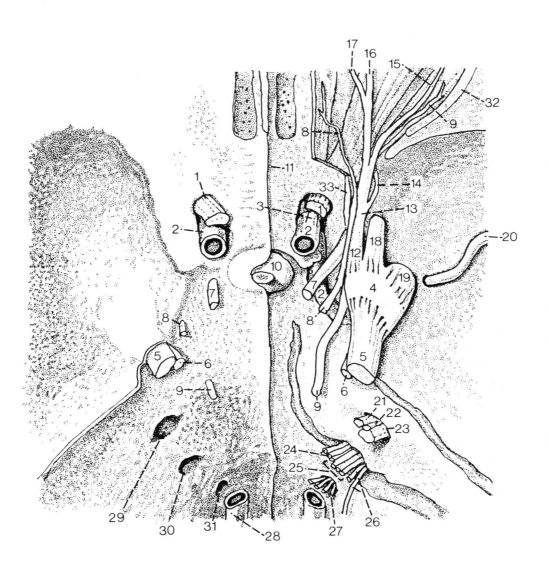

Color and label

1	Lateral sulcus (fissure of Sylvius, sylvian fissure)
2	Posterior ramus of lateral sulcus
3	Ascending ramus of lateral sulcus
4	Anterior ramus of lateral sulcus
5	Central sulcus (fissure of Rolando, rolandic fissure)
6	Precentral gyrus
7	Postcentral gyrus
8	Precentral sulcus
9	Postcentral sulcus
10	Superior temporal gyrus*
11	Superior temporal sulcus
12	Middle temporal gyrus*
13	Inferior temporal sulcus
14	Inferior temporal gyrus*
15	Superior frontal gyrus*
16	Superior frontal sulcus
17	Middle frontal gyrus*
18	Inferior frontal sulcus
19	Opercular part of inferior frontal gyrus
20	Triangular part of inferior frontal gyrus
21	Orbital part of inferior frontal gyrus
22	Orbital sulci
23	Orbital gyri
24	Olfactory bulb
25	Olfactory tract
26	Superior parietal lobule
27	Inferior parietal lobule
28	Parieto-occipital sulcus
29	Supramarginal gyrus
30	Angular gyrus
31	Lunate sulcus
32	Anterior occipital sulcus
33	Occipital gyri
34	Occipital sulci
35	Preoccipital incisure (notch)
36	Cerebellar hemispheres
37	Pons
38	Flocculus of cerebellum
39	Medulla oblongata
40	Spinal cord

*Note that these gyri may be interrupted by short transverse sulci that render them segmental or discontinuous. Gyri such as these run in a **general** direction regardless of whether they are a single gyrus or several segments of a gyrus.

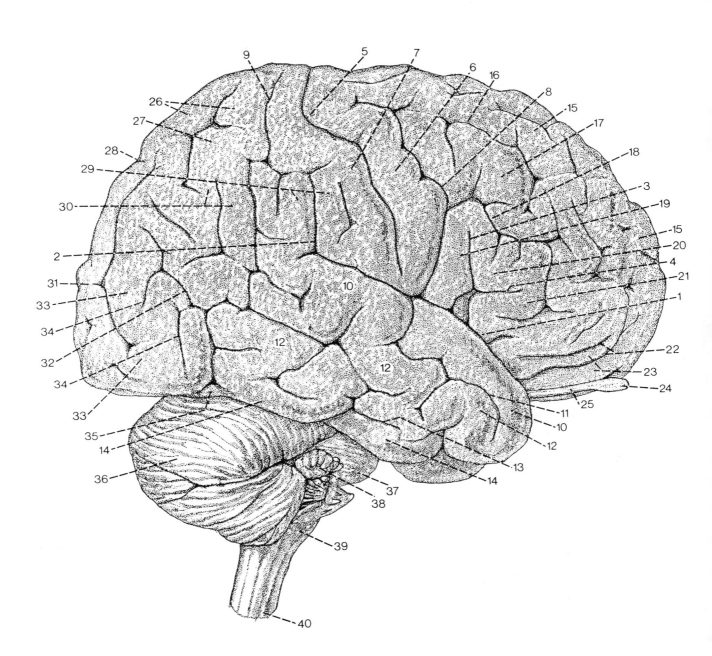

Color and label

1 Cavity of septum pellucidum
2 Corpus callosum (a small section)
3 Septum pellucidum
4 Internal capsule
5 Putamen
6 Stria terminalis and thalamostriate vein
7 Tail of caudate nucleus
8 Ventricle III
9 Tela choroidea of ventricle III
10 Pineal body
11 Brachium of inferior colliculus
12 Inferior colliculus
13 Trochlear nerve (it has already crossed the midline before it exits the dorsal surface of the midbrain)
14 Superior cerebellar peduncle (brachium conjunctivum; cut)
15 Facial colliculus
16 Vestibular area
17 Lateral aperture of ventricle IV (of Luschka)
18 Hypoglossal trigone
19 Vagal trigone
20 Obex (caudal angle of ventricle IV)
21 Fasciculus gracilis
22 Fasciculus cuneatus
23 Posterior intermediate sulcus
24 Posterior median sulcus
25 Tubercle of nucleus cuneatus
26 Tubercle of nucleus gracilis
27 Tenia of ventricle IV (line of attachment of tela choroidea roof to the rim of ventricle IV)
28 Accessory nerve (N XI)
29 Vagus nerve (N X)
30 Glossopharyngeal nerve (N IX)
31 Striae medullares of ventricle IV
32 Inferior cerebellar peduncle (restiform body; cut)
33 Middle cerebellar penduncle (brachium pontis; cut)
34 Superior medullary velum
35 Trigeminal nerve (N V)
36 Superior colliculus
37 Medial geniculate body
38 Lateral geniculate body
39 Habenular trigone
40 Internal capsule (sublenticular part)
41 Thalamus
42 Fornix (body; cut)
43 Caudate nucleus (body)
44 Lateral ventricle (left)
45 Caudate nucleus (head)

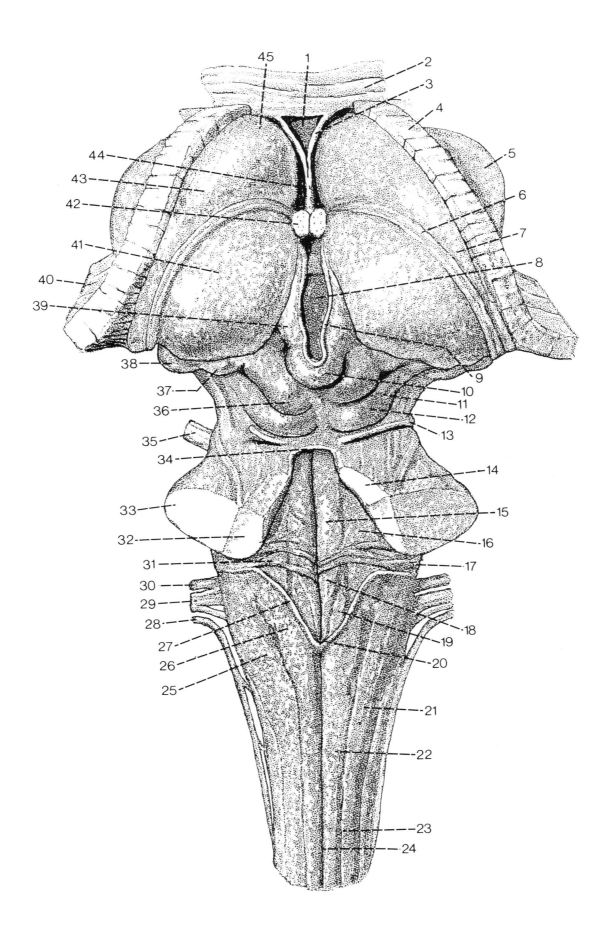

18 Arterial supply at base of brain
(After Netter with slight modification)

Color and label

1   Vertebral arteries (right and left)*
2   Internal carotid arteries (right and left)*
3   Anterior spinal artery
4   Basilar artery (note that two vertebral arteries join together
      to form the single basilar artery)
5   Posterior inferior cerebellar artery
6   Anterior inferior cerebellar artery
7   Labyrinthine (formerly: internal auditory) artery
8   Superior cerebellar artery
9   Posterior cerebral artery†
10   Posterior communicating artery
11   Middle cerebral artery†
12   Anterior cerebral artery† (note its course in the
      longitudinal cerebral fissure as it curves around
      the genu of the corpus callosum)
13   Anterior communicating artery (particularly prone to aneurysms)
14   Branch of the posterior cerebral artery
15   Pontine branches off basilar artery

These four arteries supply the brain with blood.
† These three arteries (on each side) supply the cerebral cortex.

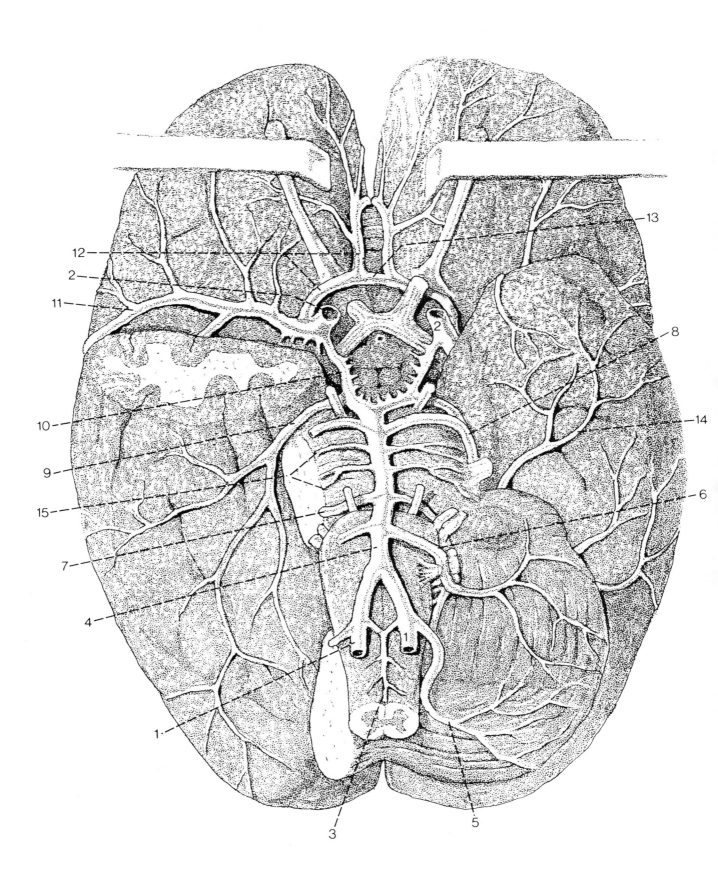

Arteries on medial surface of cerebral hemispheres and on lateral surface of cerebellum and lower brain stem

(After Wolf-Heidegger)

Color and label

1	Vertebral artery (left)
2	Basilar artery
3	Anterior inferior cerebellar artery
4	Abducent nerve (N VI)
5	Labyrinthine artery
6	Pontine branch off basilar artery
7	Posterior cerebral artery (left)
8	Oculomotor nerve (N III)
9	Posterior communicating artery (left)
10	Inferior carotid artery (right)
11	Anterior communicating artery (cut)
12	Anterior cerebral artery (right)
13	Tela choroidea of ventricle III
14	Choroid plexus of ventricle III
15	Internal cerebral vein (left; cut)
16	Great cerebral vein
17	Posterior cerebral artery (right)
18	Vestibulocochlear nerve (N VIII) with labyrinthine artery
19	Cerebellum (left hemisphere)
20	Trochlear nerve (N IV)
21	Superior cerebellar artery (left)
22	Trigeminal nerve (N V)
23	Interventricular foramen
24	Posterior inferior cerebellar artery (left)
25	Posterior spinal artery (left)
26	Genu of corpus callosum
27	Column of fornix
28	Interthalamic adhesion
29	Pineal body
30	Mesencephalon (midbrain; cut)
31	Crus cerebri (cut)
32	Hypophysis cerebri (pituitary gland)

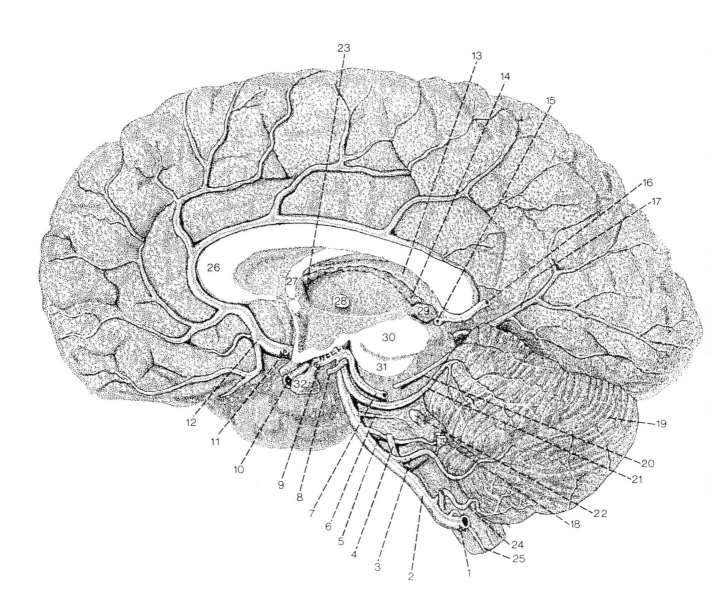

(After Neuwenhuys et al.)

Brain cut at thalamus and lower brainstem removed.

Color and label

1	Cingulate sulcus
2	Marginal part of cingulate sulcus
3	Central sulcus. An easy way to locate the central sulcus on the medial surface of the cerebral cortex is to follow the cingulate sulcus (arrows) to its marginal part (asterisk) and then go one sulcus *forward*. That sulcus will be the superior termination of the central sulcus.
4	Cingulate gyrus (Latin, *cingulum*, belt or girdle)
5	Sulcus of the corpus callosum
6	Paracentral lobule
7	Indusium griseum (Latin, gray umbrella) (remnant of the migrating hippocampus during embryonic development)
8	Precuneus lobule
9	Parieto-occipital sulcus
10	Cuneus (Latin, wedge)
11	Calcarine sulcus
12	Common stem of parieto-occipital and calcarine sulci
13	Fasciolar gyrus (connects dentate gyrus to indusium griseum)
14	Isthmus of cingulate gyrus
15	Dentate gyrus
16	Parahippocampal gyrus
17	Intralimbic gyrus of uncus
18	Limbus of Giacomini (Latin, *limbus*, border or edge)
19	Uncinate gyrus (Latin, *uncus*, hook)
20	Uncinate incisure (slit or notch)
21	Semilunar gyrus
22	Ambient gyrus (gyrus ambiens)
23	Parahippocampal gyrus (anterior part)
24	Gyrus rectus (straight gyrus)
25	Thalamus
26	Cut surface of the thalamus
27	Fornix (body)

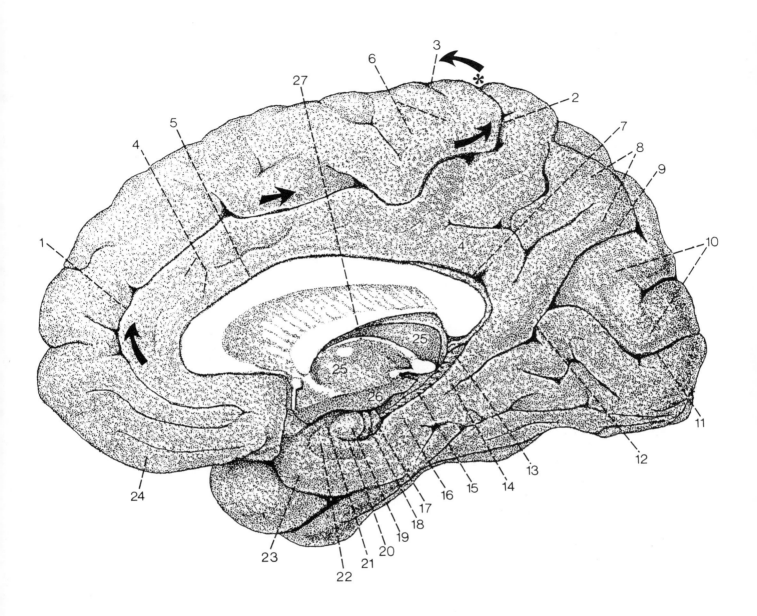

Lobes of cerebral hemisphere
(After Rohen and Yokochi)

Medial surface of right cerebral hemisphere. Front is to the left.
Midbrain cut and brain stem removed.

Color each cortical area a different color. *Label* as indicated.

F Front cortex (frontal lobe)
P Parietal cortex (parietal lobe)
O Occipital cortex (occipital lobe)
T Temporal cortex (temporal lobe)
L Limbic cortex (cingulate gyrus and
    parahippocampal gyrus)

1	Hypothalamus forming lateral wall of lower part of ventricle III
2	Optic chiasm
3	Anterior commissure
4	Genu of corpus callosum
5	Cingulate sulcus
6	Cingulate gyrus
7	Column of fornix
8	Sulcus of corpus callosum
9	Thalamus
10	Precentral sulcus
11	Precentral gyrus
12	Central sulcus (of Rolando; note that the central sulcus occupies only a short length on the medial surface)
13	Postcentral gyrus
14	Marginal part of cingulate sulcus
15	Parieto-occipital sulcus
16	Calcarine sulcus
17	Common stem of the parieto-occipital sulcus and the calcarine sulcus
18	Isthmus of cingulate gyrus
19	Parahippocampal gyrus
20	Lateral occipitotemporal gyrus
21	Collateral sulcus
22	Midbrain (cut)
23	Uncus of parahippocampal gyrus

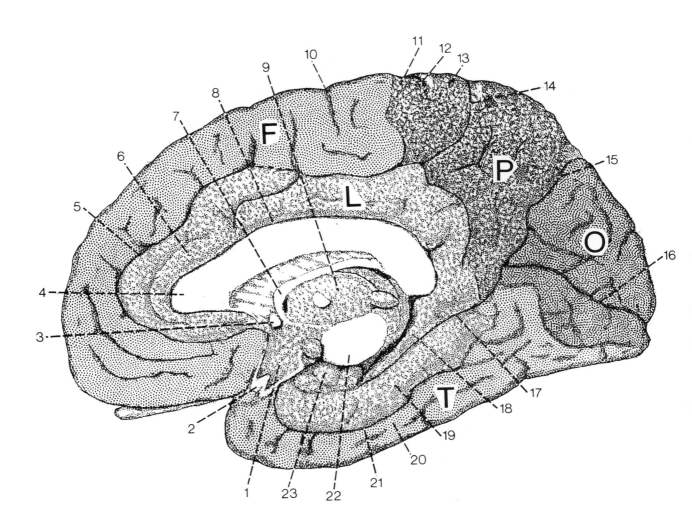

Brainstem cut at midbrain. Lower part of brainstem and cerebellum removed.

Color and label

1   Longitudinal fissure (anterior part between frontal lobes)
2   Olfactory bulb
3   Orbital gyri
4   Lateral olfactory stria
5   Inferior temporal sulcus
6   Anterior perforated substance
7   Infundibulum and tuber cinereum (Latin, funnel and gray eminence)
8   Optic tract
9   Mamillary bodies
10 Interpeduncular fossa
11 Midbrain (mesencephalon; cut)
12 Lateral occipitotemporal gyrus
13 Splenium of corpus callosum and fasciolar gyrus (the latter connects dentate gyrus of hippocampal formation with medial and lateral longitudinal stria of indusium griseum)
14 Medial occipitotemporal gyrus* (left hemisphere)
15 Occipital pole (posterior part of cerebrum)
16 Longitudinal fissure (posterior part between occipital lobes)
17 Calcarine sulcus
18 Cingulate gyrus
19 Medial occipitotemporal gyrus* (right hemisphere)
20 Occipitotemporal sulcus*
21 Preoccipital notch (incisure)
22 Collateral sulcus
23 Parahippocampal gyrus
24 Mesencephalic aqueduct (cerebral aqueduct)
25 Lateral occipitotemporal gyrus*
26 Substantia nigra
27 Inferior temporal gyrus*
28 Crus cerebri (cerebral peduncle)
29 Uncus of parahippocampal gyrus
30 Inferior temporal sulcus*
31 Optic nerve and optic chiasm
32 Middle temporal gyrus*
33 Olfactory tract
34 Orbital sulci
35 Olfactory sulcus
36 Gyrus rectus

*These gyri and sulci vary somewhat and often only approximate the shape and position that their names imply.

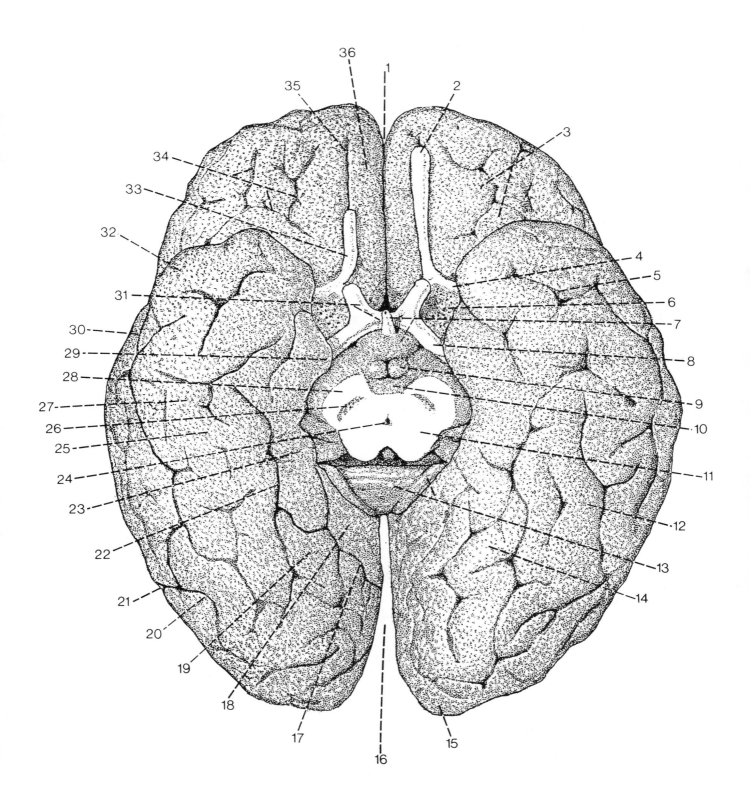

Figure A: The Three Meninges and Spinal Nerves

The spinal cord and brain are covered by three connective tissue membranes called **meninges** (Greek, membranes; singular, meninx). The innermost is the **pia mater** (Latin, *pia,* faithful, gentle, or pious; *mater,* mother). It is the thinnest of the three and faithfully covers the surface of the brain and spinal cord, extending the full depth of each fissure and sulcus (Latin, groove). The pia contains blood vessels and laterally forms two denticulate ligaments on each side of the spinal cord that help stabilize the spinal cord within the vertebral canal.

The middle meninx is the **arachnoid mater** (Greek, spider or web). It is so named because of the many tiny fibers or arachnoid trabeculae (Latin, little beams) that extend across the subarachnoid space from the pia to the arachnoid. The arachnoid space contains cerebrospinal fluid, which protects the brain and spinal cord in an aqueous environment. Enlargements of the subarachnoid space are called **cisterns** (or cisternae). The cerebrospinal fluid supports the brain and spinal cord against gravity and more evenly distributes blows and jolts to the central nervous system.

The outermost meninx is the **dura mater** (Latin, tough mother). It is fibrous and strong and extends laterally to enclose the spinal nerve roots and to ensheath each dorsal root ganglion. The dura mater becomes continuous with the epineurium of the nerve at the lateral border of the ganglion.

The inner gray matter, which contains largely neuronal somata, in cross-section forms an H or butterfly shape with a larger ventral horn (v horn) and a somewhat thinner dorsal horn (d horn).

There are 31 pairs of spinal nerves. Each spinal nerve arises by a ventral root and a dorsal root. (In the human, **anterior** and **posterior** are synonymous with **ventral** and **dorsal,** respectively.) Each root is formed by the coalescence of many dorsal and ventral root **filaments** or **rootlets.** Each spinal nerve almost immediately divides into a large **ventral ramus** and smaller **dorsal ramus** (Latin, branch). The ventral rami become **nerves** of the body such as the ulnar, median, femoral, and intercostal nerves. The dorsal rami innervate mainly the deep muscles of the back such as the erector spinae and the skin of the back. In the brachial and lumbosacral plexuses, the ventral rami become divided into ventral and dorsal **divisions.** In primitive vertebrates the ventral division supplied the ventral **flexor** (flex) muscles of the limbs and the dorsal division supplied the dorsal **extensor** (ext) muscles. This still holds true in the arm, where the radial nerve, which is derived from the dorsal division, supplies all the extensor muscles of the arm. The rotation of the limbs and the upright stance have somewhat distorted this pattern in the leg; for instance, a muscle such as the iliopsoas, which extended the hip in primitive vertebrates, but flexes the hip in humans, is still supplied by the femoral nerve, which is derived from the dorsal division of the lumbar plexus. The tibial nerve, on the other hand, is derived from the **ventral** division and supplies most of the flexors of the leg.

Figure B: Spinal Nerves, Spinal Roots, and Rami

Note that the **ventral ramus** and **dorsal ramus** each contain both **motor** and **sensory fibers.** Motor neuron 1 travels with the ventral ramus and supplies a muscle such as an intercostal or a limb muscle. Motor neuron 2 supplies a deep muscle of the back such as the erector spinae via a dorsal ramus. All limb musculature is supplied by ventral rami. Sensory neurons 3 and 4 with their unipolar perikarya in the dorsal root ganglion supply sensory fibers to both the ventral ramus (fiber 3) and dorsal ramus (4). Fiber 4 enters the spinal cord via the dorsal root and synapses in the dorsal horn upon internuncial neuron 5, which in turn synapses upon motor neuron 2. Afferent fiber 3 terminates upon neuron 6, which is a **cell of origin** of a crossed ascending tract. Fiber 7 is a descending fiber from a higher center. It ends upon interneuron 8, which in turn synapses upon motor neuron 9. Remember that the spinal **roots** contain either motor or sensory fibers and that the **rami** are **mixed** and contain both motor and sensory fibers.

Directions: Upper figure. Color each of the meninges a different color. **Color** the denticulate ligament the same color as the pia, and the trabeculae the same as the arachnoid. **Color** the gray matter another color and use a different color for the ventral and dorsal root filaments.
Lower figure. Use one color for motor neurons 1 and 2 and another for sensory neurons 3 and 4. Color the white and gray matter each separately and trace the connections involving neurons 5 and 9.

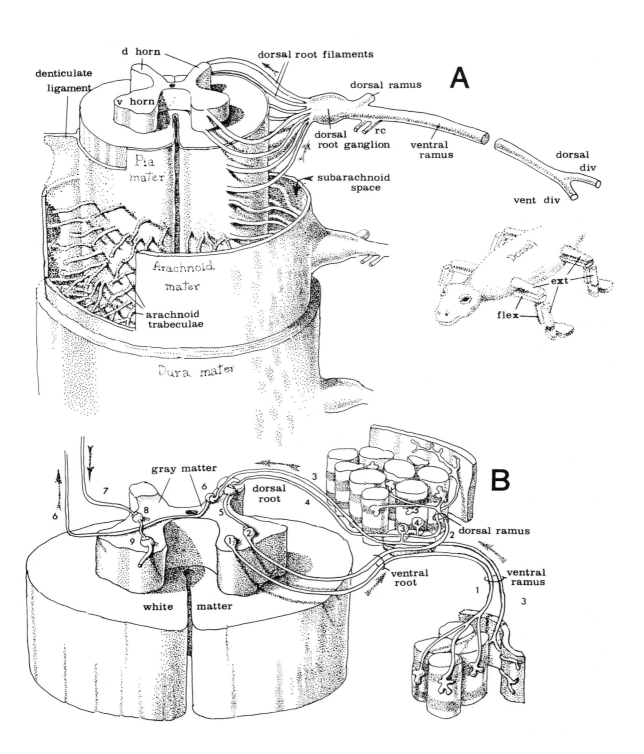

A

denticulate ligament

d horn

v horn

dorsal root filaments

dorsal ramus

dorsal root ganglion

rc

ventral ramus

dorsal div

vent div

Pia mater

subarachnoid space

ext

flex

Arachnoid mater

arachnoid trabeculae

Dura mater

B

gray matter

7

6

6

8

9

5

1

2

dorsal root

3

4

3

4

dorsal ramus

2

white matter

ventral root

ventral ramus

1

3

Color and label

1   Dura mater
2   Arachnoid mater
3   Arachnoid trabeculae
4   Pia mater
5   Denticulate ligament
6   Dorsal horn (of gray matter)
7   Ventral horn (of gray matter)
8   White matter
9   Dorsal root filaments
10   Dorsal root ganglion
11   Ventral root filaments
12   Spinal nerve trunk
13   Dorsal ramus
14   Ventral ramus
15   Communicating rami
16   Subarachnoid space

Lower Figure: White Matter and Gray Matter

The white matter consists mainly of ascending and descending myelinated axons. In the spinal cord, the white matter is divided into three *funiculi* (Latin, little rope), the ventral, lateral, and dorsal funiculi, shown on the viewer's left side. On the viewer's right side, it is apparent that each funiculus contains several tracts, or *fasciculi* (Latin, little bundles). The dorsal funiculus contains mainly two tracts, or fasciculi, the fasciculus gracilis and fasciculus cuneatus. The layers, or laminae of Rexed, in the gray matter are shown on the viewer's left side. Rexed, a Swedish neuroanatomist, divided the gray matter into 10 laminae on the basis of cell types. Layer I is most dorsal. Layer II is the substantia gelatinosa (Latin, jelly-like substance) (sg, on the right). Note that lamina IX, which contains the motor neurons, is not a lamina at all, but rather forms several columns. Lamina X contains the cells around the central canal. The ascending and descending tracts in the white matter canot be identified except by special means.

Color each of the three funiculi on the left.
Then color Lamina I, III, V, VII, and IX

Abbreviations: dorsolat fasc, dorsolateral fasciculus; dorsal fun, dorsal funiculus; dorsal sp cer tr, dorsal spinocerebellar tract; fasc cun, fasciculus cuneatus; fasc gr, fasciculus gracilis, lat fun, lateral funiculus; lat cort sp tr, lateral corticospinal tract; propriosp tr, propriospinal tract; sp th trs, spinothalamic tracts; sg, substantia gelatinosa; vent fun, ventral funiculus; and vent sp cer tr, ventral spinocerebellar tract.

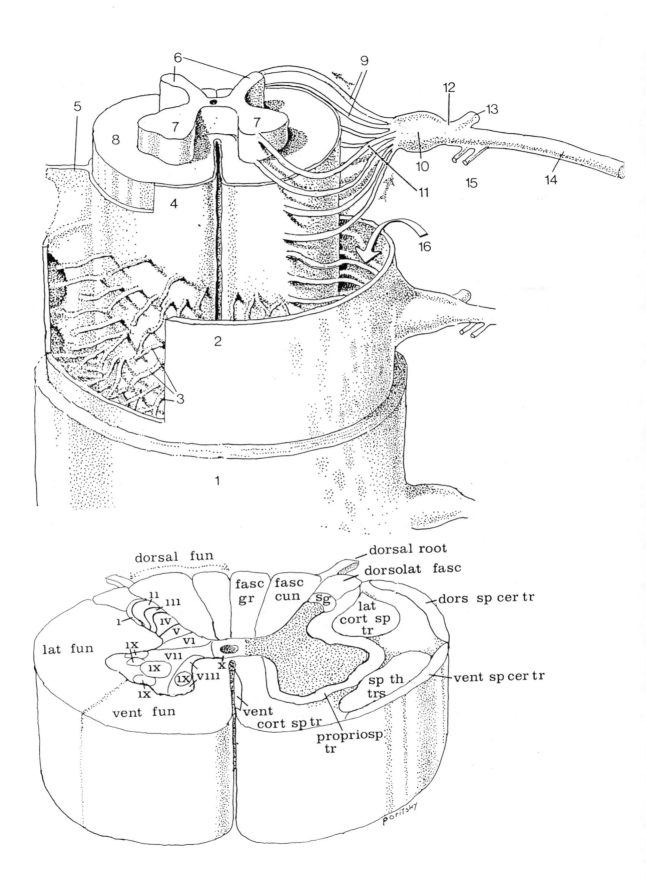

dorsal fun

dorsal root

fasc gr

fasc cun

dorsolat fasc

sg

dors sp cer tr

ll

lll

l

lV

V

Vl

lat cort sp tr

lX

Vll

x

lat fun

lX

lX

VlVlll

sp th trs

vent sp cer tr

vent fun

lX

vent cort sp tr

propriosp tr

poritsky

Spinal nerve components are the names given categories of different nerves that travel within
spinal nerves.

GSE Stands for **general somatic efferent** and includes the axons of alpha motor neurons and axons of gamma motor neurons.

GVE Stands for **general visceral efferent** and includes all sympathetic and parasympathetic fibers.

GSA Stands for **general somatic afferent** and includes pain, touch, and temperature fibers as well as fibers that convey deep pressure, joint position, muscle tension, and muscle length.

GVA Stands for **general visceral afferent** and includes all fibers, from the viscera (intestines, stomach, lungs, heart, etc.). Pain from the viscera tends to be diffuse and poorly localized. Most GVA fibers function at the subconscious level and play vital roles in the regulation of heart beat, blood pressure, breathing, intestinal motility, and digestion.

Color and label. Use boxes as color keys.

1   **Alpha motor neuron.** Its axon innervates voluntary skeletal muscles.

2   **Gamma motor neuron.** Its axon ends upon the intrafusal cells in muscle spindles. It controls their state of tension and hence their sensitivity to stretch.

3   **Sympathetic preganglionic neuron cell body.** Its axon ends upon postganglionic neuron 7. Preganglionic sympathetic neurons lie in the intermediolateral column of the spinal cord. In sacral levels S2–S4 of the spinal cord, these neurons are parasympathetic rather than sympathetic.

4   **Muscle spindle fiber** (or intrafusal fiber). Note that the gamma motor neuron supplies the contractile ends of the muscle spindle fiber, thus stretching and sensitizing the central part of the intrafusal fiber.

5   **Striated muscle cell**

6   **Gland cells.** Autonomic fibers (parasympathetic and sympathetic fibers) supply glands, smooth muscle, and the heart.

7   **Sympathetic postganglionic cell body** in a ganglion of the sympathetic chain. Its axon (14) runs into the spinal nerve. It will eventually end upon a hair follicle, a sweat gland, or a blood vessel.

8   **Sympathetic ganglion.** This is part of the sympathetic chain. These ganglia are also referred to as paravertebral ganglia.

9   **Dorsal root ganglion**

10   **Cell body (soma) of GVA fiber**

11   **Cell body of GSA fiber.** GSA fibers convey information from touch receptors, pressure receptors, and proprioceptors.

12   **Meissner's tactile (touch) corpuscle.**

13   **Intestinal wall.** GVA fiber begins with extensive arborization within the wall of the intestine.

14   **Sympathetic postganglionic fiber.** Note that this fiber re-enters the spinal nerve.

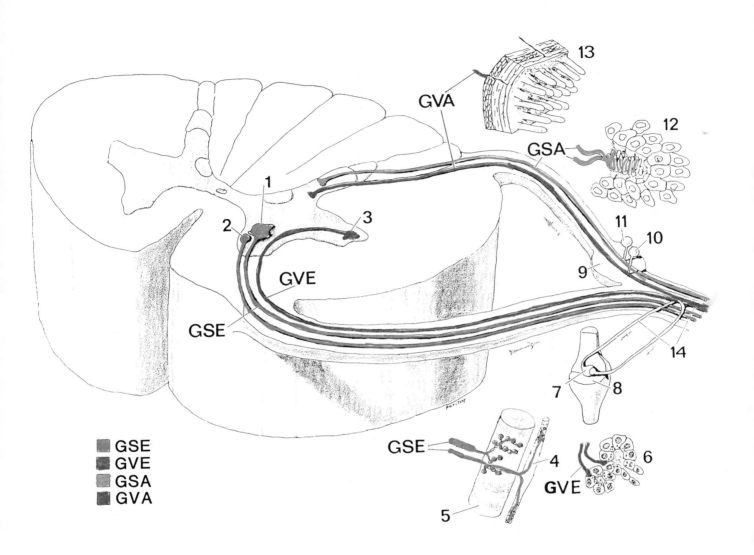

GVA

GSA

13

12

11

10

9

1

2

3

GVE

GSE

14

7   8

GSE

4

5

6

GVE

GSE
GVE
GSA
GVA

26 Arterial supply and vascular pattern to a portion of spinal cord

(After Windle)

Color and label

1   **Posterior spinal arteries.** These supply posterior one-third of spinal cord.
2   **Anterior spinal artery.** This supplies anterior two-thirds of spinal cord.
3   **Anterior medullary feeder artery.** These are variable in both position (level) and in number (average a total of 8 for the whole spinal cord) (Dommisse 1975, cited in Clemente 1985). These feeder arteries join with and supply the anterior spinal artery with additional blood. They arise from the spinal branches of the segmental arteries such as the posterior intercostal arteries.
4   **Posterior medullary feeder artery.** These join with and augment the posterior spinal arteries. They arise like the anterior medullary feeder arteries.
5   **Spinal rami** (branches) **of segmental arteries.** These enter the spinal canal bilaterally at every intervertebral level.
6   **Anterior** (ventral) **radicular branches.** These supply the ventral roots (Latin, *radix,* root).
7   **Dorsal** (posterior) **radicular branches** to dorsal roots.
8   **Sulcal** (or central) **arteries.** These average 5–9 per segment and average 210 for all 31 spinal cord segments (Tvetan 1976, cited in Clemente 1985).
9   **Coronal arteries**
10   **Superficial pial plexus**
11   **Penetrating vessels**
12   **Dorsal root ganglion** (spinal ganglion)
13   **Dorsal rootlets** (filaments) and **dorsal root**
14   **Ventral rootlets** (filaments)

References

Clemente CD (ed): Gray's Anatomy, Philadelphia, Lea & Febiger, 1985.

Dommisse GF: The Arteries and Veins of the Human Spinal Cord from Birth. Edinburgh, Churchill Livingstone, 1975.

Tvetan L: Spinal cord vascularity. III. The spinal cord arteries in man. Acta Radiol Diagn (Stockh) 17:257-273, 1976.

Windle WF (ed): The Spinal Cord and Its Reaction to Injury. New York, Marcel Dekker, 1980.

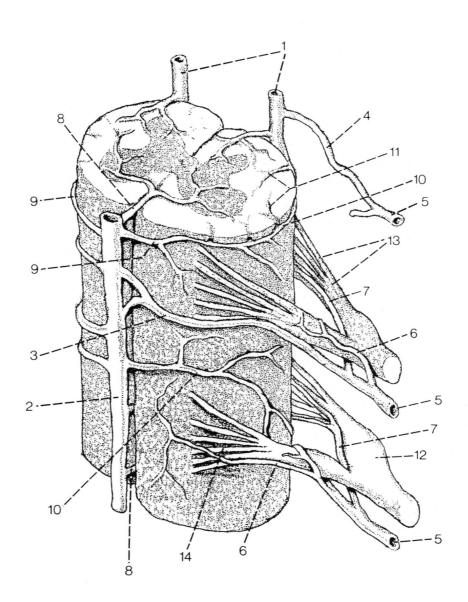

27 The cauda equina of the spinal cord
(After Benninghoff and Goerttler)

The posterior parts of the lumbar vertebrae have been removed, the dura mater cut open, and the posterior portion of the sacrum cut away to reveal the sacral canal.

Color and label

1   Dura mater (cut)
2   Subcostal nerve (T12)
3   Dorsal root (spinal) ganglion of nerve L1
4   Conus medullaris
5   Iliohypogastric nerve (L1)
6   Ilioinguinal nerve (L1)
7   Dorsal root ganglion of nerve L3
8   Dorsal ramus of nerve L3
9   Filum terminal internum
10   Dorsal root ganglion of nerve L5
11   Femoral nerve (L2, L3, L4)
12   Dural sac
13   Fibers from S1 forming sciatic nerve
14   S2 fibers forming sciatic nerve
15   S3 fibers forming sciatic nerve
16   Sciatic nerve (L4, L5, S1, S2, S3)
17   Sacral nerve (S5)
18   Filum terminale externum
19   Sacral nerve (S4)
20   Cauda equina
21   Lumbosacral trunk. Fibers from L4 and L5 forming sciatic nerve.

Benninghoff A, Goerttler K: Lehrbuch der Anatomie des Menchen, Vol. 3, 9th ed. Munich, Urban and Schwarzenberg, 1975.

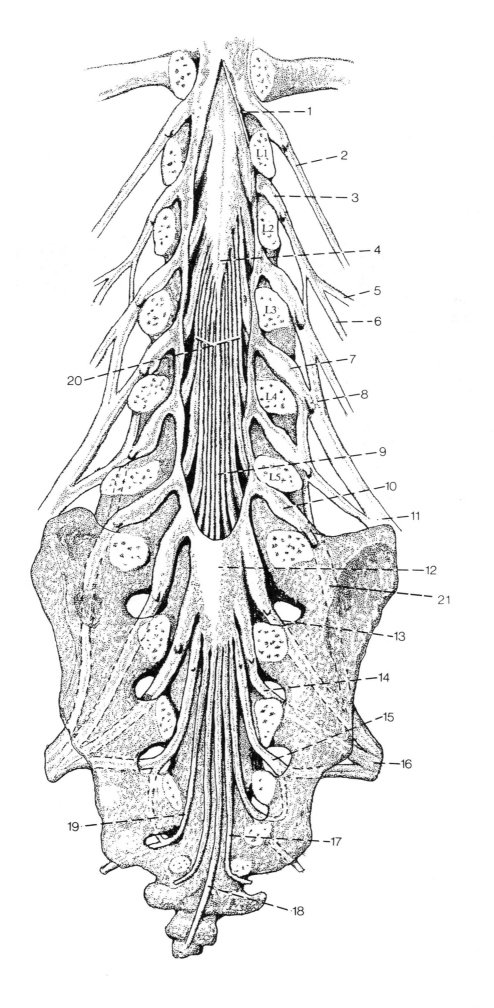

28   The alpha motor neuron

The alpha motor neuron is also called the lower motor neuron, peripheral motor neuron, and the final common pathway. Sherrington, an English physiologist (1856-1952), called it the final common pathway, because he realized that these large neurons, whose axons end directly upon muscles, are the final and only connecting link between the central nervous system and muscles, and all our mental and emotional life must be expressed through them.

The axon of each motor neuron leaves the spinal cord and travels to a muscle where it divides, sometimes into a thousand or more branches. Each branch ends upon one muscle fiber. When the alpha motor neuron fires off, each of the muscle fibers it contacts will contract.

Note the afferent fibers bringing messages from other neurons, some of which are nearby; others are as far away as the cerebral cortex. Each afferent axon at its end contains a tiny bag-like swelling, the axon terminal or *bouton terminal* (French, terminal button). Some of these axon terminals are excitatory and slightly depolarize the area of motor neuron membrane that they overlie. Other axon terminals are inhibitory and slightly hyperpolarize the underlying membrane. A single alpha motor neuron may receive as many as 30,000 axon terminals from incoming fibers. When a critical amount of membrane is simultaneously depolarized and the total resulting depolarizing current reaches a certain threshold, the motor neuron will discharge in an all-or-none fashion.

 Note the bushy protoplasmic astrocyte, which is one of the three types of neuroglial cells. Besides astrocytes, which are either protoplasmic or fibrous, neuroglia also include oligodendrocytes and microgliocytes. The bushy appearance of protoplasmic astrocytes is due to their processes wedging between and around axons, dendrites, and the processes of other glial cells. Astrocytes also send processes that form perivascular end feet that almost completely ensheathe the capillaries in the CNS.

Note the two oligodendrocytes (Greek, *oligo,* few; *dendro*, branch; *cyte,* cell; literally few branched cells). One oligodendrocyte is in a perineuronal position; the other is connected to the myelin of five afferent fibers. Each of these myelin segments had been synthesized by a single process of an oligodendrocyte spreading itself along the axon for a distance of one internode. The myelin is formed for the condensation and tight packing of the spirally wrapped oligodendrocyte cell membrane.

Color each of the structures indicated.

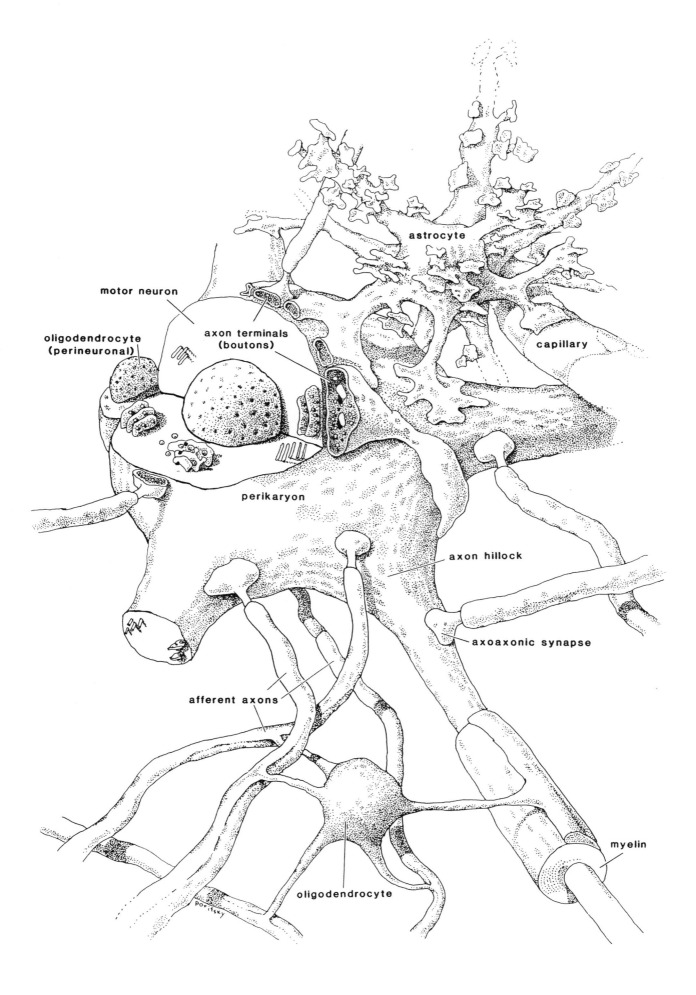

motor neuron

oligodendrocyte
(perineuronal)

axon terminals
(boutons)

astrocyte

capillary

perikaryon

axon hillock

axoaxonic synapse

afferent axons

myelin

oligodendrocyte

Etymological cartoon: Atropos

Greek: *a*, not; *tropos*, turn (she would not turn)

The deadly poison atropine is named after Atropos, one of the three Fates. In Greek mythology the three Fates spun the web of destiny for all mankind. It was Atropos who determined how long one would live and when one's life would end. She was usually depicted holding shears, which she used to cut the threads of life that suspend all mortals. She would not heed, or even turn, when beseeched by humans pleading for more life.

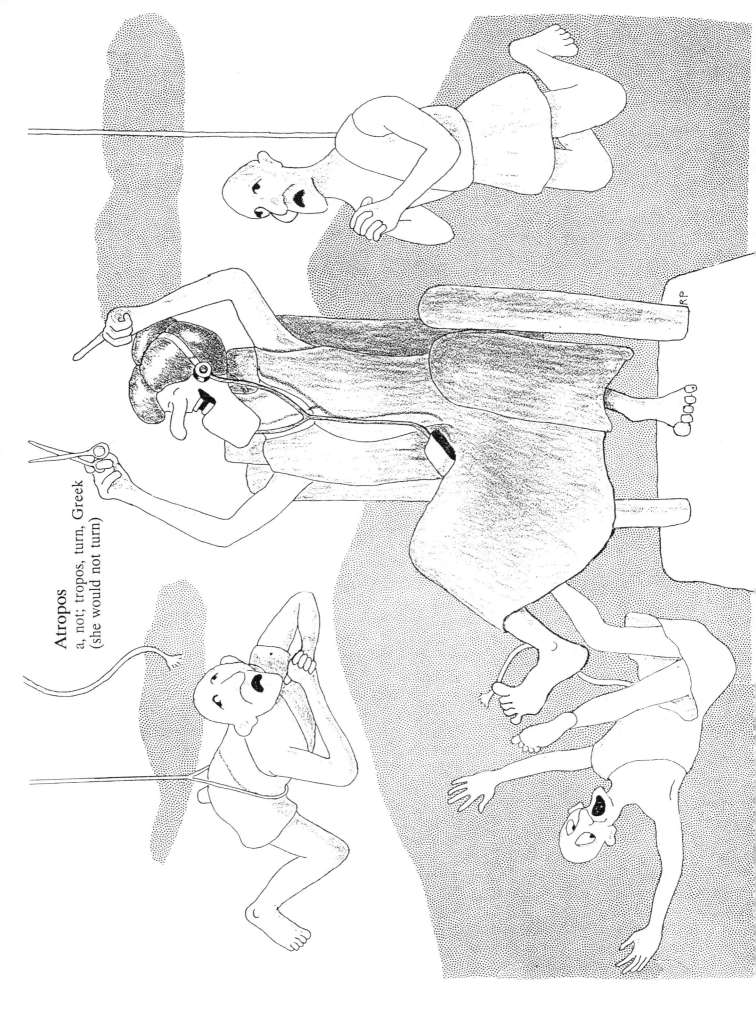

Atropos
a, not; tropos, turn, Greek
(she would not turn)

The **motor unit** consists of an alpha motor neuron, its axon, and all the muscle fibers innervated by that motor neuron. Each motor unit works as a functional unit. The force of contraction depends in large part upon the number of motor units simultaneously discharging. In addition, the frequency of impulses from each motor neuron directly affects the degree of contraction of the muscle fibers it supplies. Figure A shows an alpha motor neuron innervating 8 muscle fibers. This is a relatively small number of muscle fibers to be supplied by one motor neuron. Muscles such as the finger muscles and eye muscles have small motor units in which one motor neuron supplies only 8 or 10 muscle fibers. Because these muscles have many motor units, each of which contains relatively few neurons, these muscles are capable of performing precise and delicate movements. On the other hand, large muscles such as the gastrocnemius have motor units in which one motor neuron innervates approximately 1,800 muscle fibers. Muscles such as these–with large motor units but with fewer motor units (per unit volume)–are not able to contract with as many degrees of tension as are muscles with smaller and more numerous (per unit volume) motor units.

Color the motor unit (motor neuron, its axon, and the muscle fibers it innervates).

Figure B shows that the motor neurons that supply shoulder muscles lie higher in the spinal cord than do motor neurons that supply the more distal limb musculature. Thus the motor neurons that innervate the levator scapulae lie at cervical levels C3-C4; those to the biceps lie at C5-C6, and those to the adductor pollicis muscle in the thumb lie at C8-T1. The importance of this is evident when the spinal cord is damaged in the neck region. If the break is just above C8, the individual will lose the use of muscles in the hand, but will still have use of the more proximal muscles of the arm. If the spinal cord is damaged just below C4, only the most proximal limb muscles such as the levator scapulae would still be able to function. The loss of function is due to the interruption of descending motor fibers, which carry motor commands to the motor neurons.

Color each of the motor neurons, their fibers, and the muscles that they innervate.

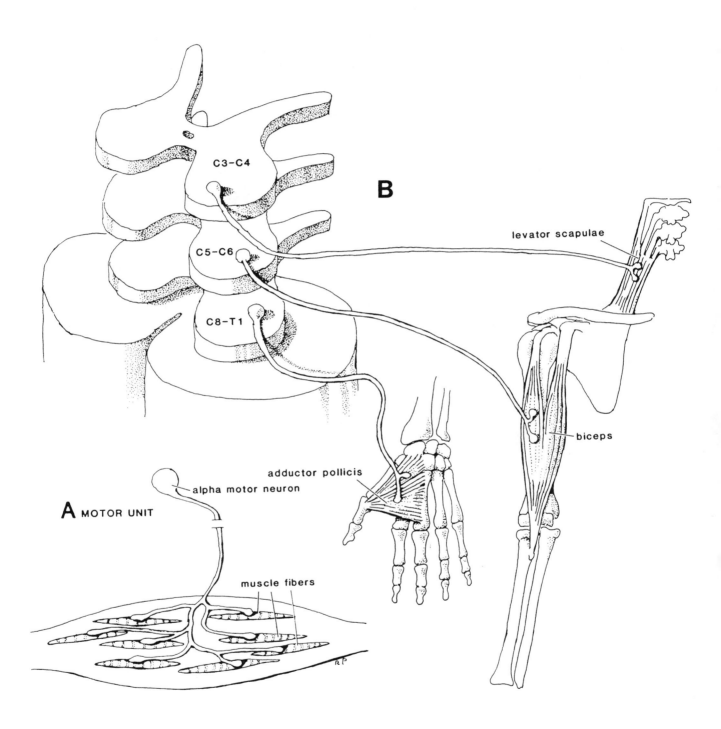

C3-C4

B

C5-C6

C8-T1

levator scapulae

biceps

adductor pollicis

alpha motor neuron

A MOTOR UNIT

muscle fibers

The muscle spindle is a length sensor. It signals information on the length of the muscle, on any change in length, and on how fast the change occurs. Figure A is a single cell (or fiber) from a muscle spindle. Each muscle spindle in man contains an average of 10 such fibers called **intrafusal fibers.** The rest of the muscle fibers–those that actually contract–are called **extrafusal fibers.** Each muscle has many spindles. The small abductor pollicis brevis has about 80 and the large latissimus dorsi over 350. However, the abductor pollicis has considerably greater density of spindles than does the latissimus dorsi. In Figure A the spindle cell is in a stretched state. In Figure B the same cell is in a shortened state. The stretching or lengthening of a spindle occurs when its muscle, such as the biceps brachii (Figure C) is lengthened. Notice that the spindle cell in Figures A and B has the annulospiral ending of a 1a afferent fiber wrapped around its central sensory portion. The annulospiral ending is very sensitive to any stretching of the central portion of the spindle cell. This central part contains a number of nuclei (not shown) and is noncontractile (it cannot contract by itself). The contractile portions of the spindle cell are at its ends and receive their motor supply from **gamma motor neurons.** Discharge of the gamma fiber will cause the contractile ends of the spindle cell to contract, which will stretch the central sensory portion with its annulospiral ending. Thus, the gamma motor neuron determines the sensitivity of the spindle by maintaining its sensory portion at the critical threshold. However, the spindle fires off not only when the muscle is lengthened, but it also discharges at a steady low frequency when the muscle is "at rest," that is, not changing its length.

Color the annulospiral ending about the spindle cell in Figure A and its afferent fiber. Its unipolar perikaryon is in the spinal (or dorsal root) ganglion and its central portion synapses directly upon alpha motor neurons of the same muscle (seen in Figure C 3). **Color** the gamma motor neuron in Figures A and B. Its perikaryon is in the ventral horn of the spinal cord gray matter in the vicinity of alpha motor neurons. Its axon leaves the spinal cord in the ventral root and travels to the target muscle in the same nerve as the alpha motor axons. Appreciate the fact that the gamma motor neuron cannot either lengthen or shorten the spindle; the length of the spindles is determined by the length of the muscle itself. The gamma motor fiber "tightens up" the central sensory part of the cell. The spindle is **not** subjected to the tension within the muscle. It is arranged **in parallel** with the extrafusal fibers, that is, with the rest of the muscle.

Figure C shows the biceps and its spindle lengthened, as occurs with extension of the elbow. The triceps extends the elbow and the biceps relaxes and is stretched. **Color** the alpha motor neuron and its fiber to the triceps. The biceps and triceps usually act as antagonistic muscles. One must relax when the other contracts.

Figures C and D show an enlarged isolated spindle cell below the biceps and the same cell within the biceps, both of which are attached to the same 1a afferent. Starting with the annulospiral endings around both spindle cells, **color** the 1a fiber centrally to the spinal cord where it divides into a number of branches. Three of the terminal branches of the 1a afferents are shown in Figure C: (1) the dorsal columns (fasciculus cuneatus), (2) an ending upon an inhibitory interneuron that inhibits the triceps alpha motor neuron, and (3) a synapse directly upon the alpha motor neuron to the same muscle (the biceps brachii). These three components, the 1a fiber, the alpha motor neuron, and the synapse between the two, constitute a two-neuron monosynaptic reflex, and are the basis for the myotatic or stretch reflex (such as tapping the patellar tendon and the resultant knee jerk). The stretch reflex is the only reflex with just one synapse.

Figure D shows the biceps contracted and its muscle spindle shortened. This occurs when its alpha motor neurons (agonists) discharge. In normal movement the contraction of any single muscle probably requires tens or hundreds of motor neurons to discharge, each causing the contraction of all the muscle fibers that it innervates, that is, its **motor unit.** When a muscle contracts, not only do the alpha motor neurons discharge but the gamma motor neurons discharge simultaneously. This **coactivation** of gamma and alpha motor neurons ensures a continuous sensitivity for the spindle so that it does not become "unloaded" or "desensitized" whenever it is shortened. This coactivation is also a means of increasing the alpha motor neuron's rate of firing and, hence, the force of contraction. In Figure D, **color** both the alpha and gamma motor neurons and their fibers. The gamma fiber is causing the ends of the spindle cell to contract and to remain sensitive.

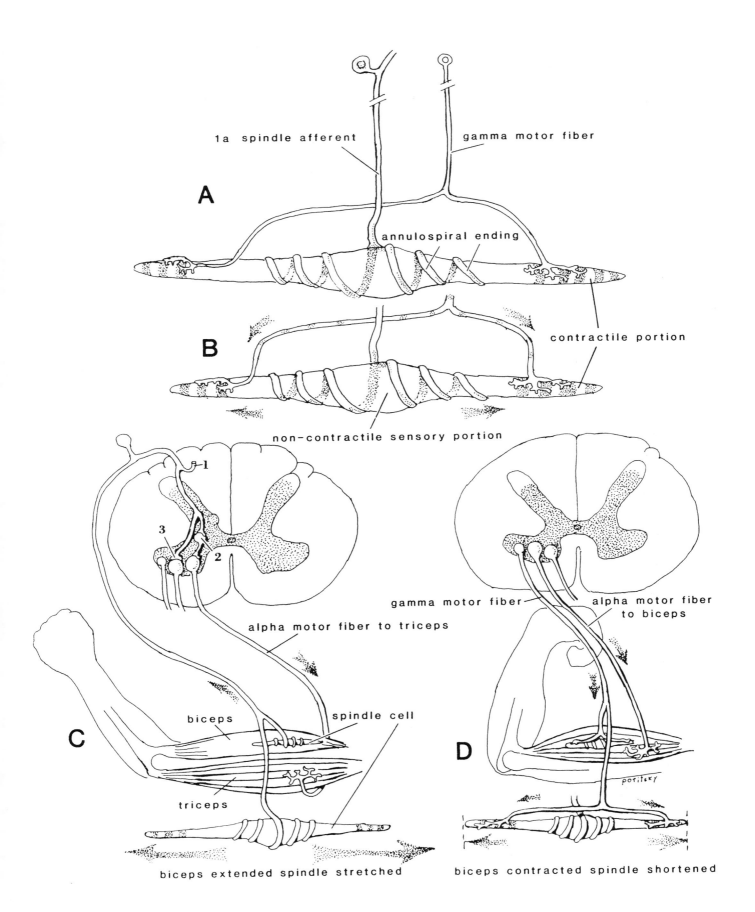

1a spindle afferent

gamma motor fiber

A

annulospiral ending

B

contractile portion

non-contractile sensory portion

1

3

2

alpha motor fiber to triceps

biceps

spindle cell

triceps

C

biceps extended spindle stretched

gamma motor fiber

alpha motor fiber to biceps

D

biceps contracted spindle shortened

poritsky

Cut out Figures 32 and 33 and attach to one another as indicated.

Neuron 1 is a **cell of origin** of **pyramidal** or **corticospinal** fiber in the "leg" region of the precentral gyrus (motor area 4). **Trace** its fiber caudally to its termination. Note how the three pyramidal fibers 1, 2, and 3 are squeezed together in the posterior limb of the internal capsule (asterisk, * on left side) between the thalamus (thal) and medial part of the globus pallidus (gp 1). Note also how the pyramidal fibers occupy the intermediate third of the cerebral peduncle in the midbrain. In the pons the pyramidal fibers are broken up into longitudinal bundles that regroup into the compact **pyramids** (pyr) in the medulla. In the lower medulla, between 75% and 90% of the fibers decussate (pyr decuss) and continue down the spinal cord as the **lateral corticospinal tract.** The remaining uncrossed fibers become the **ventral corticospinal tract.** This tract descends on the medial aspect of the ventral funiculus and ends mainly in the cervical spinal cord after first crossing to the opposite side. Fiber 1 carrying leg motor commands continues caudally to the sacral level where it synapses upon internuncial neuron (interneuron) 4, which in turn contacts alpha motor neuron 5, which sends its axon to muscle fibers in a muscle of the leg. Corticospinal neuron 2 in the "hand" region of the motor cortex is exceptional because its axon ends directly upon alpha motor neuron 6 in the cervical spinal cord instead of upon an internuncial as most corticospinal fibers do. Neuron 6 is an alpha motor neuron (or lower motor neuron) whose axon innervates muscle fibers in a muscle of the hand. Neuron 3 is a corticobulbar or corticonuclear neuron. Its fiber extends from the "face" region of the motor cortex to the opposite facial nucleus where it synapses upon facial motor neuron 6 whose axon innervates muscle fibers in a muscle of facial expression such as the orbicularis oris.

By definition, the pyramidal or corticospinal tract consists of all fibers that pass through the pyramids in the medulla. The pyramidal tract begins with cells that lie in the fifth layer of the cerebral cortex and ends in the spinal cord, where most of its fibers synapse upon interneurons that influence both alpha and gamma motor neurons. The pyramidal tract is only one of several descending motor tracts that carry "motor commands" to the lower motor neurons; however, it is the only descending tract that travels from cerebral cortex to spinal cord with no synaptic interruption. It is found only in the higher mammals and reaches its greatest development in humans. Each pyramidal tract contains about one million fibers, of which about 90% are thin with a diameter of 1-4 µm. About 90% of all pyramidal fibers are myelinated and 10% unmyelinated. Some 30,000 pyramidal fibers are very large, with diameters of 11-22 µm. These large fibers are believed to arise from the 30,000 giant Betz cells in motor area 4. These large fibers are the longest fibers, extending from the cortex to sacral levels of the cord. Neuron 1 is one such large fiber. In their course to the spinal cord, pyramidal fibers give off many collaterals to structures such as the striatum (putamen and caudate nucleus), thalamus, red nucleus, pontine nuclei, and reticular formation. Originally it was believed that pyramidal fibers arose only from the Betz cells in area 4. After more accurate counts of the number of Betz cells (30,000) and the total number of pyramidal fibers (about 1,000,000) became available, this view could no longer be held. Somewhat surprisingly, it now appears that only about one quarter of the pyramidal fibers have their origin in motor area 4, whereas the remaining three quarters of pyramidal fibers arise from the sensory area in the parietal lobe.

Directions: Trace the descending course of pyramidal fibers 1, 2, 3 using the same color. Use another color for alpha motor neurons 5, 6, and 7 and a third color for interneuron 4.

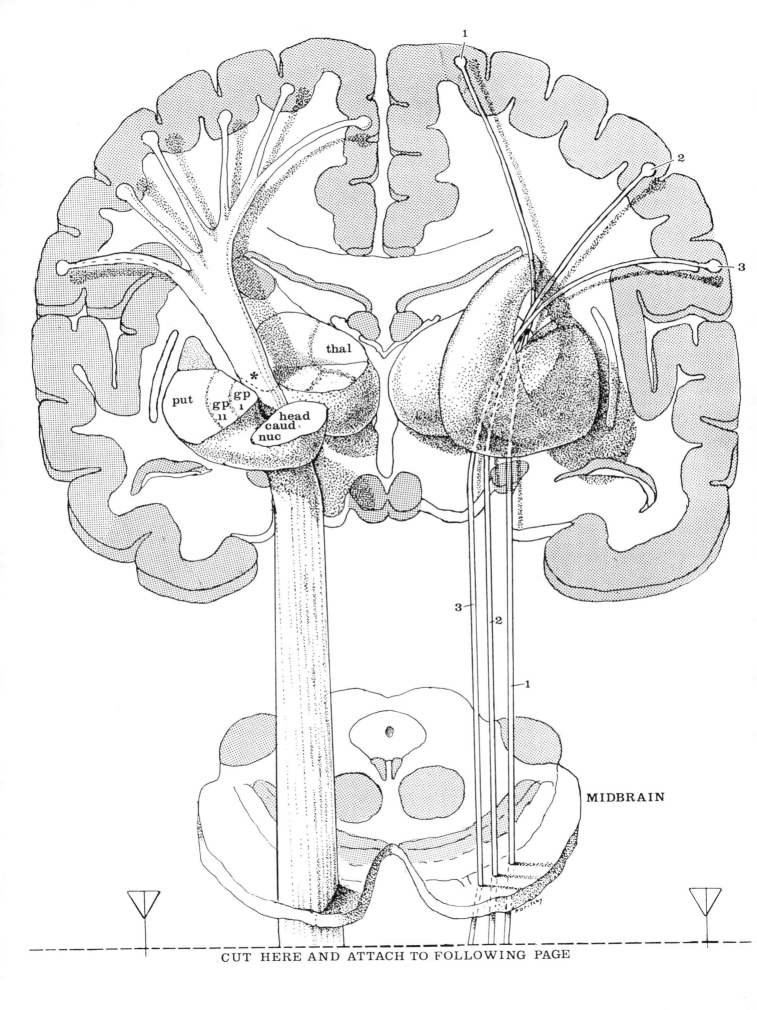

put

gp
ll

gp
l

*

thal

head
caud
nuc

MIDBRAIN

1

2

3

3

2

1

CUT HERE AND ATTACH TO FOLLOWING PAGE

The pyramidal tract *(continued)*

It is now believed that in addition to carrying "motor commands" to alpha and gamma motor neurons, the pyramidal tract also has an important sensory function: it most likely regulates the transmission of sensory information to the brain, particularly finger and hand proprioception during delicate movement such as writing or playing a musical instrument. Presumably, the "sensory" pyramidal tract component would "sharpen" or "zero in" on proprioceptive information from the hand and fingers, possibly augmenting these sensations, while at the same time suppressing sensory information from the rest of the body. This appears to be supported by the large proportion of pyramidal fibers that arise from the somatosensory cortex. Also these fibers end in the dorsal horn of the spinal cord, where presumably they could affect incoming proprioceptive and exteroceptive information. Pyramidal fibers carrying "motor commands" usually end upon interneurons in the intermediate gray matter of the spinal cord. These interneurons (or internuncials) act upon both alpha motor neurons as well as gamma motor neurons. Thus, corticospinal neurons exert their influence upon the lower motor neurons by way of an interneuron so that two synapses are involved, and the pyramidal neuron-to-alpha motor neuron path is said to be disynaptic (two synapses). In humans and the monkey, however, some pyramidal fibers act monosynaptically, that is, they end directly upon the lower motor neuron. These monosynaptic fibers end in the region of finger alpha motor neurons and are presumed to supply finger muscle motor neurons (neuron 2). Interneurons, such as 6, are considerably more structurally complex than indicated in the drawing, and have a vast intricate array of dendrites. These interneurons probably play a crucial role in all movement. Even the simplest movement requires incredible timing and coordination of all motor neurons involved. The sequence of impulses to the prime movers must be exactly right, so that, for example, the hand is moved to the desired position. The antagonist muscles must relax to just the right degree so that the hand does not overshoot its mark. The synergist muscles must stabilize and work with the prime movers, and the gamma motor neurons must maintain the correct tautness of the muscle spindle fibers so that the muscle spindles remain sensitive even as the muscle shortens. The interneurons probably play a key role in determining the exquisitely complex discharge pattern of the neurons involved. The pyramidal tract is responsible for rapid, isolated, discrete movements, especially movements of the fingers and toes. Following pyramidotomy (cutting the pyramidal tract) in monkeys, these movements are lost, although the hand and fingers can still be used for simpler movements (for example, walking). The influence of the pyramidal tract upon the gamma motor neuron helps maintain normal muscle tone. Damage to the pyramidal tract is not followed by muscle atrophy because the alpha motor neuron and its axon are still intact.

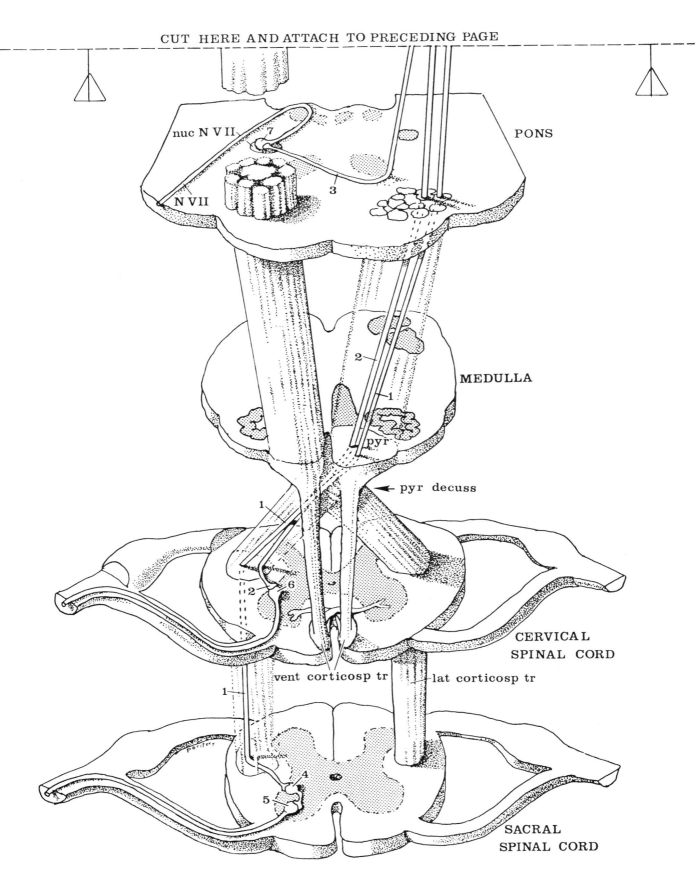

34 Etymological cartoon: Latin words used to describe parts of the nervous system

1. *Locus ceruleus*, blue place. This mass of nerve cells in the brain derives its name from its blue color.

2. *Tectum*, roof. The former name was *lamina quadrigemina*, the plate with the four bodies - that is, the four colliculi ("little hills").

3. *Vitrum*, glass. *In vitro* means "in glass" (that is, in a test tube or petri dish).

4. *Fenestra*, window. The ear has two small *fenestrae*, the oval window and the round window. Fenestrated capillaries have tiny holes in their walls.

5. *Lithos*, stone (Greek). Otoliths, or ear stones, are found in the inner ear.

6. *Lemniscus*, ribbon. This term describes a flat bundle of axons.

7. *Brachia conjunctiva*, the arms that come together. This was the old name for the superior cerebellar peduncles because the two peduncles would come together and decussate.

8. *Macula*, spot. In ancient Rome instead of calling "Here Spot, here Spot" (that is, if you had a dog with a big spot), you would call, "Veni Macula, veni Macula." Immaculate means spotless.

9. *Substantia gelatinosa*, jelly-like substance. This layer of the spinal cord gray matter, now designated layer II of Rexed, appears jelly-like because of the absence of myelinated fibers.

10. *Ampulla*, a swelling or a flask.

11. *Genu*, knee. Geniculate means bent, as in geniculate ganglion or lateral geniculate body. You may wish to genuflect when you encounter an important person such as an anatomy professor, especially before an exam. You might also wish to address him or her as "your eminence." An eminence is something that rises above its surroundings. In anatomy an eminence means a bump, and in the Church or in the palace it was a term of respect for a very important person who rose above his contemporaries.

12. *Peduncle*, little foot or stalk. The cerebellum is attached to the brain stem by six peduncles (three on each side).

13. *Operculum*, a cover or lid. The operculum of the cerebral hemisphere covers the insula.

14. *Amygdala*, almond. This mass of neurons in the temporal lobe has an almond shape.

15. *Putamen*, a shell or husk. This shell-shaped mass of neurons partially envelops the globus pallidus.

16. *Uncus*, hook. The uncinate gyrus on the temporal lobe suggests a hook.

17. *Decussate*, to intersect or to cut in the form of an X.

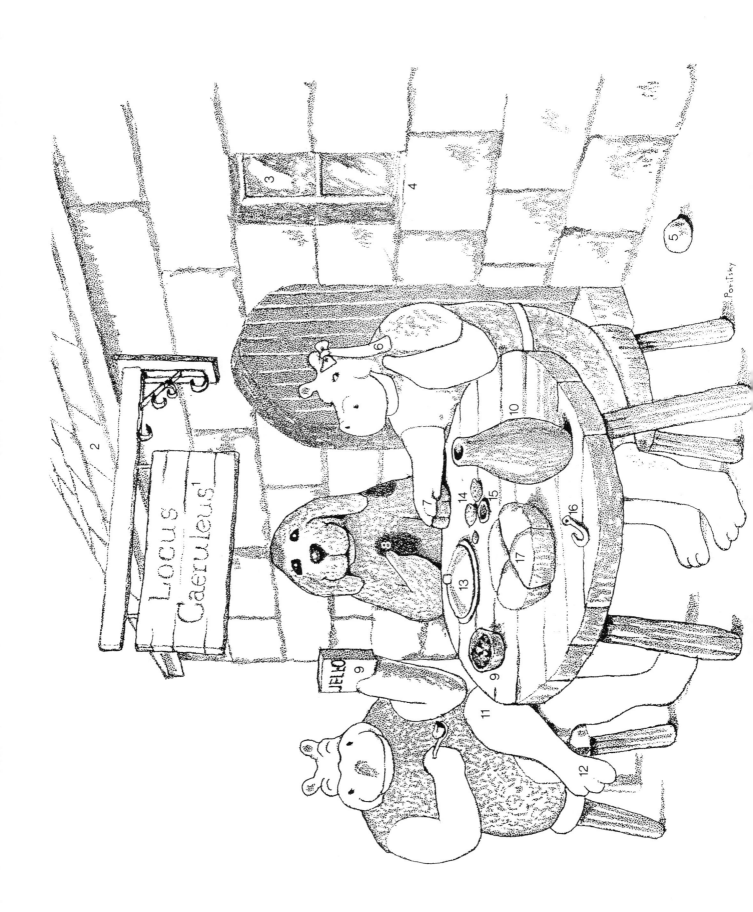

The four ventricles are fluid-filled spaces deep within the substance of the brain. Each of the two lateral ventricles lies within a cerebral hemisphere. They are called the **left** and **right lateral ventricles**. They are essentially mirror images of each other. Each lateral ventricle communicates with the **third ventricle** by a short **interventricular foramen** (of Monro). The third ventricle communicates with the fourth ventricle by way of the **mesencephalic aqueduct** (formerly called the aqueduct of Sylvius or cerebral aqueduct). The fluid within the ventricles is **cerebrospinal fluid** and is made mainly by the choroid plexus in each ventricle. Note the three horns of each lateral ventricle. The third ventricle is narrow and lies between the two thalami above and the two hypothalami below. The **fourth ventricle** is diamond-shaped and lies half in the pons and half in the medulla oblongata, with the cerebellum forming its roof. The fourth ventricle communicates with the fluid-filled **subarachnoid space** that surrounds the brain by three openings. These are the two **lateral apertures** (of Luschka) and the single **median aperture** (of Magendie). These three openings are the only paths by which cerebrospinal fluid can leave the interior of the brain and enter the subarachnoid space that surrounds the brain. Eventually the cerebrospinal fluid is reabsorbed into the large vein that arches under the skull, the superior sagittal sinus.

Color and label

1	Frontal (anterior) horn of lateral ventricle
2	Temporal (inferior) horn of lateral ventricle
3	Occipital (posterior) horn of lateral ventricle
4	Third ventricle
5	Mesencephalic aqueduct (cerebral aqueduct)
6	Fourth ventricle
7	Central canal of spinal cord
8	Spinal cord
9	Cerebellum
10	Coronal suture
11	Lambdoid suture
12	Site of interthalamic adhesion
13	Interventricular foramen (of Monro)

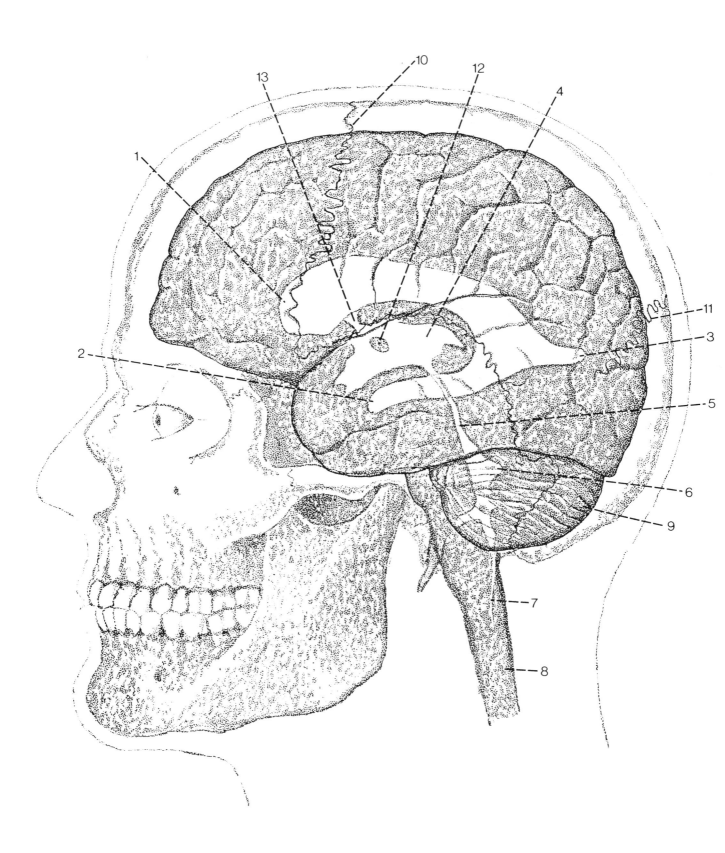

36 Ventricles of the brain: Lateral and superior views

UPPER FIGURE VIEWED FROM LEFT
LOWER FIGURE VIEWED FROM ABOVE

Color and label

1 Frontal (anterior) horn of left lateral ventricle
2 Occipital (posterior) horn of left lateral ventricle
3 Temporal (inferior) horn of left lateral ventricle
4 Frontal horn of right lateral ventricle
5 Occipital horn of right lateral ventricle
6 Temporal horn of right lateral ventricle
7 Third ventricle (ventricle III)
8 Fourth ventricle (ventricle IV)
9 Left interventricular foramen (of Monro)
10 Right interventricular foramen (of Monro)
11 Mesencephalic (formerly cerebral) aqueduct
12 Location of interthalamic adhesion
13 Central canal of spinal cord
14 Left lateral aperture of fourth ventricle (of Luschka)
15 Right lateral aperture of fourth ventricle (of Luschka)
16 Median aperture of fourth ventricle (of Magendie)
17 Impression of anterior commissure on third ventricle
18 Location of lamina terminalis in front of third ventricle
19 Optic recess of third ventricle
20 Infundibular recess of third ventricle
21 Suprapineal recess of third ventricle
22 Pineal recess of third ventricle

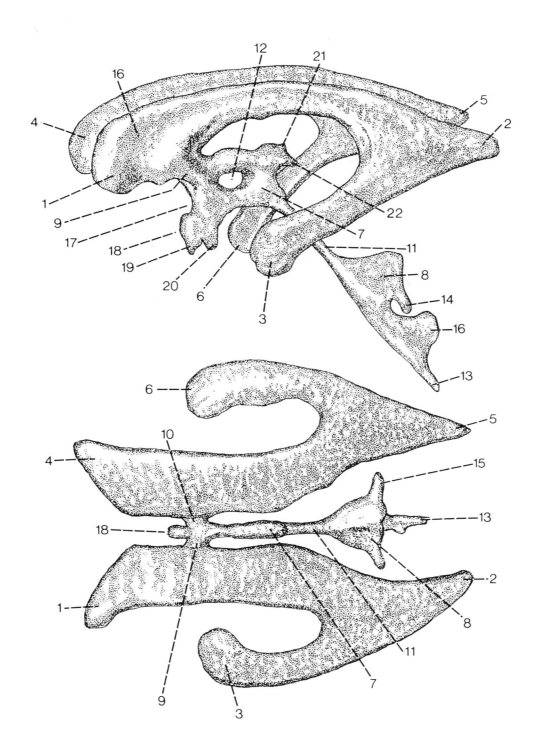

37 Ventricles of the brain: Anterior and posterior views

UPPER FIGURE VIEWED FROM FRONT
LOWER FIGURE VIEWED FROM BACK

Color and label

1 Frontal (anterior) horn of left lateral ventricle
2 Occipital (posterior) horn of left lateral ventricle
3 Temporal (inferior) horn of left lateral ventricle
4 Frontal horn of right lateral ventricle
5 Occipital horn of right lateral ventricle
6 Temporal horn of right lateral ventricle
7 Third ventricle
8 Fourth ventricle
9 Left interventricular foramen
10 Right interventricular foramen
11 Mesencephalic (cerebral) aqueduct
12 Impression of pes (paw) of hippocampus in temporal horn of right lateral ventricle
13 Central canal of spinal cord
14 Left lateral aperture of fourth ventricle
15 Right lateral aperture of fourth ventricle
16 Median aperture of fourth ventricle
17 Impression of facial colliculus in fourth ventricle
18 Impression of hypoglossal trigone in fourth ventricle
19 Location of nodulus of cerebellum in fourth ventricle

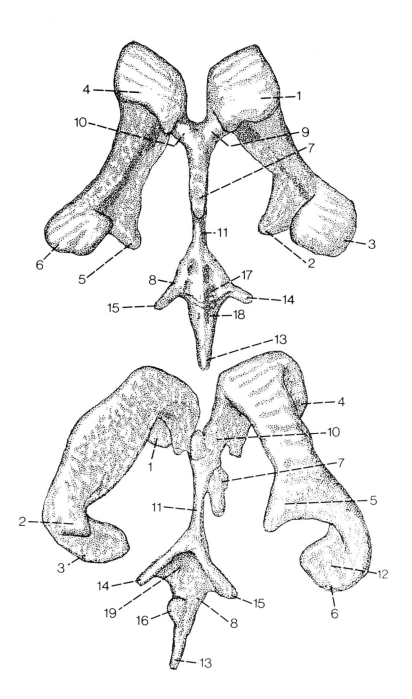

38 Brain dissection showing hippocampus and fornix

(After Netter)

Color and label

1 Frontal horn of lateral ventricle
2 Corpus callosum; genu (partially cut away)
3 Septum pellucida (right and left; note cavity or cavum between the two septa)
4 Head of caudate nucleus (partially cut away)
5 Columns of fornix (right and left)
6 Stria terminalis and thalamostriate vein
7 Digitations of hippocampus
8 Bodies of fornix (right and left)
9 Dentate gyrus (part of hippocampus)
10 Thalamus (partially cut away)
11 Fimbria of hippocampus
12 Hippocampus proper (Ammon's horn)
13 Crura of fornices (right and left)
14 Calcar avis (Latin, bird's spur) in occipital horn of lateral ventricle
15 Commissure of hippocampus
16 Splenium of corpus callosum (cut)
17 Cerebellum (seen between occipital lobes of cerebral hemispheres)
18 Head of caudate nucleus (cut surface)
19 Thalamus (cut surface)

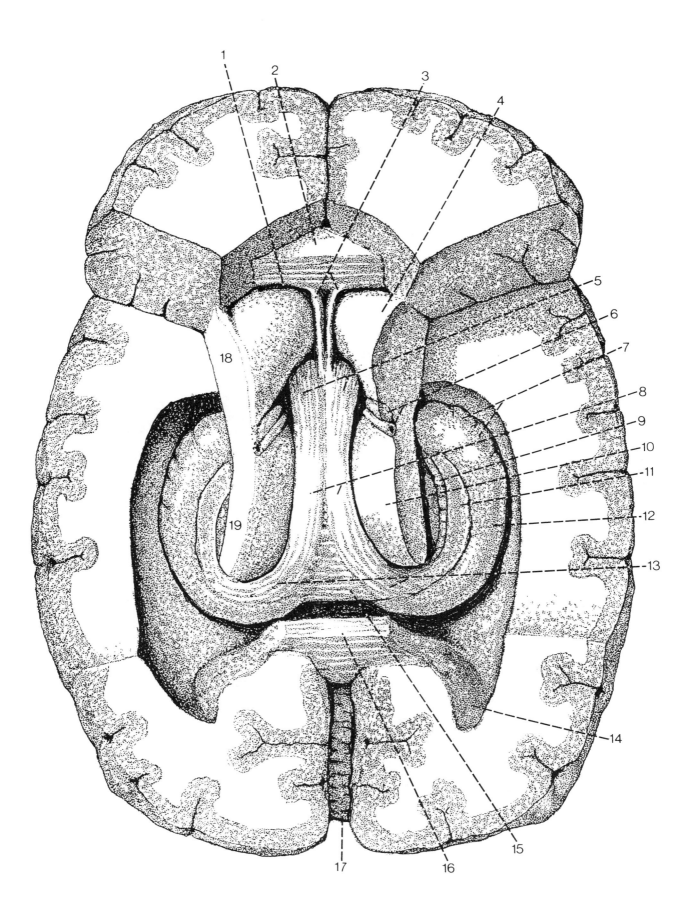

39 Etymological cartoon: Fornix

Fornix meant an arch, vault, basement, or brothel. The word fornication is derived from the prostitutes in ancient Rome plying their trade under the vaulted arches opening onto the street and in basements under public buildings. Hence, to fornicate could roughly mean "to go under the arch."

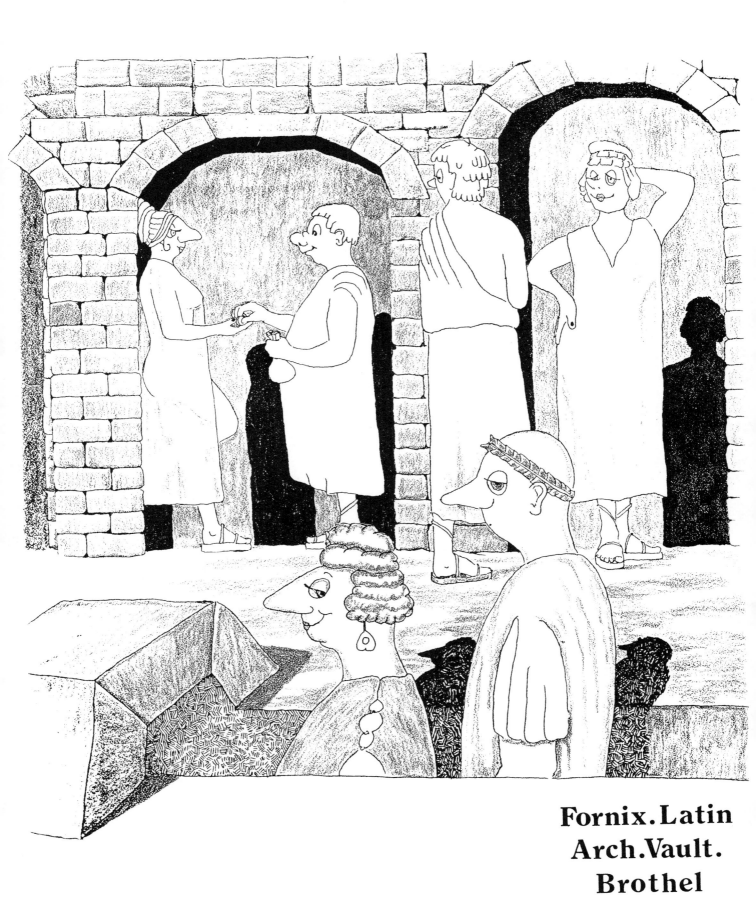

Fornix.Latin
Arch.Vault.
Brothel

40 Brain dissection to show mamillary bodies, fornix, and hippocampus After Sobotta

The lateral ventricles are opened. The right half of the corpus callosum is shown. The brain stem, thalamus, and hypothalamus are removed. The fornix is dissected free, as are the mamillary bodies, mamillothalamic tracts, and anterior commissure.

Color and label

1 Olfactory bulb (right)
2 Genu of corpus callosum (corpus callosum sectioned close to median plane)
3 Medial longitudinal stria of indusium griseum
4 Septum pellucidum
5 Lateral longitudinal stria of indusium griseum
6 Body (truncus) of corpus callosum
7 Body of fornix
8 Lateral ventricle (right)
9 Posterior horn of lateral ventricle
10 Occipital pole of right cerebral hemisphere
11 Splenium of corpus callosum
12 Mamillary bodies and mamillothalamic tracts (cut)
13 Crus of fornix
14 Posterior horn of left ventricle
15 Calcar avis projecting into posterior horn of lateral ventricle
16 Dentate gyrus
17 Pes (paw) of hippocampus
18 Digitations of hippocampus
19 Amygdaloid body
20 Anterior pole of left temporal lobe
21 Olfactory bulb and tract (left)
22 Anterior bundle of anterior commissure
23 Anterior commissure
24 Column of fornix
25 Posterior bundle of the anterior commissure (note its fan shape; this part of the anterior commissure is larger and projects mainly to the anterior parahippocampal gyrus, which has been removed).

Amygdala, hippocampus, and fornix (isolated view)

Color and label

1 Amygdaloid body (left)
2 Hippocampal digitations
3 Pes hippocampi (Latin, paw of hippocampus)
4 Dentate gyrus
5 Fimbria of hippocampus
6 Crus of fornix (leg of fornix)
7 Corpora of fornices (bodies of fornices)
8 Columns of fornices
9 Mamillary bodies
10 Mamillothalamic tract (cut; projects to anterior thalamus)
11 Fasciolar gyrus (connects dentate gyrus to medial and lateral longitudinal striae of indusium griseum)
12 Hippocampal commissure
13 Lateral longitudinal stria of indusium griseum (cut)
14 Medial longitudinal stria of indusium griseum (cut)
15 Dentate gyrus (right), named for its toothed appearance
16 Amygdaloid body (right)

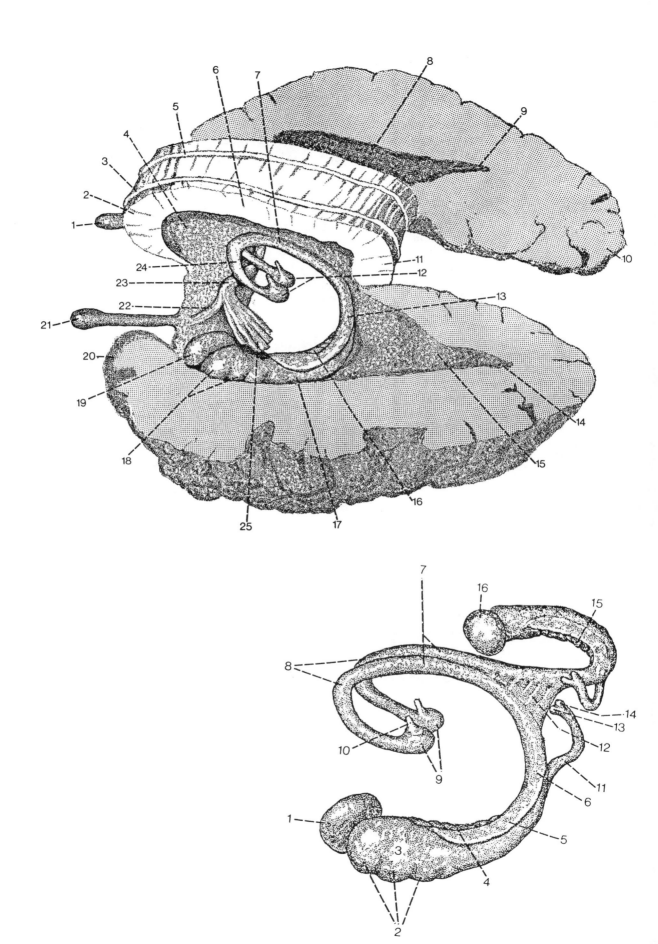

Figure A shows the relative position of these nuclear masses in a horizontally cut brain. The **caudate** (Latin, tailed) **nucleus** consists of a **head** (1), a **body** (2), and a long **tail** (3) that curves posteriorly, then inferiorly, and finally anteriorly into the temporal lobe where it approaches but does not fuse with the **amygdala** (4) (Greek, almond). Note that the head of the caudate nucleus (1) is joined to the putamen anteriorly. The **putamen** (Latin, husk, shell) and inner **globus pallidus** (Latin, pale globe) constitute the **lentiform** (Latin, lentil-shaped) **nucleus**. The **lentiform nucleus**, the **caudate nucleus,** and **claustrum** (Latin, barrier), which is a thin cellular mass lateral to the putamen, constitute the **corpus striatum** (Latin, striped body). Their striated or striped appearance is due to the numerous bundles of myelinated axons that traverse these structures. Note that the caudate nucleus and putamen are also joined by many thin cellular bridges that traverse the internal capsule (13).

Figures B and C show these structures cut by two frontal planes. The caudate nucleus and putamen constitute the **neostriatum** (Greek, *neos,* new) or simply the **striatum.** The globus pallidus is the **paleostriatum** (Greek, *paleos,* old) or simply **pallidum.** The term **basal nuclei** (formerly, basal ganglia) is often used synonymously with corpus striatum, that is, the caudate nucleus, lentiform (putamen and globus pallidus), and claustrum. Although it is often included in diagrams of the basal nuclei, the **amygdala** (or amygdaloid body) is usually not considered as one of the basal ganglia or as part of the corpus striatum. The caudate nucleus and putamen together contain an estimated 110 million closely-packed small neurons surrounding some 600,000 scattered large neurons. The globus pallidus, on the other hand, has considerably fewer cells–about 710,000–which are much larger and more widely dispersed.

Color and label

1	Head of caudate nucleus	8	Thalamus (left)
2	Body of caudate nucleus	9	Outline of right thalamus
3	Tail of caudate nucleus	10-11	Anterior limb of internal capsule
4	Amygdala	11	Genu of internal capsule
5	Putamen	11-12	Posterior limb of internal capsule
6	Globus pallidus (lateral part)	13	Cellular bridges between caudate
7	Globus pallidus (medial part)		nucleus and putamen

Color the striatum (1,2,3,5) one color, the globus pallidus (6,7) another color, and the amygdala (4) a third color.

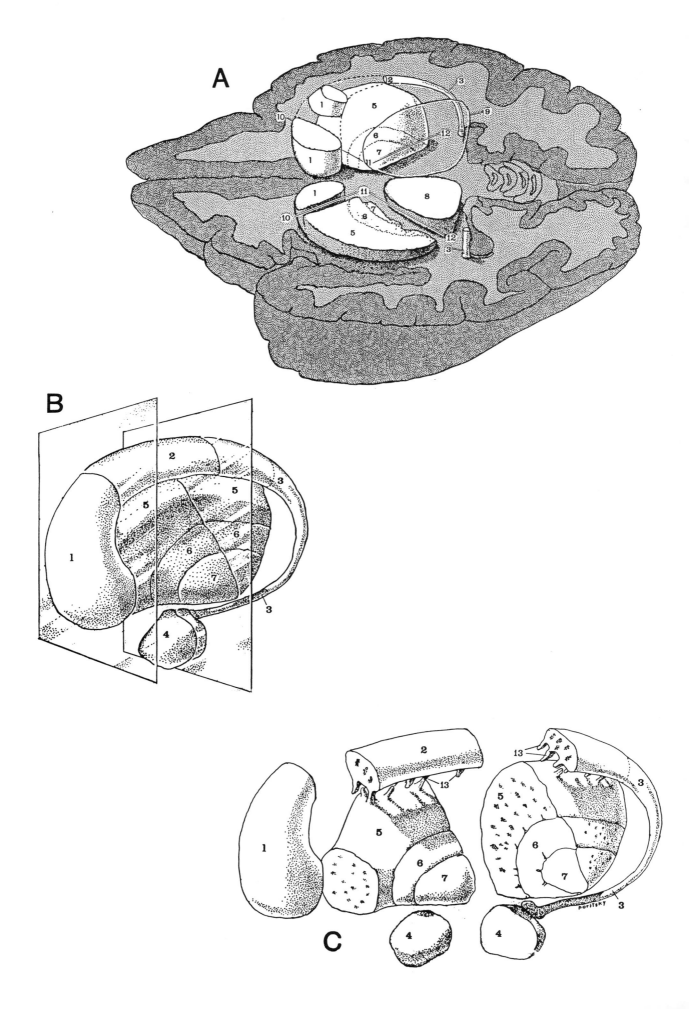

Caudate nucleus, putamen, and amygdala, exposed by opening left ventricle from the left side (After Rohen and Yokochi)

FRONT OF BRAIN TO LEFT

Color and label

1   Anterior horn of left lateral ventricle
2   Head of caudate nucleus
3   Internal capsule
4   Putamen (left, lateral side)
5   Gray matter bridges between caudate nucleus and putamen
6   Choroid plexus of lateral ventricle
7   Calcar avis (Latin, bird spur)
8   Posterior horn of left lateral ventricle
9   Tail of caudate nucleus
10   Caudal extent of tail of caudate nucleus
11   Hippocampal digitations
12   Inferior horn of lateral ventricle in temporal lobe (note narrow cleft of lateral ventricle separating amygdala from hippocampus)
13   Amygdala (lateral aspect)
14   Cut surface in temporal lobe
15   Anterior pole of temporal lobe
16   Anterior commissure (posterior part)

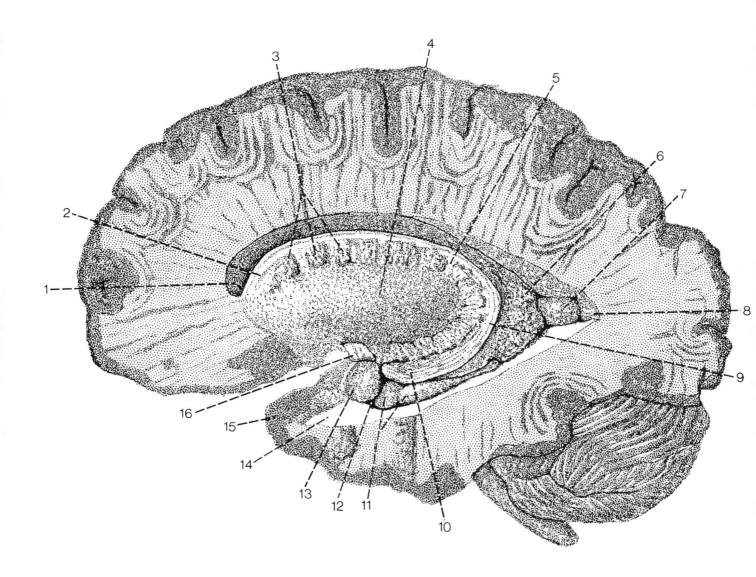

43 Caudate nucleus, thalamus, and left lateral ventricle (After Rohen and Yokochi)

Left cerebral hemisphere dissected from left side. Putamen and globus pallidus largely removed.

Color and label

1   Frontal (anterior) horn of left lateral ventricle
2   Head of caudate nucleus
3   Bridges of gray matter (nerve cell bodies) between caudate nucleus and putamen
4   Body of caudate nucleus
5   Thalamus (left lateral surface)
6   Calcar avis in occipital (posterior) horn of lateral ventricle
7   Internal capsule (posterior limb; cut)
8   Hippocampus
9   Caudal extent of tail of caudate nucleus
10   Amygdaloid body (Greek, *amygdala,* almond)
11   Temporal lobe (cut open)
12   Globus pallidus (remnant)
13   Limen (Latin, threshold) of insula. The insula is cortex hidden in the depths of the lateral fissure and covered by overlapping gyri from the frontal, parietal, and temporal lobes that form the operculum (Latin, lid or cover).
14   Anterior commissure
15   Putamen (remnant)
16   Claustrum (Latin, barrier)
17   Anterior limb of internal capsule

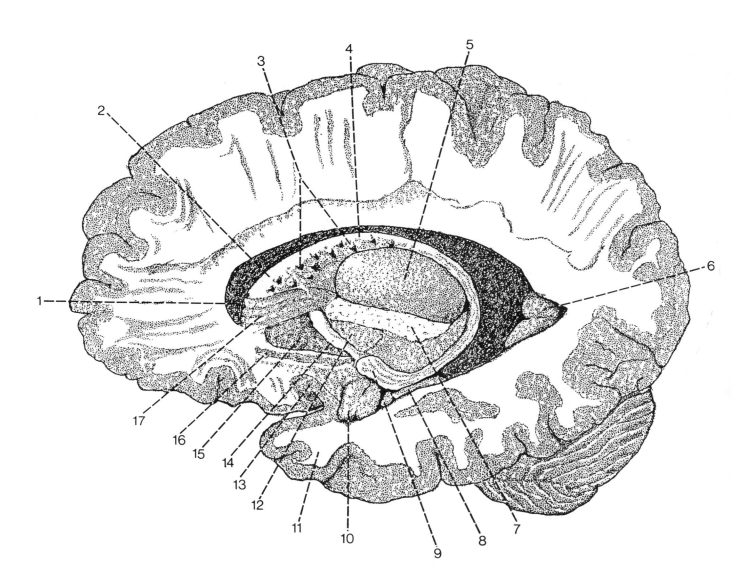

Cranial nerve motor nuclei and parasympathetic nuclei viewed within a transparent brain stem: Dorsal view

Color and label

1. Accessory oculomotor nucleus (Edinger-Westphal nucleus). This nucleus contains the parasympathetic cell bodies whose fibers travel with N III, GVE component.
2. Oculomotor nucleus (N III; GSE)
3. Nerve III fibers exiting ventrally
4. Trochlear nucleus (N IV; GSE)
5. Trochlear nerve (N IV). Note its fibers exiting dorsally and crossing to opposite side.
6. Decussation (crossing midline) of trochlear nerve
7. Motor root of trigeminal nerve (N V) exiting with mandibular nerve V3
8. Semilunar ganglion
9. Motor nucleus of trigeminal nerve (SVE). This nucleus contains the alpha motor neuron cell bodies that supply the muscles of mastication.
10. Facial nerve (SVE). It supplies all the muscles of facial expression on the same side.
11. Abducent nucleus. Its motor neuron cell bodies supply the lateral rectus muscle of eye.
12. Superior salivatory nucleus (GVE). This nucleus contains the parasympathetic cell bodies, whose fibers exit as part of facial nerve and synapse upon postganglionic parasympathetic cell bodies in the pterygopalatine ganglion and submandibular ganglion.
13. Genu (Latin, bend, knee) of intrapontine portion of facial nerve
14. Facial motor nucleus (SVE). This contains the motor neuron cell bodies, which give rise to fibers that supply the muscles of facial expression.
15. Inferior salivatory nucleus (GVE). This consists of parasympathetic cell bodies, whose fibers exit with glossopharyngeal nerve (N IX) and synapse in the otic ganglion.
16. Glossopharyngeal nerve (N IX). Note that the motor neurons in the superior part of the nucleus ambiguus send SVE fibers that travel with the glossopharyngeal nerve.
17. Vagus nerve (N X; SVE fibers). Most of the fibers of motor neurons in the nucleus ambiguus exit with vagus nerve.
18. Accessory nerve fibers (N XI; cranial part). These fibers arise from motor neurons in the caudal part of the nucleus ambiguus and join the vagus nerve; they supply muscles in the larynx, pharynx, and upper esophagus.
19. Accessory nerve (N XI). These fibers arise from the spinal accessory nucleus in the cervical spinal cord and supply the trapezius and sternocleidomastoid muscles.
20. Nucleus ambiguus. Gives rise to SVE fibers that exit with nerves IX, X, XI.
21. Spinal accessory nucleus
22. Hypoglossal nucleus (right and left; GSE). Its fibers supply all the homolateral muscles of the tongue.
23. Dorsal vagal nucleus (GVE). These neurons give rise to parasympathetic fibers that exit with nerve X. Most of the parasympathetic outflow is by way of the vagus nerve.
24. Parasympathetic fibers within the vagus nerve

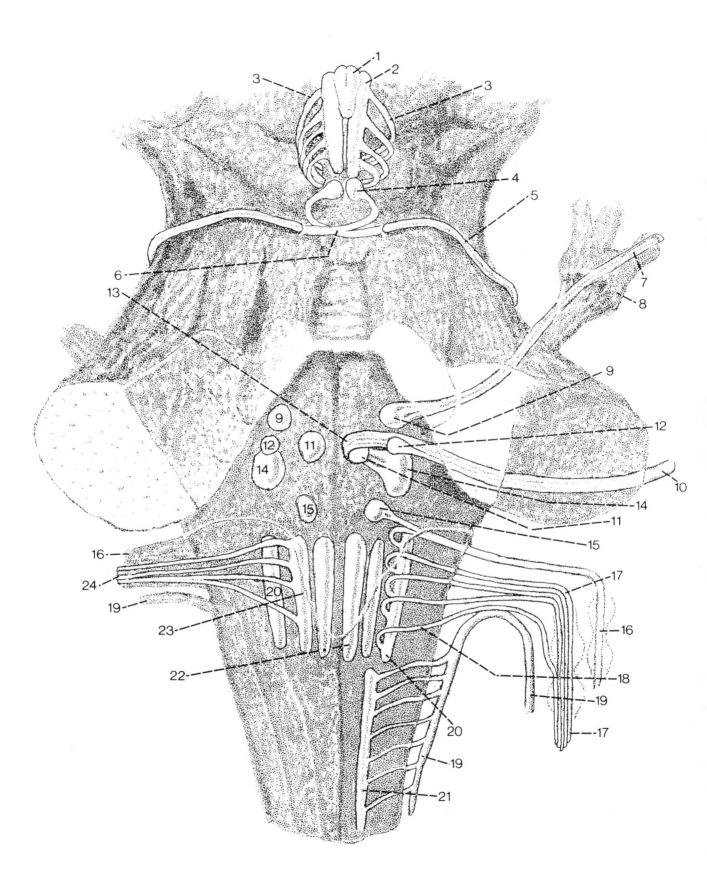

Color and label

1	Red nucleus
2	Accessory oculomotor nucleus (Edinger-Westphal nucleus). It contains preganglionic parasympathetic cell bodies whose fibers exit with nerve III.
3	Oculomotor nucleus (GSE)
4	Cerebral aqueduct (aqueduct of Sylvius; new name: mesencephalic aqueduct)
5	Trochlear nerve (N IV; GSE)
6	Trochlear nerve (N IV) (exiting dorsally and decussating)
7	Ventricle IV
8	Trigeminal motor nucleus (SVE)
9	Genu of facial nerve (intrapontine genu)
10	Abducent nucleus (GSE)
11	Superior salivatory nucleus (GVE). It contains preganglionic parasympathetic cell bodies whose fibers exit with facial nerve.
12	Choroid plexus of ventricle IV
13	Inferior salivatory nucleus (GVE). It contains preganglionic parasympathetic cell bodies whose fibers exit with nerve IX.
14	Hypoglossal nucleus (GSE)
15	Dorsal vagal nucleus (GVE). It contains preganglionic parasympathetic cell bodies.
16	Nucleus ambiguus (GVE)
17	Spinal accessory nucleus. These motor neurons give rise to fibers that supply the trapezius and sternocleidomastoid muscles via nerve XI.
18	Inferior olivary nucleus
19	Hypoglossal nerve (N XII; GSE). Supplies all the homolateral tongue muscles.
20	Accessory (spinal accessory) nerve (SVE). Fibers arising from the cell bodies in the caudal nucleus ambiguus transfer to the vagus nerve and supply muscles of the larynx.
21	Vagus nerve (SVE). Most of the fibers that arise from the nucleus ambiguus exit with the vagus nerve and supply the muscles of the palate and pharynx.
22	Parasympathetic fibers from dorsal vagal nucleus exiting with vagus nerve (GVE)
23	Glossopharyngeal nerve (N IX). These are SVE fibers from rostral nucleus ambiguus headed for muscles of the upper pharynx where they form the pharyngeal plexus with the vagus nerve.
24	Parasympathetic fibers of glossopharyngeal (GVE)
25	Abducent nerve (N VI)
26	Motor fibers of facial nerve (N VII) to muscles of facial expression (SVE)
27	Facial motor nucleus (SVE)
28	Parasympathetic (GVE) fibers traveling with facial nerve
29	Pons
30	Mandibular nerve
31	Motor fibers of trigeminal nerve traveling with mandibular nerve to the muscles of mastication (SVE)
32	Trigeminal ganglion (semilunar ganglion; gasserian ganglion)
33	Parasympathetic fibers (GVE) within the oculomotor nerve
34	Oculomotor nerve (N III; GSE)
35	Crus cerebri (cerebral peduncle) of midbrain

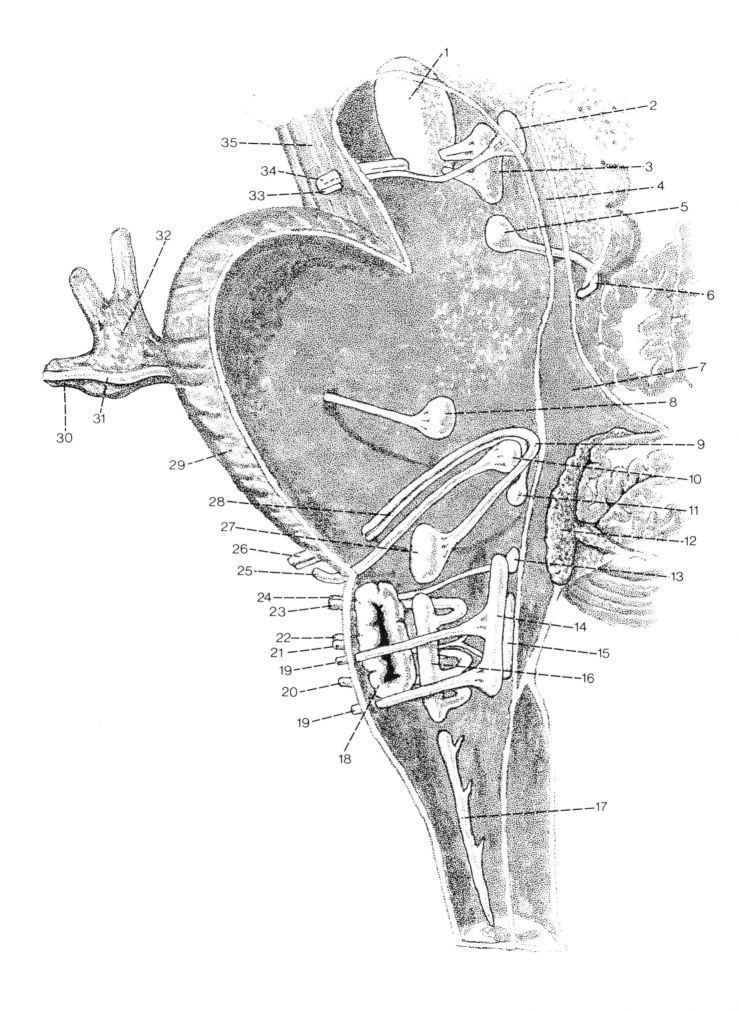

Color and label

1 Trigeminal mesencephalic nucleus (mesencephalic nucleus of V)
2 Trigeminal mesencephalic tract (mesencephalic root or tract of V)
3 Trigeminal principal sensory nucleus (new name: trigeminal pontine nucleus)
4 Trigeminal spinal tract (spinal tract of V)
5 Trigeminal spinal nucleus (spinal nucleus of V)
6 Sensory portion (portio major) of trigeminal nerve
7 Trigeminal ganglion
8 Dorsal cochlear nucleus
9 Ventral cochlear nucleus
10 Cochlear portion of vestibulocochlear nerve
11 Vestibular portion of vestibulocochlear nerve
12 Cochlea
13 Vestibular apparatus (3 semicircular ducts, utricle, saccule)
14 Superior vestibular nucleus*
15 Lateral vestibular nucleus*
16 Spinal vestibular nucleus*
17 Medial vestibular nucleus*
18 Sensory fibers of facial nerve from skin of ear entering spinal tract of V
19 Sensory fibers of glossopharyngeal nerve entering spinal tract of V
20 Sensory fibers in vagus nerve from skin of ear drum entering trigeminal
     tract of V
21 Spinal tract of V becoming continuous with dorsolateral fasciculus
     (tract of Lisseaur)
22 Spinal nucleus of V becoming continuous with substantia gelatinosa

Vestibular nuclei are shown on left side only.

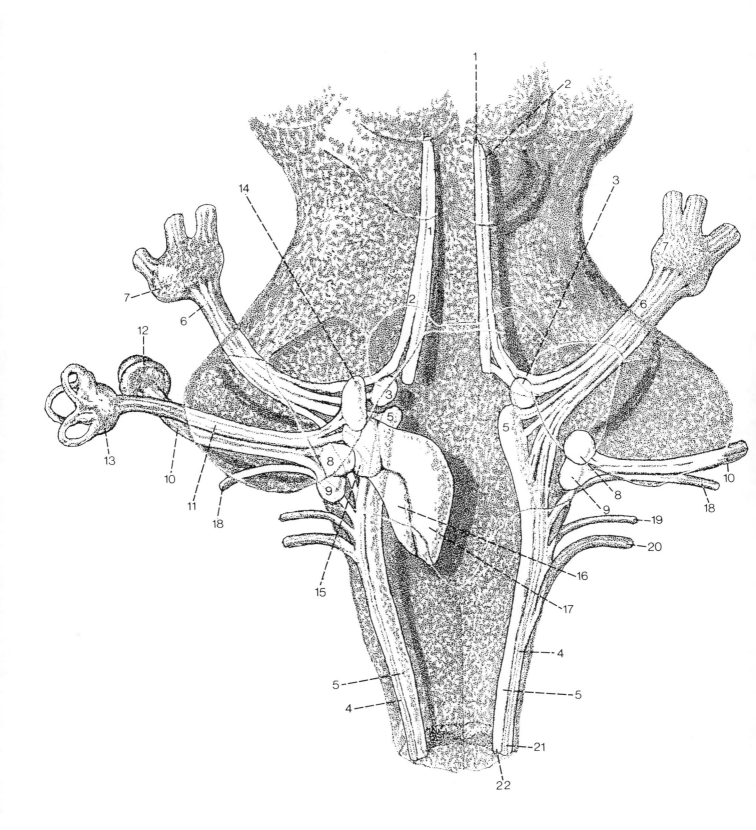

47 Cranial nerve sensory nuclei in right half of brain stem

Color and label

1   Trigeminal mesencephalic nucleus (mesencephalic nucleus of V)
2   Mesencephalic aqueduct (formerly aqueduct of Sylvius, cerebral aqueduct)
3   Trigeminal mesencephalic tract (mesencephalic root or tract of V)
4   Principal trigeminal sensory nucleus (new name: trigeminal pontine nucleus)
5   Four vestibular nuclei (included here as a single group)
6   Dorsal cochlear nucleus
7   Nucleus of solitary tract (cephalic part; taste)
8   Solitary tract (the surrounding solitary nucleus has been partially removed)
9   Solitary tract nucleus (caudal part; general sensation from pharynx and larynx)
10 Trigeminal spinal nucleus
11 Trigeminal spinal tract
12 Vagus nerve sensory rootlets entering solitary tract (taste; general sensation from pharynx and larynx)
13 Glossopharyngeal nerve sensory fiber entering solitary tract (taste and general sensation from posterior one-third of tongue)
14 Vestibulocochlear nerve
15 Facial nerve taste fibers entering solitary tract
16 Trigeminal nerve (within pons; intrapontine part)
17 Pons
18 Trigeminal ganglion
19 Cerebral peduncle (on ventral mesencephalon)
20 Red nucleus

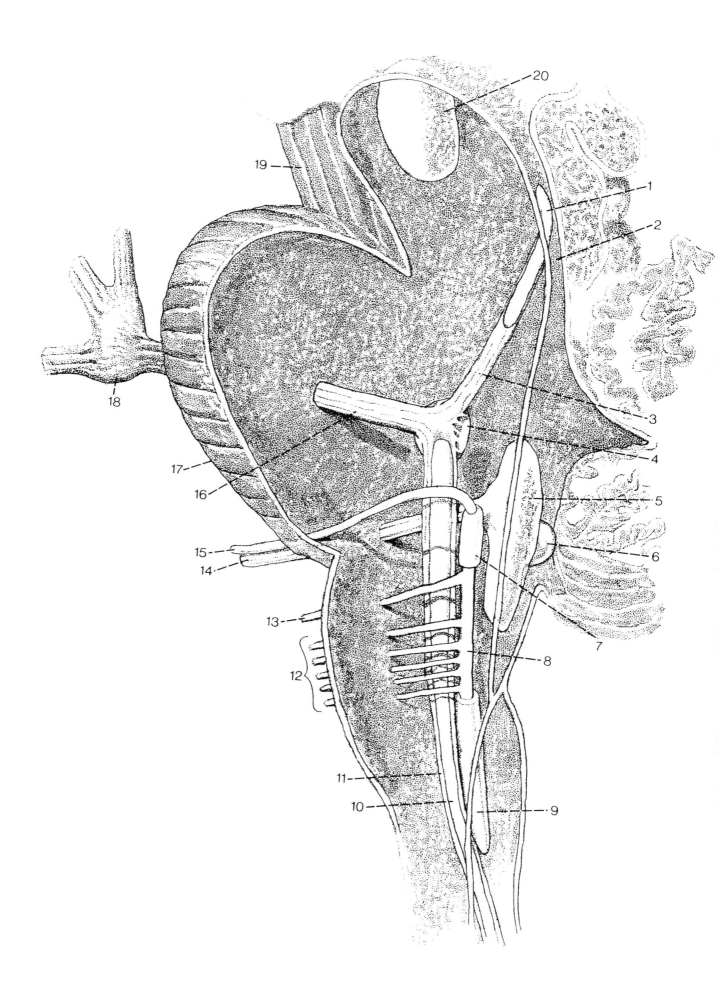

There are seven categories or **components** of fibers within all 12 cranial nerves. Some individual cranial nerves, such as the vagus, may contain five different components. Others such as the hypoglossal contain only a single component.

Directions: Use a different color for each of the components and related nuclei. Figure A (top) is a transverse section through the lower medulla and shows the relative position of the cranial nerve nuclei in terms of their components. The three more medial **motor nuclei** contain the cells of origin of the three motor components (neurons 1, 2, 3). The three more lateral **sensory nuclei** serve as terminal, integrative, and relay stations for the four **sensory** components. One nucleus, the nucleus of the solitary tract, receives the fibers of two components; thus there are seven components and only six nuclei at this level. Note that the cell bodies of the four sensory components (4,5,6,7) lie outside the brain in ganglia.

In Figure A, locate neuron 1 in the GSE (general somatic efferent) nucleus. Four cranial nerves, III, IV, VI, and XII, carry GSE fibers and supply head muscles that are derived from the myomers of somites in the embryo. The only somatic (or myomeric) muscles in the facial region are those of the tongue (nerve XII) and the extrinsic eye muscles (nerves III, IV, VI).
Color neuron 1 and the GSE nucleus in Figure A and, in Figure B, the nuclei of nerves III, IV, VI, and XII.

Return to Figure A and locate neuron 2 in the SVE (special visceral efferent) nucleus. These motor neurons supply muscles that are derived from the branchial or gill arches and are called branchiomeric muscles (see Figure 82). SVE fibers leave the brain stem in the following nerves: V, VII, IX, X, and XI. Note the position of the SVE nucleus in relation to the GSE nucleus. Note also how the fiber of 2 first curves medially and dorsally before exiting, as do the fibers of VII, IX, and X before they exit. The SVE fibers all tend to exit more laterally on the brain stem than do the GSE fibers, which exit ventrally (with the exception of nerve IV, which exits dorsally). The perikarya of SVE motor neurons lie in the following SVE nuclei: motor nucleus of V (Motor Nuc V), facial motor nucleus (Nuc VII), nucleus ambiguus (Nuc Ambig), and spinal nucleus of XI (Sp Nuc XI).
Color neuron 2 in Figure A and the above-mentioned SVE nuclei in Figure B.

Return to Figure A and locate neuron 3 in the GVE (general visceral efferent) nucleus, which contains preganglionic parasympathetic cell bodies and represents the following GVE nuclei: Edinger-Westphal (EW) nucleus (new name: accessory oculomotor nucleus), superior salivatory nucleus (ss), inferior salivatory nucleus (is), and dorsal nucleus of X (Dor Nuc X). The nerves containing preganglionic parasympathetic fibers are III, VII, IX, and X.
Color GVE neuron 3 and each of the GVE nuclei.

GVA (general visceral afferent) includes conscious sensations from the pharynx and larynx which end in the caudal part of the solitary nucleus, as well as subconscious impulses involved in a wide range of pulmonary, cardiovascular, and digestive reflexes that arise in the thorax and abdomen, and terminate in both the dorsal nucleus of X and in the nucleus of the solitary tract. GVA fibers travel within nerves IX and X and their somata lie in the inferior ganglia of both nerves.
Color GVA neuron 4 and the GVA nucleus (nucleus of solitary tract) in Figure A and the **caudal** part of the nucleus of the solitary tract (Nuc Solit Tr) in Figure B.

Taste is SVA (special visceral afferent) and travels in three nerves, VII, IX, and X. All taste fibers end centrally in the rostral part of the nucleus of the solitary tract.
Color SVA neuron 5 and the SVA nucleus in Figure A and the rostral part of the nucleus of the solitary tract in Figure B.

Cutaneous face sensation and proprioception from the jaw muscles and the lips, cheek, and tongue musculature are designated GSA (general somatic afferent) and travel centrally within nerve V. GSA impulses end in the three sensory nuclei of nerve V, the mesencephalic nucleus of V (Mesen Nuc V), the principal (or main) sensory nucleus of V (Pr Sen Nuc V), and the spinal nucleus of V (Sp Nuc V).
Color neuron 6, GSA nucleus, and the three sensory nuclei of V.

Fibers from the inner ear are SSA (special somatic afferent). These travel centrally within the VIII nerve. They end centrally in the four vestibular nuclei, the superior vestibular nucleus (sv), the medial vestibular nucleus (mv), the inferior vestibular nucleus (iv), and the lateral vestibular nucleus (1v); and in the two cochlear nuclei, the dorsal cochlear nucleus (d) and the ventral cochlear nucleus (v).
Color the SSA neuron and the vestibular nuclei and cochlear nuclei.

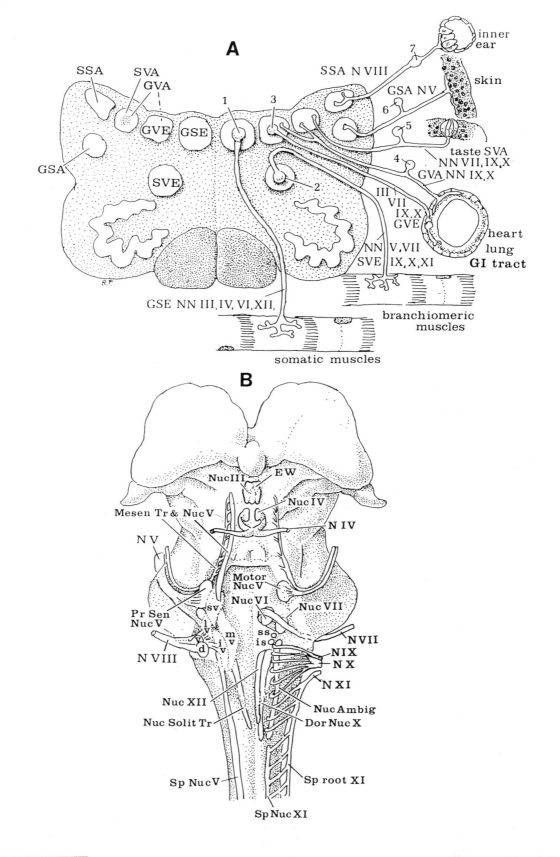

A

SSA   SVA   GVA

GVE GSE

GSA

SVE

1   3

2

SSA N VIII

GSA NV

inner ear

skin

taste SVA
NN VII, IX, X
GVA NN IX, X

6

5

4

III
VII
IX, X
GVE

NN V, VII
SVE IX, X, XI

7

heart
lung
GI tract

GSE NN III, IV, VI, XII,

branchiomeric
muscles

somatic muscles

B

NucIII   EW

Mesen Tr & Nuc V

Nuc IV

N IV

N V

Motor
Nuc V

Nuc VI

Nuc VII

Pr Sen
Nuc V

sv

N VIII

l
v

m
v

d

i
v

ss

is

N VII

N IX

N X

N XI

Nuc XII

Nuc Solit Tr

Nuc Ambig

Dor Nuc X

Sp Nuc V

Sp root XI

Sp Nuc XI

Figure A based upon and modified from Brodal A: Neurological Anatomy in Relation to Clinical Medicine, 3rd ed. New York, Oxford University Press, 1981, Figure 7-1.

Figure B based upon and modified from Nieuwenhuys, Voogd, van Huijzen: The Human Central Nervous System. A Synopsis and Atlas. Berlin, Springer-Verlag, 1978, Figure 93.

49 and 50 Touch, proprioception, pain, and temperature pathways

Directions: Cut out Figures 49 and 50, carefully align them, and tape them together so that the tracts continue uninterrupted from one page to the other. Starting with 1 in the lower left, **color** the course of this afferent fiber, which carries either discriminative touch* or vibratory sense from receptors in the leg, such as Meissner's corpuscles and pacinian corpuscles. Fiber 1 is the peripheral process of this first-order (or primary) afferent neuron and can extend well over a meter in length if it runs from the big toe to the dorsal root ganglion of spinal nerve L5. Cell body 2 is the unipolar perikaryon of this neuron lying in the dorsal root ganglion. The central process 3 turns medial upon entering the spinal cord and ascends in the dorsal columns forming a tract or fasciculus, the **fasciculus gracilis (FG)**. **Trace and color** the ascent of fibers 1–3. Note 3 remains dorsal, medial, and homolateral (not crossed). It ends in the **nucleus gracilis** where it synapses upon second-order neuron 7. Fiber 4 carries either proprioception, discriminative touch,* or active touch† from the arm. Its cell body is 5 and its central process 6 turns medial in the spinal cord and ascends as the more lateral **fasciculus cuneatus (FC)**. Follow fiber 6 upward until it too terminates on neuron 8 in another nucleus in the medulla, the **nucleus cuneatus**. Thus the dorsal columns (or dorsal funiculus) are composed of the central processes of first-order sensory neurons, whose unipolar perikarya reside in dorsal root pattern ganglia. Note the orderly pattern of fibers, with those from the leg being most medial, the thoracic fibers lateral to those, and arm fibers most lateral. This orderly projection of fibers within the dorsal columns forms a **somatotopic projection** or lamination (layering).

Locate neurons 7 and 8 in the nucleus gracilis and nucleus cuneatus. These second-order neurons are the cells of origin of the **internal arcuate fibers (IAF)**, which become the **medial lemniscus (ML)**. Note that the fibers in the medial lemniscus decussate as internal arcuate fibers, form the ribbon-like medial lemniscus, and ascend until they reach the **ventral posterior lateral nucleus** (or nucleus ventralis posterolateralis, VPL) of the thalamus, where they end as synapses upon neurons 9 (leg) and 10 (arm). Neurons 9 and 10 project fibers to the somatosensory cortex. **Trace and color** fibers 7, 8, 9, 10.

Conscious proprioception from the leg was formerly believed to ascend entirely in the dorsal columns. However, recent research has shown leg proprioception to ascend as follows: fiber 12 (lower left) from leg joint receptors or leg muscle spindles passes its cell body 13 and becomes central process 14, which ascends in the fasciculus gracilis up to the thoracic spinal cord level, where it ends and synapses upon neuron 15 in the nucleus thoracis (formerly, nucleus dorsalis of Clarke). Neuron 15 gives rise to the dorsal spinocerebellar tract (DSCT). A collateral (Coll) of fiber 15 synapses in nucleus Z on neuron 16. This neuron sends fiber 16, which joins the medial lemniscus and ends in the nucleus VPL on neuron 17. Neuron 17 projects to the leg region of the somatosensory cortex. **Color and trace** fibers 12–17.

Locate leg pain fiber 18 on the lower right. Trace it to its unipolar soma, 19, where its central process, 20, enters the spinal cord via the dorsal root and synapses upon neuron 21 in the gray matter of the dorsal horn. Neuron 21 is a cell of origin of the spinothalamic tract (STT) that carries sharp pain up the spinal cord to the thalamus. The numerous collateral fibers normally given off by fiber 21 are not depicted here. Note that fiber 21 decussates in the anterior white commissure, usually within one spinal cord segment of its cell of origin. Sharp pain fiber 21 ends in the VPL nucleus of the thalamus, where it synapses upon thalamic neuron 22, which projects to the leg region of the somatosensory cortex. **Trace and color** sharp pain fibers 18–22.

Discriminative touch is used here to signify touch that can identify patterns drawn on the skin plus the ability to distinguish two points simultaneously touching the skin as two points rather than as one point. This ability is believed to ascend the cord in both the lateral white column (funiculus) and the dorsal column.

†*Active touch* is used here to indicate touch that depends upon movement. This ability to determine size, shape, and texture of objects relies upon movement of the fingers (or toes) and is also called stereognosis (Greek, solid knowledge). This sense of active touch ascends within the dorsal columns and is the only somatosensory modality that travels exclusively within the dorsal columns. Sensory modalities such as vibratory sensation (tuning fork), which were once thought to travel only within the dorsal column, are now believed to ascend up the cord in the lateral white matter as well as in the dorsal columns.

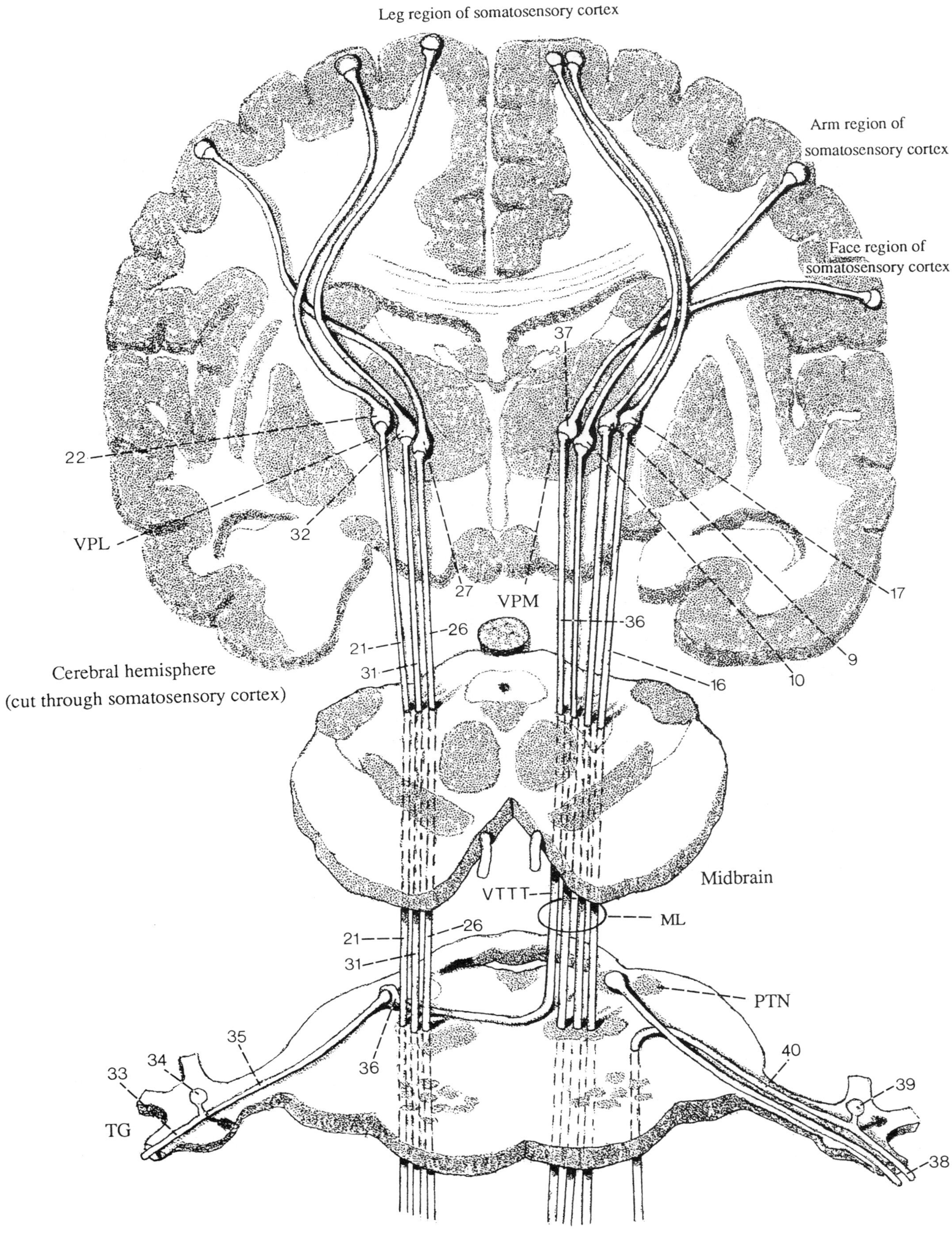

Leg region of somatosensory cortex

Arm region of somatosensory cortex

Face region of somatosensory cortex

37

22

VPL

32

27   VPM

26

21

31

16

17

9

10

36

Cerebral hemisphere
(cut through somatosensory cortex)

Midbrain

VTTT

ML

21   26

31

PTN

35

36

40

34

33

39

TG

38

Locate fiber 23 in the cervical spinal cord. It carries sharp pain from the arm to its soma, 24, where it becomes central process 25, which enters the cord and synapses upon neuron 26, which gives rise to fiber 27, which ascends in the spinothalamic tract (STT). Note again the somatotopic layering or lamination; in this tract the higher body parts (arm) are more medial rather than more lateral because this is a crossed tract, and the more cephalic fibers join the tract on its inward or medial aspect. Fiber 26 ends in the thalamus upon thalamic neuron 27, which projects to the arm region of the somatosensory cortex. **Trace and color** arm pain fibers 23–27.

Return to the lumbosacral spinal cord on the lower right and locate fiber 28, which brings light touch from leg. This is tested by gently stroking the skin with a wisp of cotton. **Trace and color** fiber 28, its soma 29, its central process 30, neuron 31 and its fiber 31 that ascends in the spinothalamic tract, and, finally, thalamic neuron 32, which projects to the leg region of the somatosensory cortex. There is a similar pathway for light touch from the arm that also ascends in the spinothalamic tract. It is not shown in this diagram. Recent evidence has shown that there is not one tract for pain and another for touch, as formerly believed, but rather that touch and pain ascend intermixed in the anterolateral funiculus.

Afferent fiber 33 carries discriminative touch from encapsulated endings in the face. **Trace and color** fiber 33, its soma 34 in the trigeminal ganglion, and its central process 35 that ends upon neuron 36 in the principal trigeminal nucleus. Neuron 36 sends its axon across the midline, where it ascends in the ventral trigeminothalamic tract, which terminates in nucleus VPM of the thalamus (nucleus ventralis posteromedialis). VPM neuron 37 projects its fiber to the face region of the somatosensory cortex. Afferent fiber 38 brings in pain or temperature from the face. Its cell body is 39, and its central process 40 descends in the trigeminal spinal tract and synapses upon neuron 41 in the trigeminal spinal nucleus.

In pathway diagrams such as this, bear in mind that what is shown on one side is also present on the other side. Also, tracts and their fibers cross the midline in an oblique longitudinal direction, not transversely, as is usually and conveniently depicted in diagrams. Pathway diagrams are highly simplified in that the vast numbers of collateral fibers and their connections, most of which are still unknown, are not shown. Ongoing neuroanatomical research necessitates constant revision and updating of maps of the nervous system.

Color and label (where appropriate)

DR	Dorsal root	VPL	Nucleus ventralis posterolateralis
DRG	Dorsal root ganglion	VPM	Nucleus ventralis posteromedialis
FG	Fasciculus gracilis	STT	Spinothalamic tract
FC	Fasciculus cuneatus	TG	Trigeminal ganglion (semilunar ganglion)
NG	Nucleus gracilis	PTN	Principal trigeminal nucleus
NC	Nucleus cuneatus	TSN	Trigeminal spinal nucleus
IAF	Internal arcuate fibers	VTTT	Ventral trigeminothalamic tract
ML	Medial lemniscus	TST	Trigeminal spinal tract
DSCT	Dorsal spinocerebellar tract	TSN	Trigeminal spinal nucleus
Coll	Collateral fiber to nucleus Z	DC	Dorsal columns (dorsal funiculus)
Z	Nucleus Z		

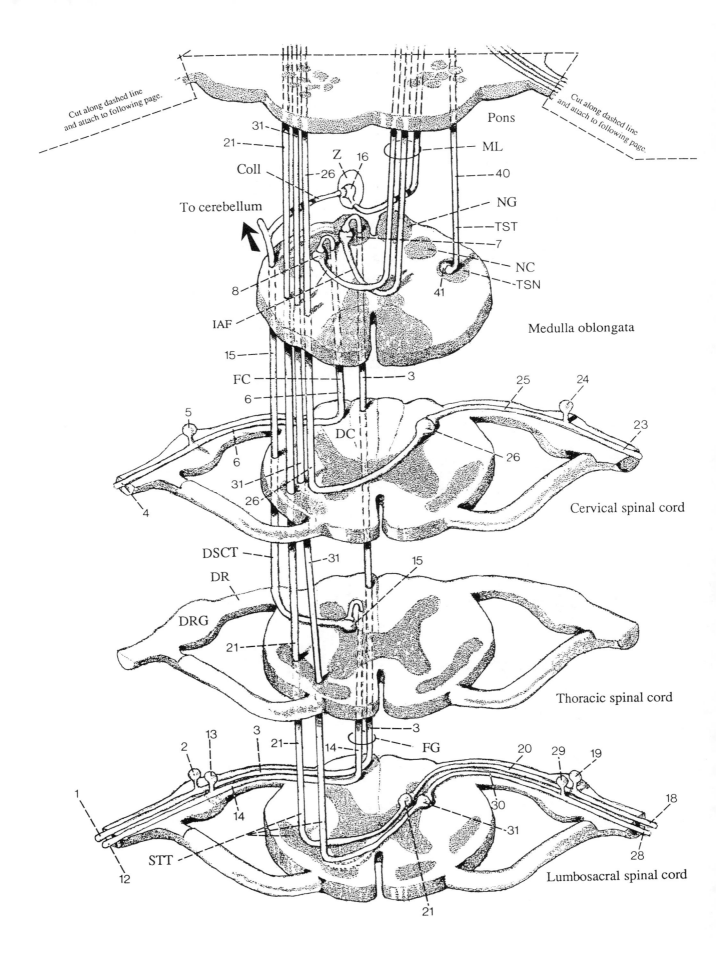

Cut along dashed line and attach to following page.

Cut along dashed line and attach to following page.

Pons

31

21

ML

Coll

Z 16

26

40

To cerebellum

NG

TST

7

8

NC

TSN

41

IAF

Medulla oblongata

15

FC

3

6

25 24

DC

5

23

6

26

31

4

26

Cervical spinal cord

DSCT

31

DR

15

DRG

21

Thoracic spinal cord

3

2 13 3

21 14

FG

20 29 19

1

14

30

18

STT

31

12

28

21

Lumbosacral spinal cord

Stereognosis (Greek, literally "solid knowledge," from *stereos*, solid, and *gnosis*, knowledge) is the ability to identify objects by touch. This ability depends upon several kinds of sensory receptors, such as Meissner's corpuscles, which are touch (or tactile) receptors (shown on opposite page), plus the brain's extraordinary ability to combine information from various receptors, some of which respond to slight deformation of the skin on the fingertips, others to joint movement, and still others to pressure. Presumably the parietal cortex, in close cooperation with certain thalamic nuclei, processes incoming tactile and proprioceptive information and "internally reconstructs" the object being examined by one's fingers, so that the individual can readily identify the object touched. This ability also employs movement of the fingers. Meissner's tactile corpuscles are particularly abundant in the tips of the fingers, where an average of one in every four dermal papillae contains one (Figure B).

In Figure C the zigzag course of the receptor axon is shown as it winds its way among the shelf-like connective tissue cells that form the bulk of the corpuscle. Several nerve fibers are found in each corpuscle. Whether these are actually separate fibers or all branches of the same parent fiber is not known.

Note the collagen fibers that connect the corpuscle to the overlying epidermis. Because of the arrangement of these collagen fibers, the slightest movement in the epidermis, such as might occur in feeling a coin, would cause a displacement of the corpuscle and a discharge of its receptor axon. Meissner's corpuscles alone cannot inform one as to the size or dimension of the object being held. This depends on other receptors, particularly the joint receptor, which provides information on just how far the fingers are flexed and extended as the fingertips probe the object. Knowledge of the extent of finger movement is essential in gauging the diameter of a coin. This allows you to distinguish a dime from a penny solely by feeling it with your fingers.

Stereognosis is believed to ascend in the cuneate fasciculus and medial lemniscus to the thalamus, where the input is processed and then relayed to the parietal cerebral cortex, where the identity and nature of the object are recognized. Damage to any part of this pathway such as the cuneate fasciculus, medial lemniscus, or parietal cortex will result in **astereognosis**, that is, the **inability** to recognize objects by touch.

Color the receptor axon in Figure C and the Meissner's corpuscle in Figure B.

Figure C is based upon and modified from Andres and von Düring: Morphology of cutaneous receptors. In Iggo A (ed): Handbook of Sensory Physiology, Vol. II: Somatosensory System. Berlin, Springer-Verlag, 1973, Figure 10, page 16.

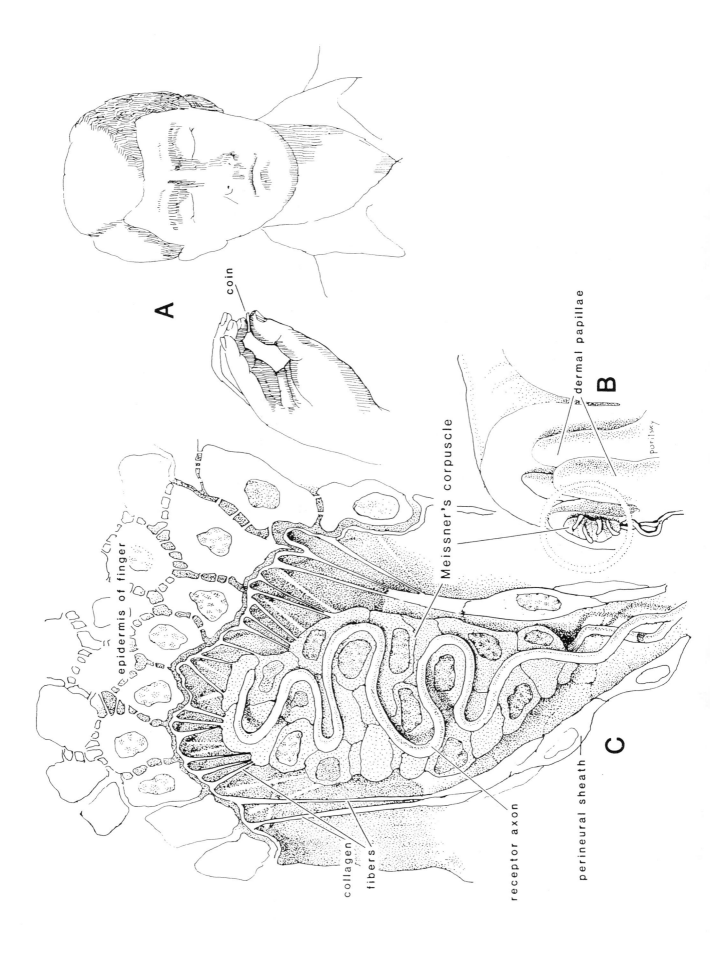

A

coin

B

dermal papillae

papillary

C

epidermis of finger

Meissner's corpuscle

collagen
fibers

receptor axon

perineural sheath

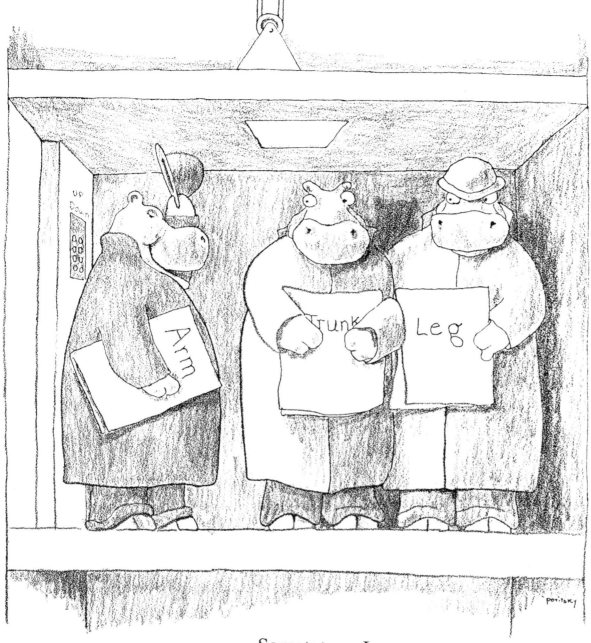

Somatotopy I

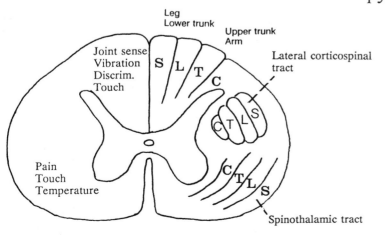

Cross-section of the spinal cord shows a somatotopic projection in both ascending and descending tracts. S, L, T, and C stand for sacral, lumbar, thoracic, and cervical. Sacral and lumbar nerves supply the leg and lower trunk. Thoracic and cervical nerves supply the upper trunk, arm, and neck. (After Brodal, 1981.)

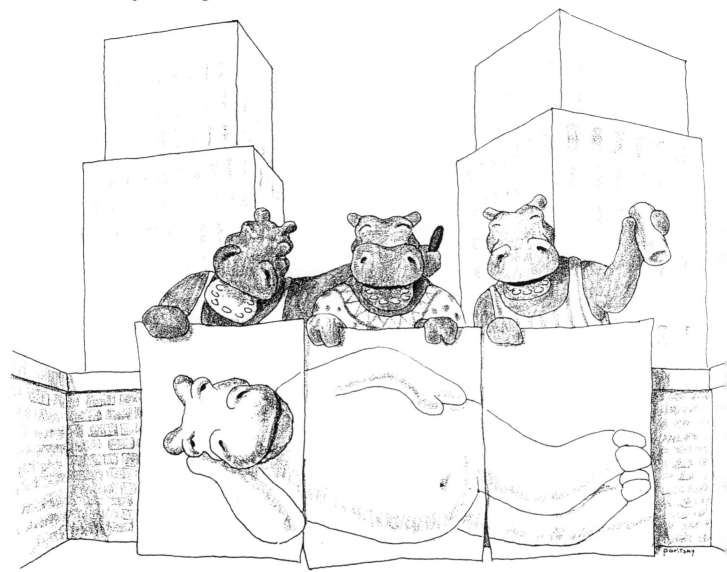

Somatotopy II

(Greek, *soma*, body; *topos*, place)

Somatotopy is a new term used to describe the somatotopic or orderly projections of tracts up and down the neural axis. Fibers that relate to each part of the body have a position next to fibers from adjacent body parts, so that a cross-section of an ascending sensory tract, such as the posterior funiculus, or of a descending motor tract, such as the pyramidal tract, presents a crude image of one-half of the body. (Technically, the hippos should be displaying only half a hippo when they reach the roof.)

The spinothalamic tract and the transmission of pain

There are two kinds of pain. One is the fast, sharp pain associated with a pinprick. The other is the slow, dull, diffuse, burning or aching pain that tells us that we have been injured and have suffered tissue damage. The sustained action of the slow pain does not let us forget that we have been hurt. The fast sharp pain, which tells us exactly where the pain is, travels within the spinothalamic tract and is diagrammatically shown by neurons 1, 2, and 3 on the opposite page. Neuron 1 is a small unipolar primary (or first-order) neuron residing in a dorsal root ganglion (5). Its peripheral process (6) runs in a spinal nerve (7) and has pain receptors at its endings (8). Pain receptors are called nociceptors, a term derived from the Latin *nocere,* which means to harm.

Fast pain is carried by the A-delta fibers, which are thinnest of the myelinated fibers. Slow pain is carried by the very thinnest fibers, the C fibers, which are unmyelinated. Fast pain fiber 1 enters the spinal cord (9) via the dorsal root (10) and synapses upon neuron 2, which is an STT neuron (spinothalamic tract neuron) or sometimes simply called a "tract cell." These STT or tract cells lie mainly in lamina I and lamina V of the dorsal horn gray matter. The STT cells are the cells of origin of the spinothalamic tract. Axons of the STT neurons cross the midline in the ventral white commissure and form a bundle of axons in the opposite anterolateral quadrant of white matter. This bundle is the spinothalamic tract (11). Its name indicates that it begins in the spinal cord and it ends in the thalamus. The axon of SST cell 2 ends upon neuron 3 in the ventral posterolateral nucleus of the thalamus (12). Neuron 3 projects to the somatosensory cortex (4) on the anterior margin of the parietal lobe. It is at the cortical level that the pain stimulus is interpreted and analyzed in terms of the exact location and nature of the injury.

It is now believed that there are two parts to the spinothalamic tract: a neospinothalamic tract (13) and a paleospinothalamic tract (14). The neospinothalamic tract ends in the lateral thalamus (as indicated by axon 2), whereas the paleospinothalamic tract ends in the medial thalamus, specifically with certain nuclei in the thalamus called the intralaminar nuclei (15). On the basis of these two sites of endings of the spinothalamic tract, plus evidence from clinical, behavioral, and physiological observations, it is now felt that the neospinothalamic pathway carries the fast, sharp pain and the paleospinothalamic pathway carries the slow, dull pain. The neospinothalamic tract is phylogenetically more recent. It conducts more rapidly with relatively little spread of impulses to adjacent structures along the way. The paleospinothalamic tract is phylogenetically older. It conducts slower with considerable stimulation of adjacent structures along the way, such as the reticular formation.

The intralaminar thalamic nuclei, which receive the paleospinothalamic fibers, project to widespread areas of the cerebral cortex (16). Thus it appears that the neospinothalamic tract carries the discriminative and localized aspect of pain to the lateral thalamus, where it is relayed to the somatosensory cortex. The paleospinothalamic tract is believed to carry the unpleasant affective quality of pain to the medial thalamus, which in turn relays it to widespread areas of the cerebral cortex and certain subcortical structures. The paleospinothalamic tract also appears to be responsible for the state of arousal along with resultant emotional and behavioral responses that pain brings forth.

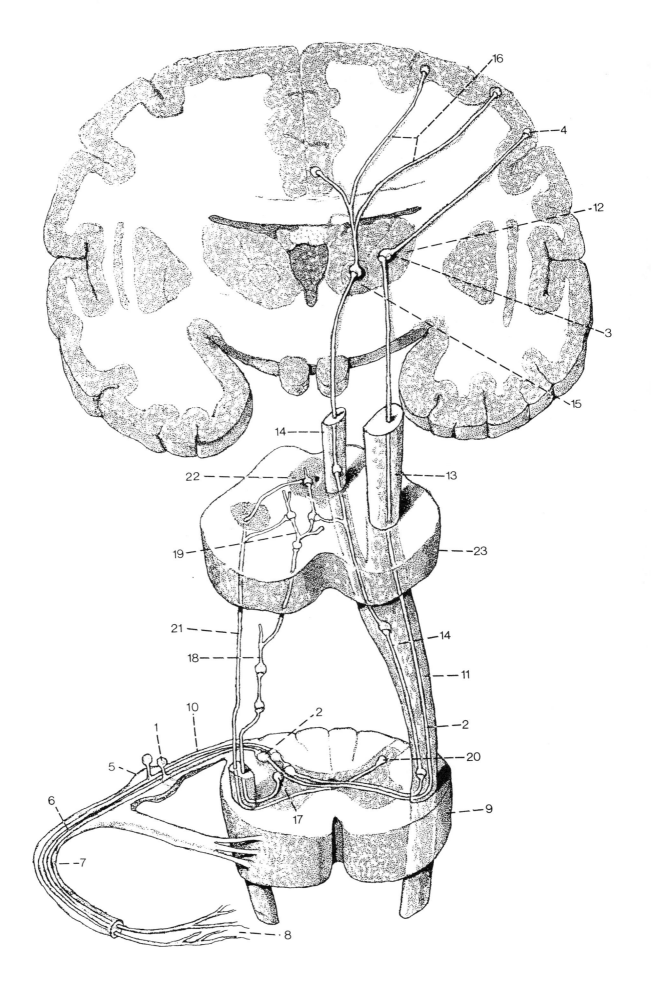

The spinothalamic tract and the transmission of pain *(continued)*

In addition to the spinothalamic tract, two other tracts carry pain. These are the spinoreticular tract and spinomesencephalic tract. Recently another pain pathway has been found in cats and monkeys. This newly discovered tract travels in the dorsolateral white matter and is called the dorsolateral spinothalamic tract (not shown here). Spinoreticular fibers arise from cell bodies mainly in laminae VII and VIII (17) and ascend in the anterolateral quadrant (18) on both sides, intermingling with spinothalamic fibers. Note they are both crossed (not shown) and uncrossed (18). Spinoreticular fibers end in the reticular formation (19) in the medulla and pons. Reticulothalamic fibers (not shown) project to the medial thalamus.

Spinomesencephalic tract fibers appear to parallel the spinothalamic fibers. They arise from cell bodies in laminae I and V (20), cross the midline, ascend in the opposite side (21), and end on neurons in the periaqueductal gray (22) in the mesencephalon (23). Although it has been shown that the periaqueductal gray is involved in both the transmission of pain as well the suppression of pain, its exact role, as well as the role of the spinomesencephalic tract, is largely unknown.

Color and label

1   A-delta pain neuron
2   Spinothalamic tract neuron (STT cell)
3   Thalamic neuron in ventral posterolateral (VPL) nucleus
4   Cortical neuron
5   Spinal ganglion
6   A-delta pain fiber
7   Spinal nerve
8   Nociceptors (pain receptors)
9   Spinal cord
10   Dorsal root
11   Spinothalamic tract
12   Ventral posterolateral nucleus (VPL) of thalamus
13   Neospinothalamic tract
14   Paleospinothalamic tract
15   Central lateral nucleus of the intralaminar complex
16   Thalamocortical fibers
17   Spinoreticular tract cell
18   Spinoreticular fiber
19   Reticular formation
20   Spinomesencephalic tract cell
21   Spinomesencephalic tract fiber
22   Periaqueductal gray
23   Mesencephalon (midbrain)

Redrawn with modification after Snyder S: Opiate receptors and internal opiates. Scientific American 236(3):44-56, 977; and Young PA: The anatomy of the spinal cord pain paths: A review. Journal of the American Paraplegic Society 9:28-38, 1986.

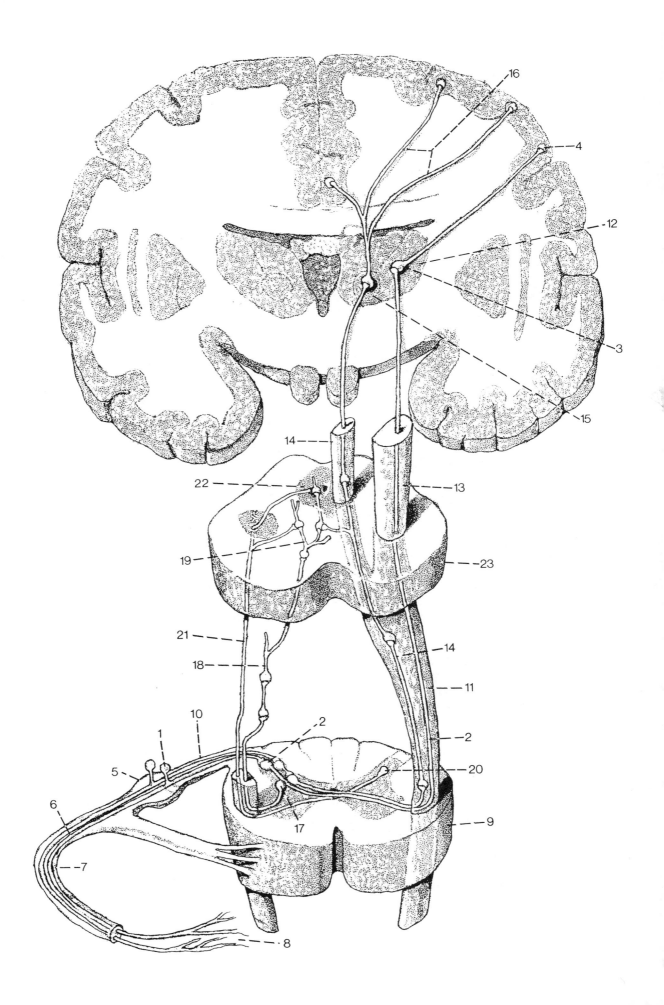

A wound (or lesion) that severs one side of the spinal cord (a hemisection) will interrupt both ascending and descending tracts. Degeneration of ascending tracts will occur *above* the lesion and degeneration of descending tracts will occur *below* the lesion (Figure B). This is due to the cell body's functioning as the trophic* *center* of the neuron and all its processes, both axon and dendrites.

If an axon is cut, the distal segment will degenerate. The isolated segment breaks up into a series of membrane-bound spheres beginning near the point of damage and proceeds distally until the whole distal segment has degenerated. The myelin likewise breaks down and is removed by scavenger cells. This degeneration from the point of damage distally is **antegrade or wallerian degeneration** and invariably occurs to axons separated from their cell bodies, both within the central nervous system as well as in peripheral nerves. (Augustus Volney Waller was a 19th-century English physiologist.)

Locate neuron 1 in the lower left. It carries discriminative touch. Follow its central process as it ascends to the level of the lesion. The portion of fiber 1 above the lesion degenerates, and discriminative touch, which is carried up the ipsilateral dorsal columns, will be lost on the *same side* of the body *below t*he level of the lesion (Figure C). However, since touch ascends on both sides of the spinal cord, touch will be impaired but not totally lost.

Locate pain fiber 2 and trace it into the spinal cord, where it synapses upon neuron 3, which crosses to the opposite side and ascends on the contralateral side. Above the level of the lesion the distal segment of neuron 3, separated from its trophic cell body, degenerates. Fast pain will be lost on the *opposite side* of the body *below* the level of the cut. Because slow pain ascends on both sides of the cords, slow pain will persist.

Locate descending motor fiber 4 in Figure B. Its cell body is at a higher level not shown in the drawing. **Follow** fiber 4 caudally to the lesion, below which point its fiber degenerates. Because of this, alpha motor neurons below the lesion are unable to receive motor commands from the brain, and this part of the body is paralyzed. This type of paralysis affects the upper motor neuron but leaves the alpha motor neuron intact. Therefore, this type of paralysis is not characterized by the immediate flaccidity in voluntary muscles that follows damage to the alpha motor neuron or to its axon.

Clearly it is important to know which tracts have **crossed** and which tracts have **not crossed** in determining loss of function following hemisection (half cut) of the cord. **Fast pain** will be lost on the **opposite side**, because fast pain pathways cross soon after entering the cord. However, **slow pain** will continue to be perceived (see Figure 53). **Motor function** will be lost on the **same side**, because descending motor fibers once in the cord remain homolateral. The same is true of **discriminative touch** and **proprioception**, which ascend on the *same side* of the cord and likewise will be lost on the *same side* of the body.

Trophein (Greek) means to nourish or sustain and refers in this case to the apparent sustaining action or influence that the cell body exerts upon its processes. Without this sustaining factor, the axons and dendrites separated from their cell body degenerate. In addition to maintaining their component processes, neurons exert a trophic action upon nonnervous structures such as taste buds. A neural "trophic action" appears to play a crucial role in amphibian limb regeneration; a certain amount of nerve appears to be essential for an amputated newt limb to regenerate. If the nerves are removed from an adult newt limb, it will not regenerate following amputation. The identity of this trophic substance or influence remains unknown.

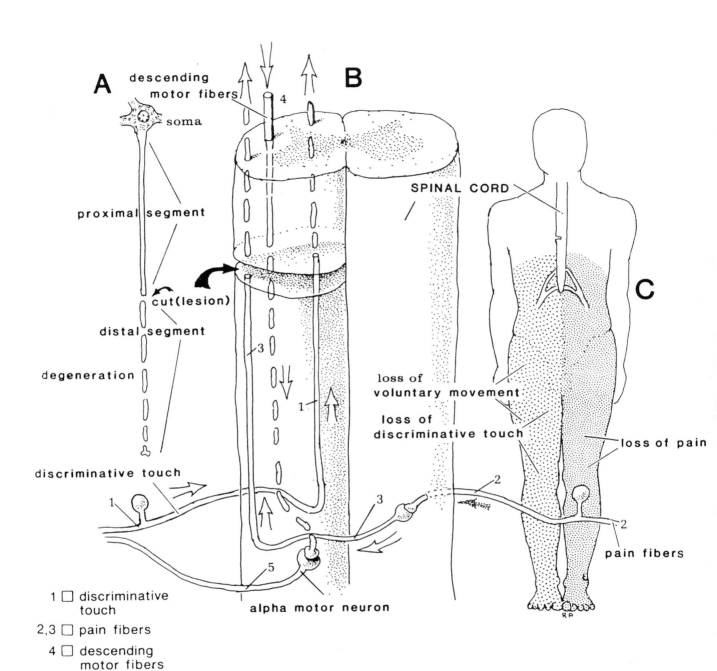

A

descending motor fibers

soma

proximal segment

cut (lesion)

distal segment

degeneration

discriminative touch

1

B

4

SPINAL CORD

3

1

loss of voluntary movement

loss of discriminative touch

3

5

alpha motor neuron

C

2

loss of pain

2

pain fibers

1 ☐ discriminative touch

2,3 ☐ pain fibers

4 ☐ descending motor fibers

On the right side, the drawing shows one neuron for each of the functional components carried in these three cranial nerves. On the left side, the nuclei associated with these nerves are depicted as longitudinal columns in the medulla. The drawing of the brain stem on the upper right indicates the level of the medulla through which the section passes. The position of these columns of cell bodies is characteristic of each of these six cranial nerve components. For example, the hypoglossal nucleus lies medial and dorsal, a position also occupied by the more rostral **general somatic efferent (GSE)** nuclei of nerves III, IV, and VI.

The **hypoglossal nerve (XII)** begins with cell bodies that lie in a longitudinal column of cells in the medulla. This column of cells is the **hypoglossal nucleus** (1). Note that the hypoglossal nerve emerges as a series of rootlets (2) between the olive and the pyramids. Each hypoglossal nerve supplies all the tongue muscles on the same side, that is, homolateral tongue musculature. Each hypoglossal nucleus receives corticonuclear fibers from the cerebral cortex. These corticonuclear fibers (or corticobulbar fibers) originate mainly in the opposite cerebral cortex (3), but the medial portion of the hypoglossal nucleus receives homolateral corticonuclear fibers (4) as well. Because the tongue muscles develop embryologically from somites, the motor neurons and their axons that comprise the hypoglossal nerve are classified as GSE. Damage to the hypoglossal nerve will cause the tongue to deviate to the paralyzed side when protruded.

The **accessory nerve (XI)** has two origins, a cranial one (5) in the caudal part of the nucleus ambiguus (6) and a spinal one (7) in the accessory nucleus, which lies at levels C2-C5 in the spinal cord (not shown). The **nucleus ambiguus** (6) lies lateral and somewhat ventral to the hypoglossal nucleus. It is actually not a compact cellular column as the drawing suggests, but a scattered collection of motor neurons, difficult to define in cross-section, hence its name, the "ambiguous nucleus." The axons that arise from the nucleus ambiguus travel with cranial nerves IX, X, and XI, and supply the muscles of the soft palate, pharynx, and larynx. These muscles are derived from branchial arches three, four, and six and their motor axons are classified as **special visceral efferent (SVE)**. Notice that axons emanating from somata in the caudal part of the nucleus ambiguus (5) exit with the cranial part of the accessory nerve (8), transfer to the vagus nerve, and eventually supply the muscles of the larynx. Accessory nerve fibers from the spinal component leave the skull, receive additional fibers from spinal nerves C3 and C4, and supply the sternocleidomastoid and trapezius muscles. Damage to the accessory nerve will result in an inability to fully elevate the arm because the trapezius muscle rotates the scapula when the arm is elevated beyond horizontal. Also there will be some difficulty in turning the head toward the unaffected (normal) side and in ventrally flexing the head from the supine position due to paralysis of the sternocleidomastoid muscle.

The **vagus nerve (X)** has five functional components, GSA, SVA, GVA, SVE, and GVE. It has two ganglia, a superior (9) and an inferior (10), that contain the somata of its afferent fibers. Vagal **general somatic afferent (GSA)** fibers carry cutaneous sensation from the skin of the ear drum to the

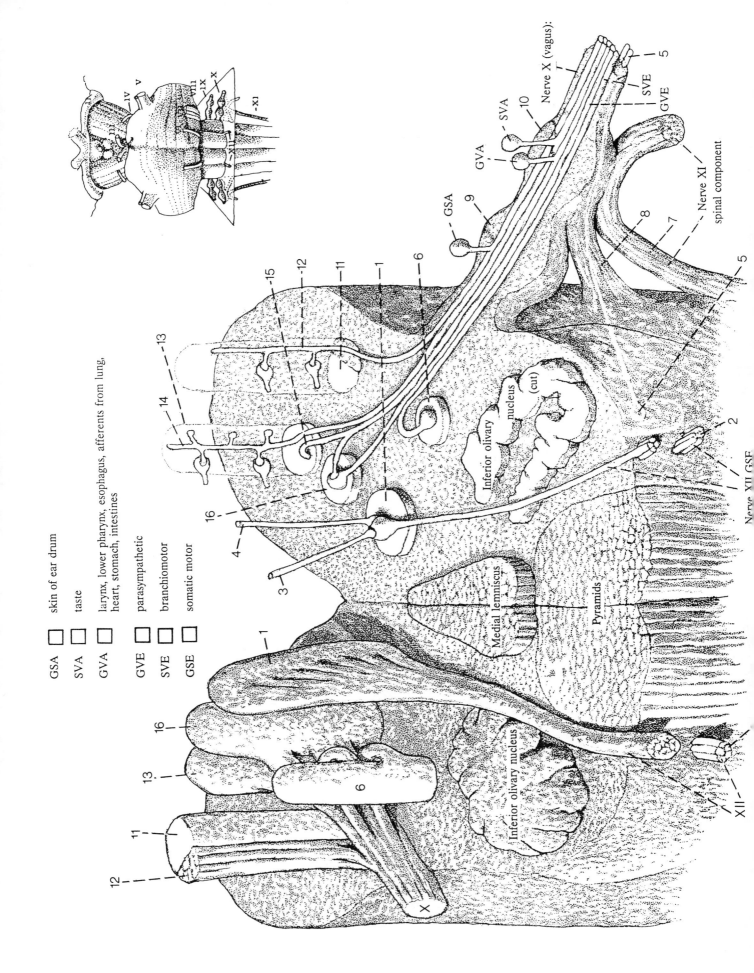

GSA skin of ear drum

SVA taste

GVA larynx, lower pharynx, esophagus, afferents from lung, heart, stomach, intestines

GVE parasympathetic

SVE branchiomotor

GSE somatic motor

Nerve X (vagus):

SVE
GVE
SVA
GVA
GSA

Nerve XI
spinal component

Nerve XII GSE

Inferior olivary nucleus (cut)

Medial lemniscus

Pyramids

Inferior olivary nucleus

trigeminal spinal nucleus (11) by way of the trigeminal spinal tract (spinal tract of V) (12). **Special visceral afferent** (SVA) fibers in the vagus nerve carry taste from taste buds on the posterior tongue and epiglottis to the rostral part of the nucleus of the **solitary tract** (13). Notice that the solitary nucleus surrounds the solitary tract (14), thus giving it its isolated or solitary appearance. **General visceral afferent** vagal fibers (GVA) include pain fibers from the mucosa of the larynx, lower pharynx, esophagus, stomach, and intestines. Hunger and nausea are also conveyed by the vagus nerve.

The great majority of GVA fibers within the vagus nerve operate at the subconscious level and play vital roles in the regulation of heart beat, blood pressure, breathing, and digestion. These include fibers from chemoreceptors and pressure receptors in the great vessels such as the aorta. These receptors monitor the chemical composition and pressure of the blood. GVA fibers within the vagus also relay impulses from stretch receptors in the lung. These stretch receptors respond to distention of the air passages in the lung and upon full distention fire off impulses that inhibit the inspiratory breathing center in the medulla, thus stopping inspiration. Vagal GVA fibers end in the caudal part of the solitary nucleus (15), in the dorsal vagal nucleus (16), and in various other autonomic centers in the medulla.

Vagal SVE fibers come from motor neurons in the nucleus ambiguus (6). These fibers supply all the muscles of the larynx, and together with the glossopharyngeal nerve, with which it forms the pharyngeal plexus, the vagus nerve supplies practically all the muscles of the pharynx as well.

Finally, the vagus nerve carries the great outflow of the parasympathetic system, which is designated as **general visceral efferent** (GVE). The GVE fibers arise from preganglionic parasympathetic cell bodies in the dorsal vagal nucleus (formerly, the dorsal motor vagal nucleus), travel widely throughout the thorax and abdomen, and eventually synapse upon postganglionic parasympathetic neurons in ganglia near or within the walls of the heart, lungs, stomach, and intestines. Vagal parasympathetic stimulation is responsible for the peristaltic wave in the esophageal smooth musculature, the secretion of gastric glands and motility in the stomach, relaxation of the pyloric sphincter, and peristalsis in the intestine.

Damage to the vagus nerve produces such symptoms as palpitations, increased pulse, constant vomiting, slowing of respiration, and a sense of suffocation. Because of vagal innervation of the eardrum, a plug of wax in the ear can produce an "ear cough," and syringing of the ear may produce vomiting and even cardiac inhibition. Unilateral paralysis of the soft palate will be noted when the patient says "ah." The normal side will be elevated, the paralyzed side will have a lower arch, and the uvula will be pulled to the normal side. This is due to the unopposed action of the normal levator veli palatini. A permanently constricted pylorus may result from complete absence of vagal control.

Color each of the functional components of nerves XII, XI, and X.

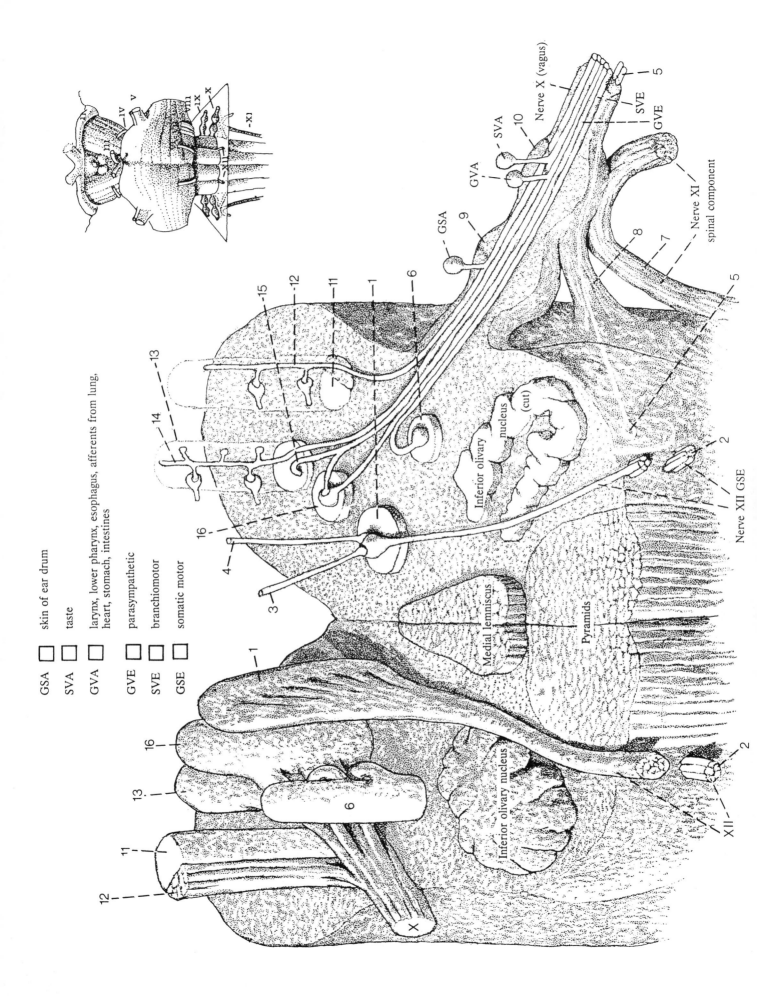

GSA — skin of ear drum

SVA — taste

GVA — larynx, lower pharynx, esophagus, afferents from lung, heart, stomach, intestines

GVE — parasympathetic

SVE — branchiomotor

GSE — somatic motor

Nerve X (vagus)

GVA
SVA
GSA

SVE
GVE

Nerve XI
spinal component

Nerve XII GSE

Inferior olivary
nucleus
(cut)

Medial lemniscus

Pyramids

Inferior olivary nucleus

XII

The **glossopharyngeal nerve (IX)**, like the vagus nerve with which it is closely associated, has the same five functional components. It also has two ganglia, a superior and inferior, which contain the unipolar somata of its afferent fibers. It emerges from the medulla by several rootlets lateral to the olive and directly rostral and in line with the vagus and accessory nerves. It contains the following functional components:

A few **special visceral efferent** (SVE) fibers arising from the rostral part of the nucleus ambiguus (1) and supplying the stylopharyngeus muscle; **general visceral efferent** (GVE; preganglionic parasympathetic) fibers originating from the inferior salivatory nucleus (2) and synapsing in the otic ganglion, which relays secretory impulses to the parotid gland. Taste fibers (**special visceral afferents, SVA**) leading from taste buds on the posterior one-third of the tongue and the palatal arches, and ending centrally in the rostral third of the solitary nucleus (3). These taste fibers have their somata in the inferior ganglion (6). A few **general somatic afferent** (GSA) fibers with somata in the superior ganglion (7) conveying pain, touch, and temperature from the skin of the ear and terminating in the spinal nucleus of V (8). Finally, **general visceral afferent** (GVA) fibers, some of which carry impulses that reach the level of consciousness and others that remain at the subconscious level; the former group includes pain and temperature from the posterior one-third of the tongue and upper pharynx, and pain from the middle ear; the latter (subconscious) group includes afferents from the carotid sinus and carotid body.

All the visceral afferents have their somata in the inferior ganglion. Some of the GVA fibers in the glossopharyngeal nerve enter the solitary tract and end in the solitary nucleus (10). However, GVA fibers from the posterior one-third of the tongue and the upper pharynx carrying pain and probably touch and temperature as well, or possible collaterals of these fibers (11), end in the spinal nucleus of the V. Afferents from the carotid body and the carotid sinus, or collaterals (12) of fibers that end in the solitary nucleus, terminate in the dorsal nucleus of X (13). Thus an

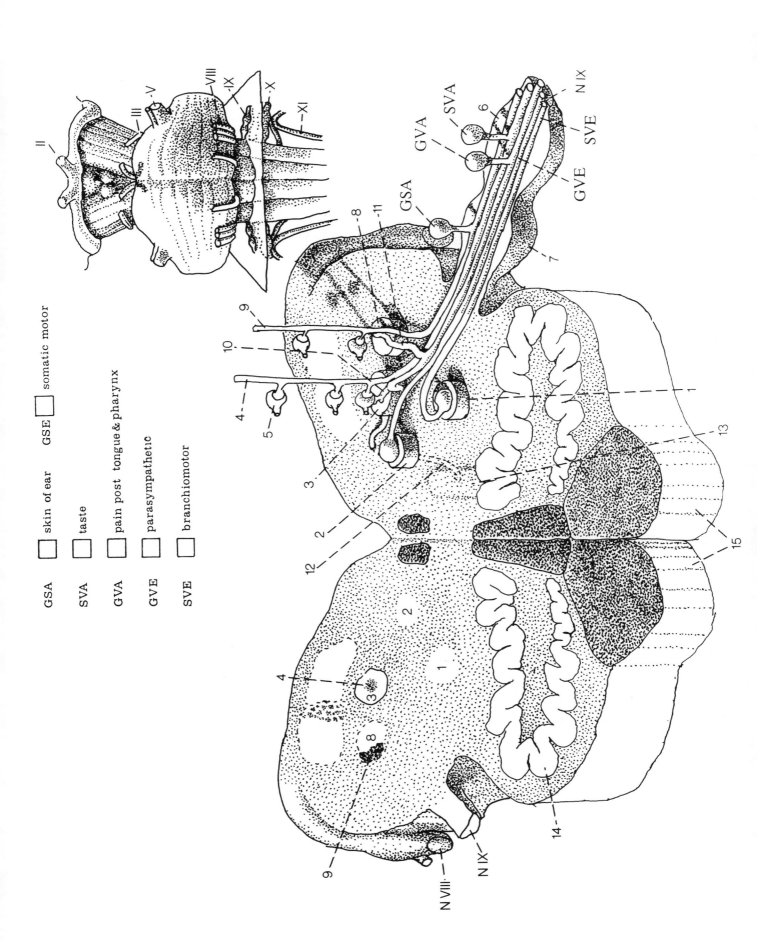

increase in arterial pressure will be registered by the carotid sinus, whose afferent fibers will cause the preganglionic parasympathetic neurons in the dorsal vagal nucleus to send inhibitory impulses via the vagus nerve to the heart (acetylcholine depresses the heartbeat), and the arterial pressure will be correspondingly lowered. The carotid body responds to hypoxia and conversely is able to bring about an increase in blood pressure, heart rate, and respiratory rate should the oxygen level decrease.

Damage to the glossopharyngeal nerve will result in a loss of all sensation from the posterior one-third of the tongue, the palatal arches, the palatal tonsil, and the upper pharynx. The **gag reflex,** which is an urge to retch or heave when the mucosa of the pharynx is touched, is lost on the afflicted side following damage to the glossopharyngeal nerve.

Directions: Using a different color for each functional component, color the soma and fiber of each of the five neurons that represent the five components of the glossopharyngeal nerve. The figure of the brain stem at the right and transecting plane indicate the level of the section.

Color and label

1 Nucleus ambiguus
2 Inferior salivatory nucleus
3 Nucleus of solitary tract
4 Solitary tract
5 Second-order taste cells
6 Inferior ganglion of nerve IX
7 Superior ganglion of nerve IX
8 Trigeminal spinal nucleus
9 Trigeminal spinal tract
10 GVA fiber to caudal nucleus of the solitary tract
11 GVA fiber from tongue and upper pharynx to spinal nucleus of V

12 GVA fiber from carotid body or carotid sinus descending to dorsal vagal nucleus
13 Dorsal vagal nucleus (below this section
14 Inferior olivary nucleus
15 Pyramids

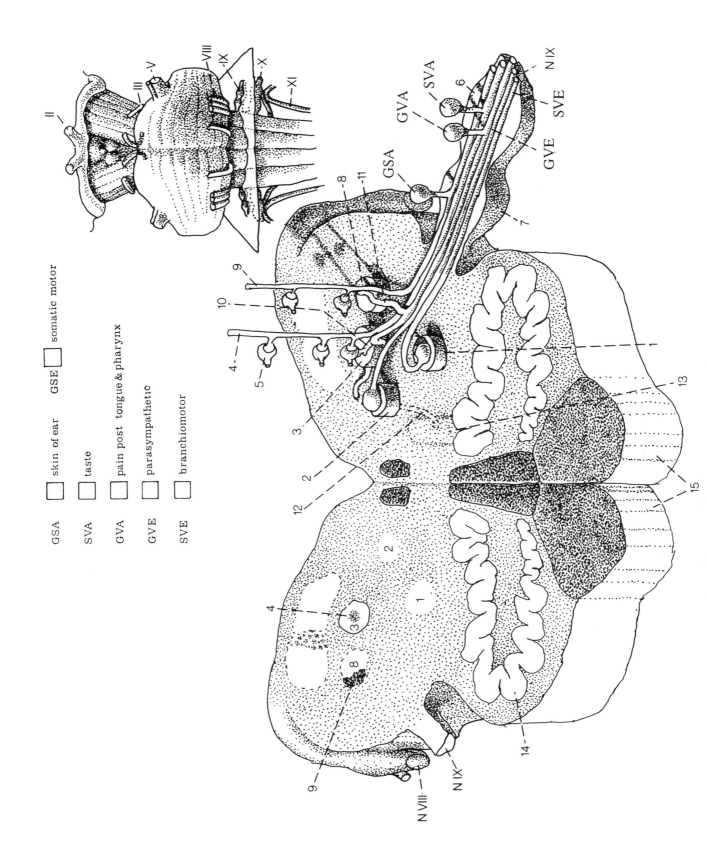

"Open your mouth and say Ah"

The soft palate is pulled up and back by the levator veli palatini muscle. This happens in speech and in swallowing. The nerve fibes to the levator veli palatini originate from cell bodies in the rostral part of the nucleus ambiguus, which lies in the medulla oblongata. Normally the two levator muscles pull equally on the soft palate, the uvula remains vertical, and the palatoglossal and palatopharyngeal arches on the two sides are symmetrical. If one vagus nerve is damaged, the normal levator veli palatini muscle will pull its half and arches higher than the paralyzed side and the uvula will point to the normal side.

Color and label

1   Levator veli palatini muscle
2   Vagus nerve (N X)
3   Lesion in right vagus nerve
4   Palatoglossal arch
5   Palatopharyngeal arch

MLF

NUCLEUS
AMBIGUUS

INFERIOR
OLIVARY

PYRAMIDS

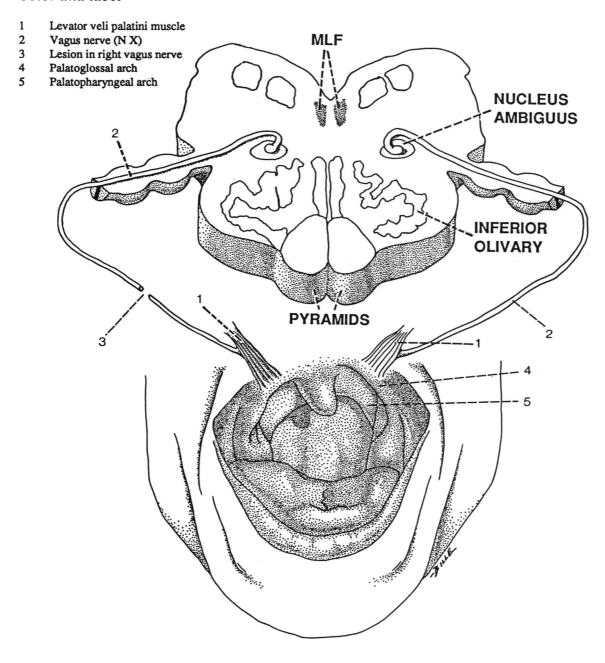

Color and label

1   **Pinna** (Latin, feather, wing) or auricle (Latin, little ear)
2   **Cartilaginous walls of ear canal**
3   **Ear canal** (external auditory meatus). It contains ceruminous glands that produce the orange-brown ear wax or cerumen. Water trapped "in the ear" after swimming is actually in the ear canal. Ear wax may tend to prevent the water from exiting if the water is lodged beyond the ear wax.
4   **Bony walls of ear canal.** Fortunately the diameter of the bony part of the ear canal is smaller than the thickness of the little finger. This prevents one from damaging the delicate ear drum with one's fingernail when scratching. The ear canal is about 2.5 cm long and actually acts as a resonator for sound waves that have frequencies between 2,000 and 4,000 cycles per second– the critical range for human speech. Thus it amplifies these sound waves.
5   **Umbo of eardrum.** The eardrum or tympanic membrane is shaped like a blunt cone, with the deepest point called the umbo. The outside of the eardrum is skin and is supplied by sensory fibers from both nerves V and X (an object pushing against the eardrum may produce a cough). Umbo is Latin for a raised ornament on a shield.
6   **Middle ear cavity.** It is lined with a mucous membrane that covers the walls, ossicles, ligaments, and nerves. Under certain conditions mucus may accumulate in the middle ear to the point that the movement of the ear drum and ossicles is impeded. **Otitis media** is a general term for inflammation of the middle ear. Nerve IX supplies sensory fibers to the middle ear and inner surface of the eardrum.
7   **Internal jugular vein**
8   **Round window.** Closed by a membrane that acts as a pressure release for pressure wave in the perilymph in the inner ear.
9   **Vestibule.** This is a fluid-filled cavity within the temporal bone. The vestibule contains both the membranous utricle and saccule.
10   **Auditory tube (eustachian tube).** This connects the middle ear with the nasopharynx. When the tube dilates, air is allowed either in or out, thus equalizing with the ambient air pressure.
11   **Nasopharynx**
12   **Malleus** (Latin, hammer). Its lower end is connected to the central umbo of the tympanic membrane.
13   **Incus** (Latin, anvil). It articulates with both the malleus and stapes through tiny synovial joints.
14   **Lateral semicircular canal**
15   **Posterior semicircular canal**
16   **Anterior semicircular canal**
17   **Facial nerve** (N VII). Cut
18   **Internal acoustic (auditory) meatus**
19   **Vestibulocochlear nerve** (N VIII)
20   **Cochlea** (Latin, snail). A snail-like tubular spiral within the temporal bone
21   **Footplate** (or base) of stapes (Latin, stirrup). It covers the oval window. Sound-induced vibrations of the footplate cause pressure waves in the perilymph in the vestibule.

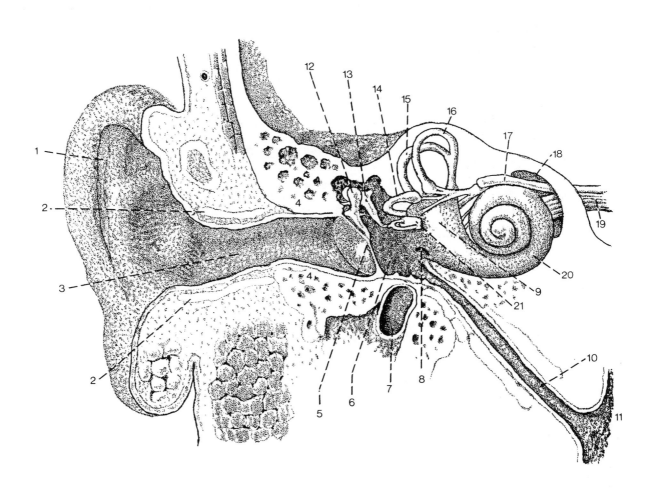

Color and label

1 **External auditory meatus** (ear canal)

2 **Tympanic membrane** (eardrum)

3 **Middle ear cavity** (tympanic cavity). This is filled with air that can only enter and leave through the eustachian tube. It is lined with mucous membrane that covers both the walls and ear ossicles. Sensory innervation is by nerve IX.

4 **Malleus.** Its lower end is connected to the center of the eardrum. Sound waves entering the ear canal cause the eardrum to vibrate. These sound-induced vibrations are carried across the middle ear cavity by the 3 ear ossicles.

5 **Incus.** The 3 ear ossicles are joined by 2 synovial joints. However, the malleus and incus vibrate as a single unit. The longer length of the malleus in relation to the incus gives a leverage advantage. (The end of the malleus moves more, whereas the end of the incus moves less but has greater force.)

6 **Base (footplate) of stapes on oval window.** The eardrum is about 15 times greater in area than the footplate of the stapes. This difference in area plus the ossicle leverage advantage results in an increase in pressure at the oval window that is about 15 times greater than that at the eardrum.

7 **Opening of vestibule into scala vestibuli.** Sound-induced pressure waves from the vibrating base of the staples set off fluid pressure waves in the perilymph which enter the scala vestibuli where they cause the membranous walls of the cochlear duct to be deflected.

8 **Scala vestibuli.** The snail-like cochlea is divided into 3 spiral compartments or scalae (Latin, staircase or ladder). The scala vestibuli and scala tympani are filled with perilymph, which has a high sodium content. The scala media or cochlear duct is filled with endolymph, which has a high potassium content. Arrows pointing UP, that is, toward the apex, indicate course of the scala vestibuli.

9 **Scala tympani.** Arrows pointing DOWN indicate course of the scala tympani. In cross-section, the 3 scala each occupy the following amount of the circular cochlea: scala vestibuli, about 150°; the cochlear duct, about 30°, the scala tympani, about 180°.

10 **Round window.** This is covered by a membrane that moves directly opposite to the movements of the stapes footplate. When the footplate moves in, the round window membrane pushes out, and vice versa. This allows the sound-induced fluid pressure waves to travel up the cochlea. Because fluid (perilymph and endolymph) is essentially incompressible, and the cells and membranes are mainly fluid, plus the fact that the fluid-filled inner ear is encased in unyielding bone, it is essential that the membrane across the round window act as a pressure release. (The new names for the oval window, which is under the footplate, and the round window are fenestra vestibuli and fenestra tympani, respectively.)

11 **Cochlear duct.** Filled with endolymph, it is part of the membranous labyrinth and is joined to the vestibule by the ductus reuniens. It contains the organ of Corti.

12 **Spiral ganglion.** This consists of the bipolar cell bodies that supply sensory fibers to the hair cells in the organ of Corti. The cell bodies lie in the bony spiral lamina. Their central processes form the cochlear portion of nerve VIII.

13 **Cochlear portion of the vestibulocochlear nerve**

14 **Basal turn of cochlea**

15 **Second turn of cochlea**

16 **Apex of cochlea with helicotrema,** which is the small opening between scala vestibuli and scala tympani

17 **Facial nerve (N VII)** (a small portion)

18 **Internal auditory meatus.** Contains nerves VII and VIII.

19 **Facial nerve in facial canal.** Note its proximity to the middle ear cavity.

20 **Vestibular part of nerve VIII**

21 **Superior and inferior vestibular ganglia**

22 **Superior semicircular canal**

23 **Tensor tympani muscle** (a portion)

24 **Tendon of tensor tympani muscle.** It attaches to the malleus and dampens its vibration during loud sounds and probably during chewing and speaking.

25 **Auditory tube (eustachian tube).** Normally it is collapsed so that air does not freely pass between the middle ear and nasopharynx. Chewing and yawning usually open the tube enough to allow the air pressure in the middle ear to equalize with that of the outside air.

26 **Superior petrosal sinus.** A vein enclosed by dura mater.

27 **Temporal bone**

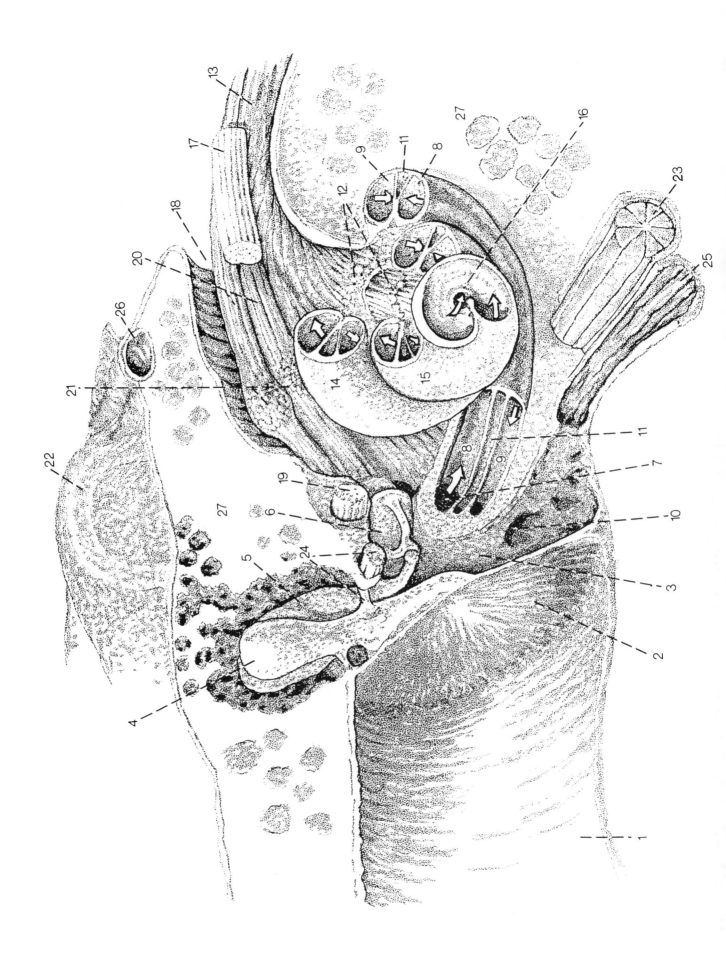

The Latin *tragus*, borrowed from the Greek *tragos*, means billy goat. Ancient anatomists used it as a name for the little bump on the ear that sometimes sprouts a little tuft of hair in older men, suggestive of the beard that goats grow. The word tragedy is derived from goat's song (*tragos*, goat, *oide*, song). One explanation is that the goat's song was the bleating of the goat about to be sacrificed in a religious ritual. Another theory is that the chorus in the earliest dramas wore goat skins when they sang or chanted. In either case, it appears that it was not a happy occasion for the goat.

Tragus
Billy goat

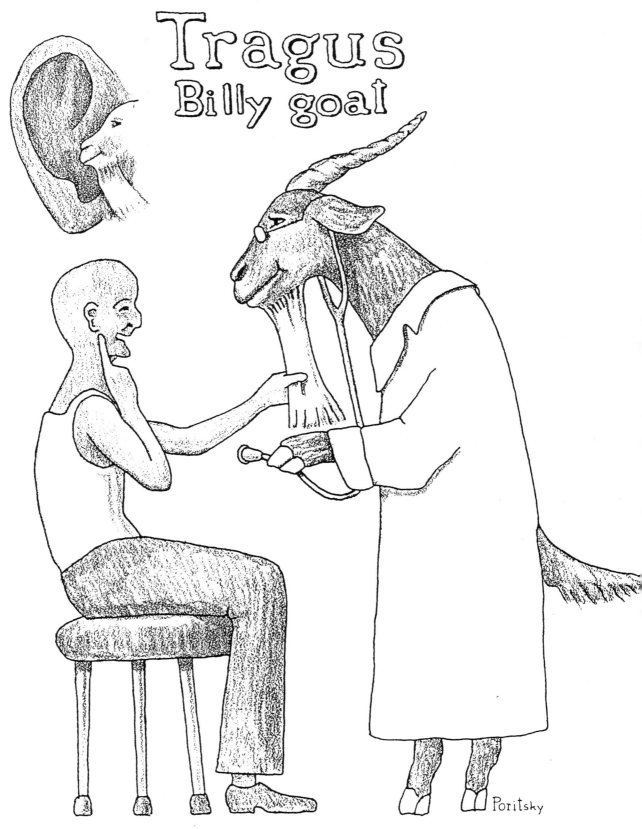

Dr Tragus: What seems to be the trouble, old timer?

Old timer: I'm growing one of these in my ear.

Poritsky

MEDIAL VIEW

Color and label

1	Anterior semicircular duct
2	Posterior semicircular duct
3	Lateral semicircular duct
4	Common crus of anterior and posterior semicircular ducts
5	Utricle (Latin, little uterus)
6	Saccule (Latin, little sac). The utricle and saccule both lie within a small cavity, the vestibule.
7	Ampulla (Latin, flask, bottle) of the anterior semicircular duct
8	Ampulla of lateral semicircular duct
9	Ampulla of posterior semicircular duct
10	Endolymphatic sac
11	Superior and inferior vestibular ganglia
12	Superior division of vestibular nerve
13	Inferior division of vestibular nerve
14	Cochlear nerve
15	Nerve to posterior ampulla
16	Endolymphatic duct arising from the utriculosaccular duct, which joins the saccule and utricule
17	Ductus reuniens. This joins the saccule to the vestibular end of the cochlear duct.
18	Spiral ganglion. This contains the bipolar cell bodies of the cochlear nerve.
19	Cochlear nerve fibers. These arise from cell bodies in the spiral ganglion. Those nerves to the right have all been cut.
20	Basal turn of cochlear duct
21	Middle turn of cochlear duct
22	Apical one-half turn of cochlear duct

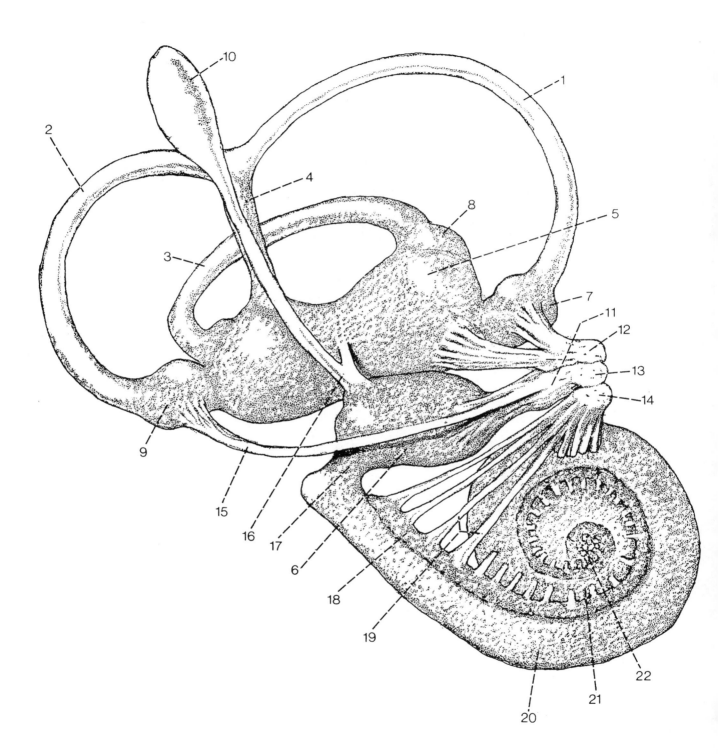

62 Membranous labyrinth of left inner ear, cut open

MEDIAL VIEW

Color and label

1   Utricle. Cut open to show its continuity with each of the 3 semicircular ducts and its macula (a position and motion sensor).

2   Saccule. Cut open to reveal its macula (saccular macula).

3   Macula utriculi (utricular macula). The macula (Latin, spot) of the utricle lies predominantly in a horizontal plane. It is stimulated both by tilting the head and by accelerating or decelerating in a horizontal direction such as speeding up or stopping suddenly in a car.

4   Saccular macula. The macula of the saccule lies in a vertical plane and responds to vertical acceleration and deceleration, such as starting and stopping in a fast elevator.

5   Crista (Latin, ridge) and cupula (Latin, little cup) in ampulla of anterior semicircular duct. Ampulla and utricle have been cut open to reveal opening of anterior semicircular duct into utricle.

6   Crista and cupula of lateral semicircular duct within its ampulla seen through its opening into utricle

7   Crista of posterior semicircular duct within its ampulla (crista ampullaris)

8   Cupula on posterior crista. Turning the head (angular acceleration) will cause the endolymph within the semicircular duct to move either toward the ampulla (ampullopetal) or away from the ampulla (ampullofugal). The moving endolymph will cause the cupula to bend one way or the other. Deflection of the cupula by endolymph moving in an ampullopetal direction will excite the hair cells on the crista. Ampullofugal deflection will hyperpolarize the hair cells and inhibit their firing off.

9   Utricle cut open. The small bony cavity that holds both the utricle and saccule is the **vestibule.** The terms vestibular function and vestibular dysfunction, however, refer not only to the utricle and saccule but to the 3 semicircular ducts as well.

10   Vestibular end of cochlear duct. This abuts on the fenestra vestibuli (round window).

11   Spiral ganglion

12   Afferent nerve fiber from bipolar neurons in spiral ganglion. There are also efferent fibers that arise from cell bodies in the superior olivary nucleus.

13   Cochlear duct, basal turn

14   Anterior semicircular duct

15   Lateral semicircular duct

16   Posterior semicircular duct

17   Endolymphatic duct. This lies within the cranial cavity adjacent to the dura mater.

18   Nerve to posterior crista ampullae (cut)

19   Upper division of vestibular nerve

20   Lower division of vestibular nerve

21   Cochlear nerve

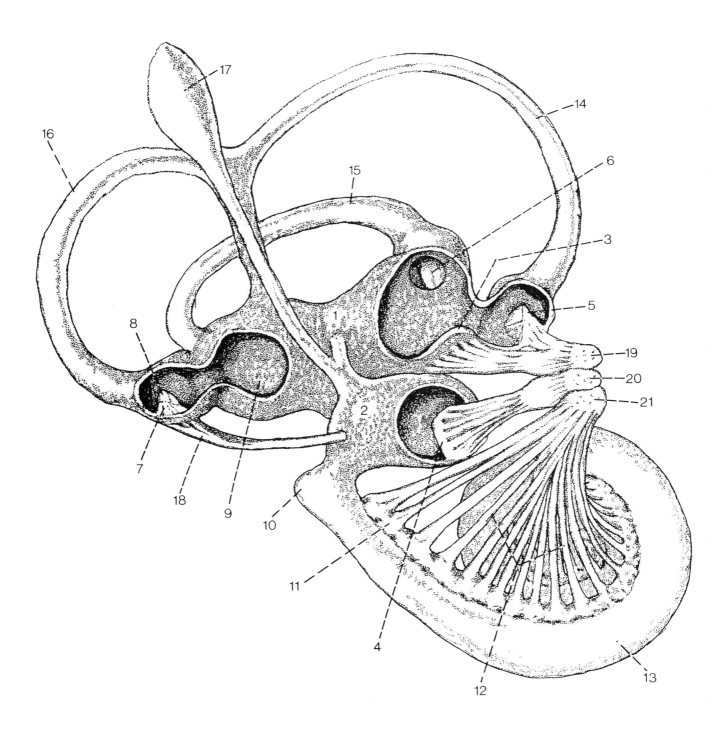

Color and label

1   Modiolus (Latin, hub, axle) (cut in upper figure). This is a small cone-shaped part of the temporal bone in the center of the cochlea. Its center contains numerous tunnels for the cochlear nerve and spiral ganglion.

2   Spiral bony lamina (basal turn). It is filled with small radial tunnels that convey the peripheral processes of the spiral ganglion neurons. The spiral bony lamina is wide at the basal turn and narrow at the apical turn.

3   Spiral bony lamina (middle turn)

4   Spiral ganglion (basal turn). This contains the cell bodies of the bipolar neurons that convey impulses from hair cells in the organ of Corti to the cochlear nuclei in the brain stem (pons). The average number of ganglion cells is 30,000.

5   Spiral ganglion (middle turn). The peripheral processes have been cut.

6   Spiral ganglion (apical one-half turn)

7   Basilar membrane (basal turn). The basilar membrane is narrow at the basal turn and wide at the apical turn.

8   Basilar membrane (middle turn). The organ of Corti (not shown) sits upon the basilar membrane.

9   Peripheral processes of spiral ganglion cells. These make synaptic contact with the inner and outer hair cells.

10   Cochlear nerve fibers (N VIII). These are the central processes of the spiral ganglion cells. There are also efferent fibers that arise from cell bodies in the superior olive. These outgoing fibers probably allow one to "zero in" and concentrate on certain frequencies and "tune out" extraneous noise. The number of fibers in the cochlear nerve is about 31,000.

11   Holes in bony spiral lamina for nerve fibers (peripheral processes of ganglion cells)

12   Wall of cochlea (cut). This varies from thick bony walls to thin membranous walls in places where the spiral turns are close to each other.

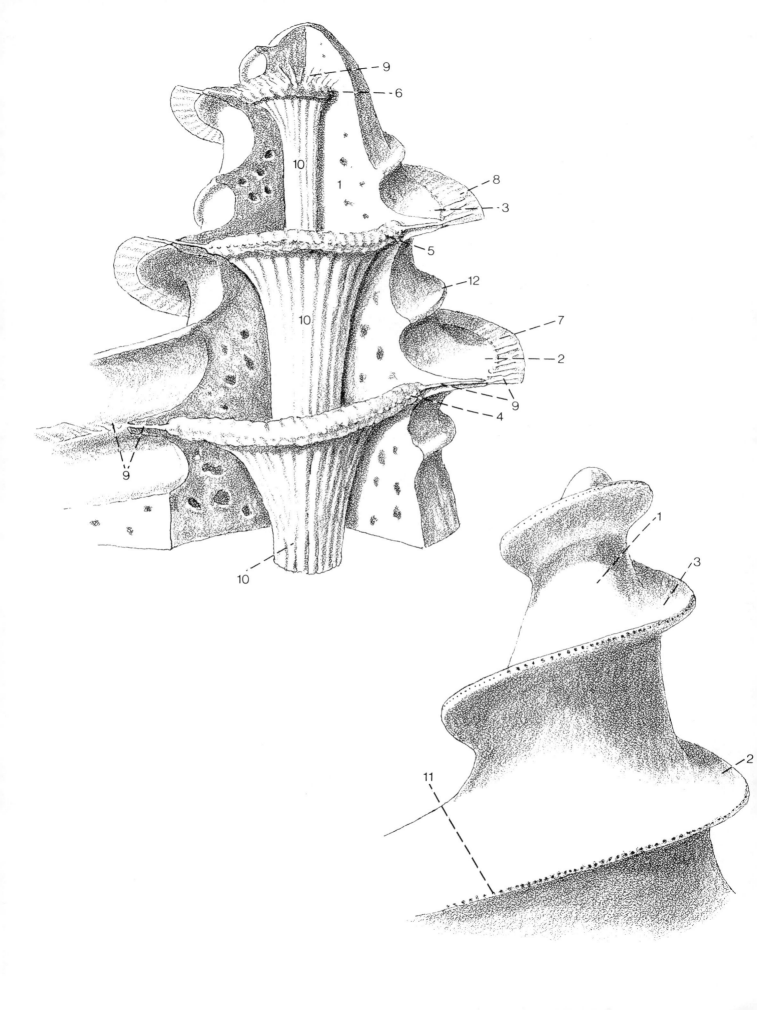

64 Organ of Corti
(After Kessel and Kardon)

Color and label

1   Spiral ganglion. These bipolar neurons lie in the bony spiral lamina. Their peripheral processes contact the inner and outer hair cells. Their central processes make up the cochlear portion of nerve VIII along with efferent fibers that arise in the superior olivary nucleus.

2   Bony spiral lamina (lamina spiralis osseous)

3   Internal spiral sulcus. Lined with inner sulcus cells

4   Inner supporting (phalangeal) cell

5   Inner hair cells. There are about 3,500 inner hair cells. Note their stereocilia form 3 straight rows and, and unlike the outer hair cells, they do not adhere to the tectorial membrane. There is just one row of inner hair cells.

6   Inner pillar cell. Note its expansive apical surface that extends between inner and outer hair cells and overlies outer pillar cell. There are about 6,000 inner pillar cells.

7   Nerve fiber traversing spiral tunnel. Nerve fibers lose their myelin upon exiting the bony spiral lamina.

8   Spiral tunnel (of Corti). Contains perilymph.

9   Spiral artery

10 Outer pillar cell. These number about 4,000. Their apical process is largely covered by the inner pillar cell apical process and extensive cuticular plate.

11 Basilar membrane. Consists of radial fibrils covered by cells on its scala tympanic surface.

12 Outer supporting (phalangeal) cells. These support the outer hair cells and number about 20,000.

13 Spiral ligament. The basilar membrane extends from central bony spiral lamina to the outer spiral ligament.

14 Tectorial membrane cut and partially removed. A gelatinous, ribbon-like structure. The tallest stereocilia of the outer hair cells are attached to its undersurface. It is attached medially to the vestibular lip of the spiral limbus, which contains the interdentate cells that secrete the membrane, and externally its outer border is attached to the surfaces of outer hair cells

15 Inner spiral sulcus cells

16 Stereocilia of inner hair cells. They form 3 straight rows, with the shortest toward the modiolus and the tallest toward the periphery.

17 Cuticular plate of inner pillar cell

18 Stereocilia of outer hair cells. These have a W or V formation.

19 Outer hair cells. These number about 20,000. The first (basal) turn of the cochlea has 3 rows of outer hair cells (and outer phalangeal cells), the second turn 4 rows of both, and the third half turn 5 rows of both.

20 Phalangeal process. Their free apical surfaces interlock tightly with the cuticular plates of hair cells, and together they form the rigid reticular lamina.

21 Border cells of Hensen

22 Cells of Claudius

23 Outer spiral sulcus

24 Phalangeal plate of outer pillar cell

25 Vestibular lip of spiral limbus

26 Spiral limbus

27 Tympanic lip of spiral limbus

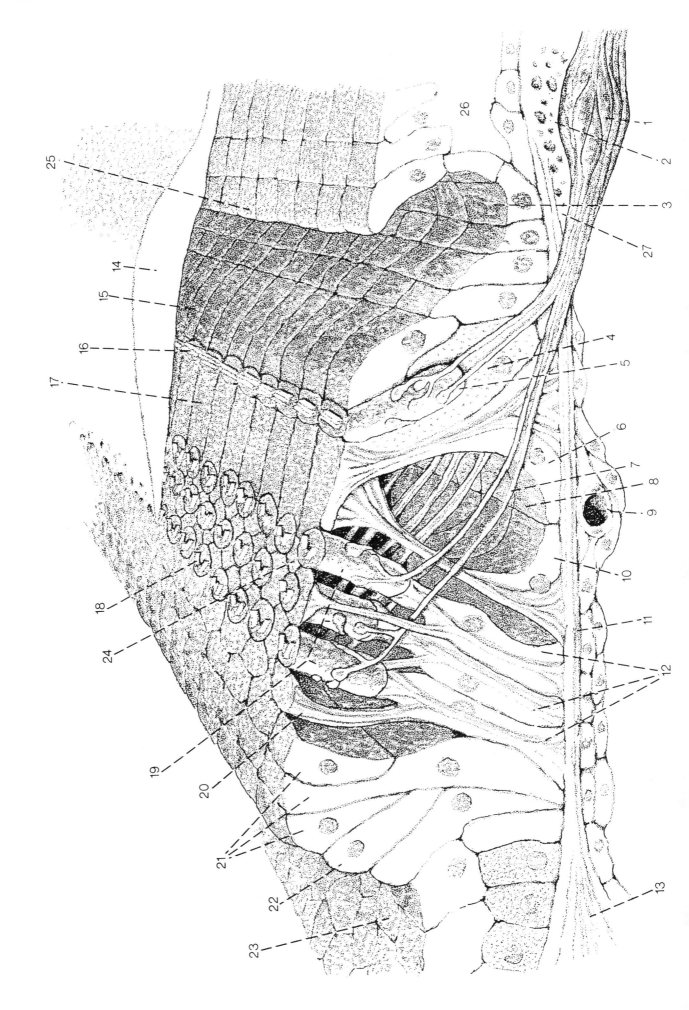

65 Inner ear hair cells and phalangeal cells (isolated phalangeal cell on right)

Color and label

1   Basilar membrane
2   Outer phalangeal cell (supporting cell of Dieter)
3   Nerve fibers (afferent and efferent; ensheathed by phalangeal cells)
4   Nerve endings (afferent and efferent)
5   Outer hair cells
6   Cuticular plate (free surface of hair cell; bathed in endolymph)
7   Phalangeal plate (free surface of phalangeal process; forms tight junctions with cuticular plates of hair cells; together they form rigid reticular lamina)
8   Stereocilia (actually 3 rows of stereocilia; tips of tallest row are embedded in tectorial membrane, which is not shown here)
9   Phalangeal process
10   Perilymph in scala tympani (high in sodium)
11   Perilymph in spaces between phalangeal cells, hair-cell bodies, and nerve fibers
12   Endolymph in cochlear duct (high in potassium)

Arrows indicate orientation of figures on the following page.

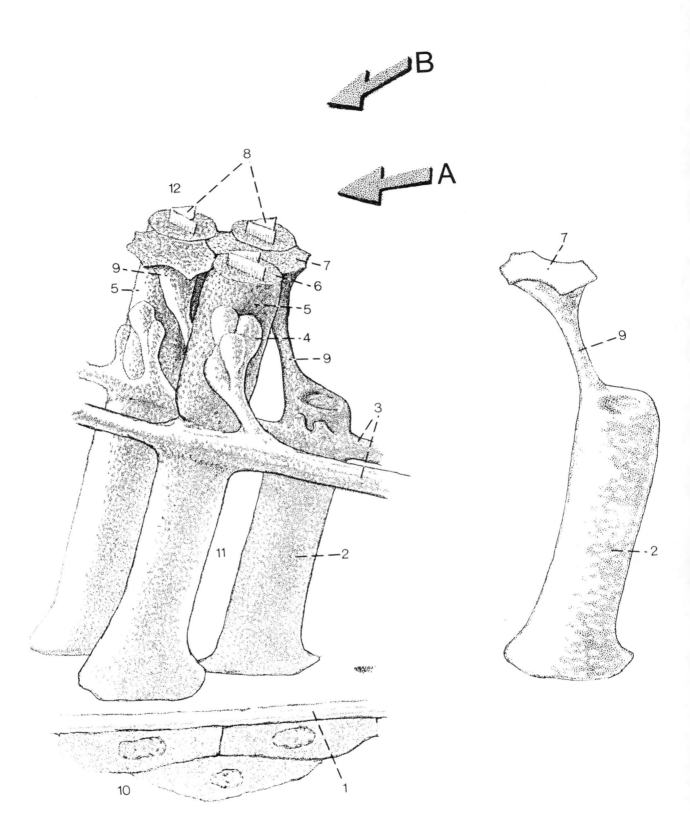

LOOKING OUT FROM CENTRAL MODIOLUS

Color and label

1   Cuticular plate (apical free surface) of outer hair cell
2   Tectorial membrane (raised in upper figure; absent in lower figure)
3   Stereocilia. Note their W or V configuration, whose open end faces the central modiolus. The stereocilia, which number about 100 for each outer hair cell, form 3 rows of different height. The tips of the tallest row are embedded in the tectorial membrane. The rising and falling of the basilar membrane and tectorial membrane cause the stereocilia to bend back and forth (in a radial direction). This deflection will excite the nerve endings on the hair cells. The stereocilia of the inner hair cells are not attached to the tectorial membrane and are apparently deflected by the drag of the endolymph.
4   Phalangeal plate of outer phalangeal cell (supporting cell)
5   Holes in tectorial membrane for tips of stereocilia
6   Fragment of broken stereocilium
7   Microvilli on apical surface of phalangeal plate

A

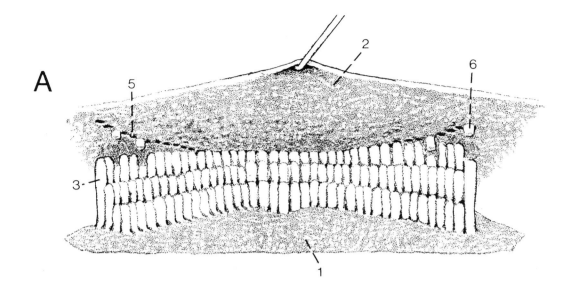

B

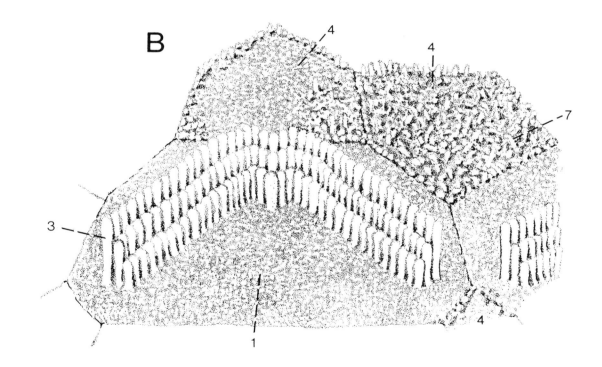

Vibrations of the footplate (base) of the stapes set off pressure waves in the perilymph of the inner ear. These pressure waves travel up the scala vestibuli (10) where they push against the vestibular membrane (9) (also called Reissner's membrane) and the endolymph within the cochlear duct (scala media). Pressure waves in the endolymph cause the basilar membrane (1) to be thrown into a series of traveling waves, much like those that travel back and forth on a taut clothesline when it is struck. These traveling waves start at the base and travel up the basilar membrane toward the apex (8). A pure musical sound from a tuning fork with no harmonics (overtones), if viewed with a stroboscopic light that flashed on and off with exactly the same frequency as the tuning fork, would give a pattern something like that in the upper left figure. If viewed from the top, the basilar membrane assumes the form of a series of depressions (3) and bumps (4) that appear to be standing still because the stroboscopic light catches them in exactly the same position of each vibration with each flash of light.

As the waves move up the basilar membrane toward the apex they steadily increase in size until they reach a certain spot where the basilar membrane is displaced the most (5). Hair cells at this point will be stimulated maximally and their nerve fibers will fire at the greatest rate. As the traveling wave moves up the basilar membrane, hair cells along the way (3,4,18,19) will also be stimulated, but not to the same degree as those at 5.

The basilar membrane rises (4) and falls (3) as the traveling wave passes through it. This up-and-down movement will cause the stereocilia of the hair cells to deflect outward when the basilar membrane goes up (19) and inward when the basilar membrane goes down (18). The membrane across the round window (14) acts as a pressure release, thus allowing pressure waves to travel within the fluid-filled cochlea. This is essential, because the endolymph and the perilymph are surrounded by hard, unyielding bone, and, like water, they cannot be compressed. Each time the footplate of the stapes pushes in at the oval window, the membrane across the round window bulges out, and vice versa.

The basilar membrane is narrowest at the base (1 in upper left) and widest at the apex (7). Conversely, the bony spiral lamina (2), which, together with the basilar membrane, forms the floor of the cochlear duct, is widest at the base and narrowest at the apex. Somewhat surprisingly, this results in high-frequency sounds, which have short traveling waves, to be confined to the basal region of the cochlea. Low-frequency sounds, on the other hand, set off traveling waves that move farther along the basilar membrane. The lower the frequency or pitch, the further its traveling wave moves toward the apex. Thus it appears that each frequency of sound has its own place on the basilar membrane, and that the basilar membrane resonates to incoming sound like a piano with its dampening pedal lifted. The "place" principle, however, is only part of the mechanism by which pressure waves in the air are converted into nerve impulses. The cochlear nerve carries volleys of nerve impulses and these volleys faithfully reproduce the frequency of the sound waves impinging on the eardrum. Thus it appears that the volley principle or "telephone theory" also operates in hearing. A single nerve fiber cannot fire off at a rate greater than 300 times per second. Most of the sounds in everyday speech have frequencies between 2000 and 3000 cycles per second (or Hertz, Hz). Frequencies greater than 300 Hz are carried by volleys of impulses by many nerve fibers, with impulses from the hair cells at the site of maximum displacement firing off at the greatest rate. Therefore the ear appears to have a **place** for each frequency as well as **volleys** of impulses that faithfully convey the original frequency of the perceived sound.

Color and label

1	Basilar membrane	11	Scala tympani (filled with perilymph)
2	Spiral bony lamina	12	Nerve cell bodies
3	Depression in basilar membrane caused by traveling wave	13	Nerve fibers (cut)
		14	Membrane across round window
4	Elevation in basilar membrane caused by traveling wave	15	Round window of middle ear (filled with air)
5	Point of maximum displacement on basilar membrane	16	Spiral ligament
		17	Inner and outer pillar cells and supporting cell
6	Basilar membrane (inactive part)		
7	Basilar membrane (apical inactive part)	18	Hair cell (stereocilia bending in)
8	Apex of cochlea	19	Hair cell (stereocilia bending out)
9	Vestibular membrane	20	Tectorial membrane
10	Scala vestibuli (filled with perilymph)		

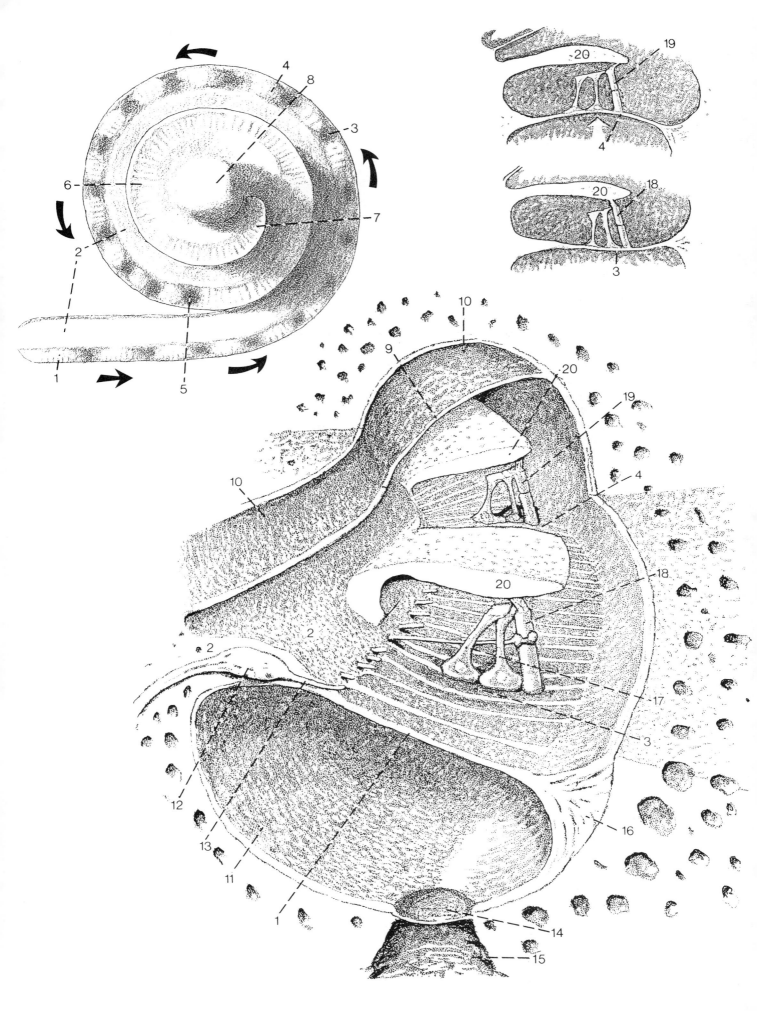

Color and label

1	Spiral ganglion. This contains the bipolar neuron cell bodies whose central processes form the cochlear (auditory) portion of the vestibulocochlear nerve (N VIII).
2	Cochlear (auditory) nerve*
3	Dorsal cochlear nucleus
4	Ventral cochlear nucleus
5	Trapezoid body (ventral acoustic stria)
6	Dorsal acoustic stria
7	Superior olivary nucleus (complex)
8	Lateral lemniscus: 60% of its fibers carry impulses from the opposite ear, 40% from the homolateral ear.
9	Nucleus of the lateral lemniscus (collections of somata along the course of the lateral lemniscus)
10	Decussating fibers. The two pathways are connected to each other by numerous fibers that cross the midline to the opposite side.
11	Nucleus of inferior colliculus
12	Brachium of the inferior colliculus
13	Medial geniculate body (nucleus) (part of thalamus)
14	Auditory radiation (acoustic radiation)
15	Primary auditory cortex on superior temporal gyrus (Heschl's gyri; area 41 of Brodmann)
16	Cochlear duct
17	Superior colliculus
18	Pineal body (gland)
19	Lateral geniculate body
20	Thalamus

Auditory is synonymous with acoustic. The *Nomina Anatomica*, which is the official list of Latin anatomical names, uses *acoustic*.

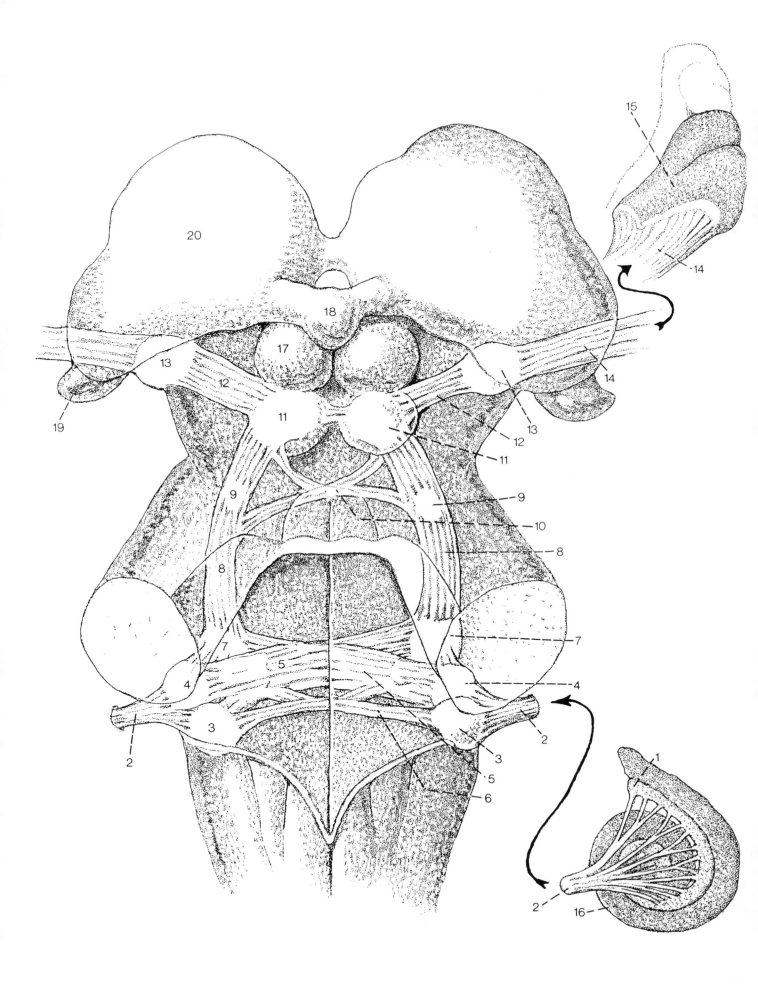

The auditory (or cochlear) nerve portion of the vestibulocochlear nerve (N VIII) consists of the central processes (1) of the bipolar neurons whose somata (25) comprise the spiral ganglia the cochlea. The peripheral processes (6) of these neurons make synaptic contact with the inner (7) and outer hair cells (8) of the organ of Corti. Incoming impulses arising from the hair cells are brought to the pontomedullary junction, where each afferent fiber (1) divides into a dorsal branch and a ventral branch, which end in the dorsal (13) and ventral (14) cochlear nuclei, respectively. The two cochlear nuclei project second-order fibers (2a-2e) mainly to the region of the opposite lateral superior olive (15), the medial superior olive (16), and a more medial nucleus of the trapezoid body (17). In the human, the lateral superior olive and nucleus of the trapezoid body are poorly developed. The second-order fibers that arise from the two cochlear nuclei traverse the midline of the brain and converge upon the opposite superior olivary complex by three routes: a dorsal acoustic stria (18), an intermediate stria (not shown), and a much larger ventral acoustic stria or trapezoid body (19). Note that some second-order fibers (2d) end in the superior olivary complex, whereas others turn rostral (2a, 2b, 2c) and continue without interruption within a flattened band, the lateral lemniscus (20). Some neurons in the ventral cochlear nucleus project to the ipsilateral superior olive (2e), but not as many as project to the opposite superior olive. Thus the central auditory pathways at the level of the lateral lemniscus and above carry impulses that are largely from the contralateral ear (about 60% contralateral, with 40% from the ipsilateral ear). Damage to one lateral lemniscus will result in a hearing impairment to both ears, but the opposite ear will be more severely affected.

Groups of somata along the course of the lateral lemniscus comprise the nucleus of the lateral lemniscus, most of which project up to the ipsilateral inferior colliculus (3e), but some project to the opposite inferior colliculus (3d). Recent investigation in the chimpanzee has demonstrated second-order fibers extending from the cochlear nucleus all the way to the contralateral medial geniculate body (2c). Up to the level of the inferior colliculi, the two auditory pathways freely communicate with each other by fibers that cross the midline. Beyond this point they do not appear to communicate. The commissure of the inferior colliculus is one such interconnection (3h). Some neurons in the inferior colliculus are sensitive to the time interval that occurs when the sound strikes one ear before the other. The sound will reach the ear facing the sound source before it reaches the ear facing away from it. These neurons fire off in response to one ear receiving the stimulus before the other. They are also able to detect the length of this interval, thus allowing the animal to determine the direction of the sound.

Other neurons in the inferior colliculus respond if the sound is louder at one ear than at the other. This, too, is a means of determining the source of the sound. The inferior colliculus appears to be a center where differences between the ears with respect to stimulus time and stimulus intensity are recorded, thus playing an essential role in locating the origin of the sound in space. Neurons in the inferior colliculus project laterally to the medial geniculate body by a short tract, the brachium (Latin, arm) of the inferior colliculus (22). The fibers within the brachium of the inferior colliculus are mainly from the ipsilaterial inferior colliculus, but there is some projection from the contralateral inferior colliculus (3g). Neurons within the medial geniculate body (23), which is a nucleus of the thalamus, project by the auditory radiation (24) to the auditory cortex (25). This area of the cortex lies on the superior surface of the superior temporal gyrus and is buried within the sylvian fissure.

One or two short transverse gyri, Heschl's gyri, mark the auditory cortical area that was designated area 41 by Brodmann. Usually the left side contains one long Heschl gyrus and the right, two shorter ones. According to Brodmann's scheme, area 41 (Heschl's gyri) is the primary auditory cortex surrounded by areas 42 and 22, the auditory association cortex. From animal studies, it is evident that the auditory cortex is essential for distinguishing different temporal patterns, such as one long tone followed by three short ones from three short tones followed by one long one. Bilateral ablation of the auditory cortex completely abolishes this ability in animals. In addition to the ascending auditory pathways just described, there is a descending auditory system that parallels the ascending one (not illustrated in drawing). It begins in the auditory cortex and ends in the opposite cochlea.

Another feature of the central auditory pathways is that there is an orderly projection of fibers with respect to frequency from the cochlea to the auditory cortex, with fibers that respond best to high frequencies at one position and those to low frequency at another position. This arrangement is referred to as a **tonotopic** (or cochleotopic) projection.

Directions: Using a different color for each order, color the central auditory pathways:
1 means first order; 2a-2e, second order; 3a-3i, third order; 4a-4b, fourth order; and 5, fifth order.

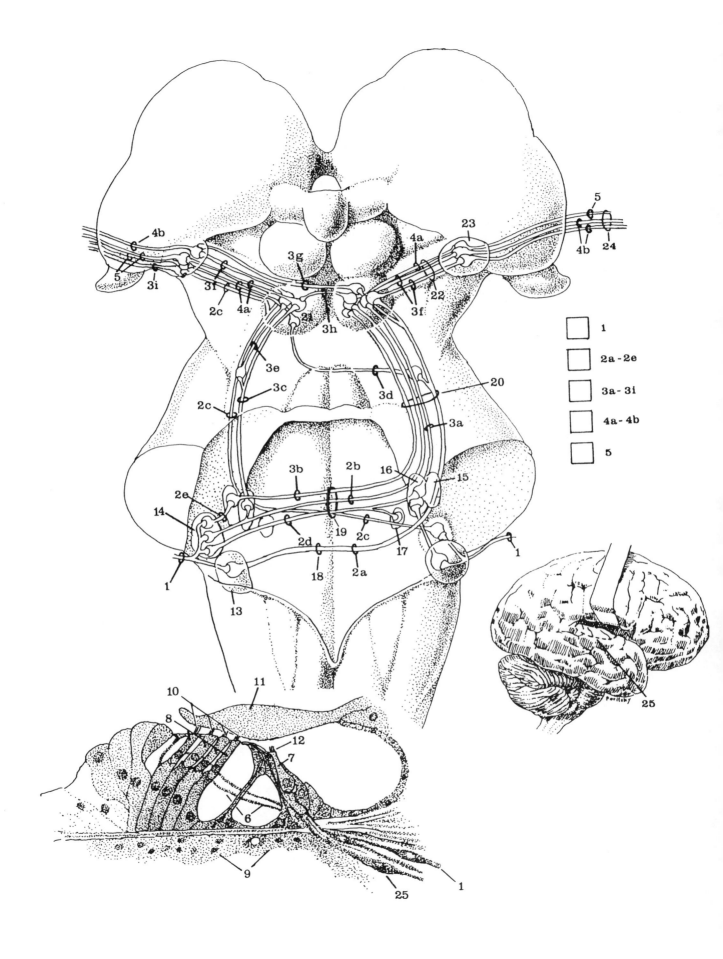

Each semicircular duct in the inner ear has a round dilated portion near the utricle called the ampulla (Latin, flask, bottle). Within each ampulla there is a crista (Latin, ridge, crest) that runs transversely to the flow of endolymph within the duct. The crista is saddle-shaped with a narrow central isthmus (2) and two wider planar regions at either end (4 on right, 12 seen through transparent cupula on left). The crista contains receptor or hair cells that have cilia (3) that are embedded into the overlying gelatinous cupula (1). The cupula (1), which is cut and removed on the right, extends from the crista completely across the ampulla to the opposite side, where it is attached (8). Thus movement of the endolymph whenever the head turns (turning the head is angular acceleration) will cause the cupula to bulge like a sail rather than bend like a swinging door as originally believed. Gelatinous strands (6) extend from the lower sides of the cupula outward, where they join the longest cilium (7) (the kinocilium) of the peripheral hair cells.

Color and label

1	Cupula (cut)
2	Isthmus of crista
3	Cilia of hair cells embedded in cupula
4	Flat end of crista (planar end)
5	Cilia of hair cells on crista (cut)
6	Gelatinous strands from cupula
8	Attachment of cupula to membranous walls of ampulla
9	Semicircular duct opening into ampulla
10	Wall of ampulla (membranous labyrinth)
11	Trabeculae in perilymphatic space
12	Planar end of crista seen through cupula

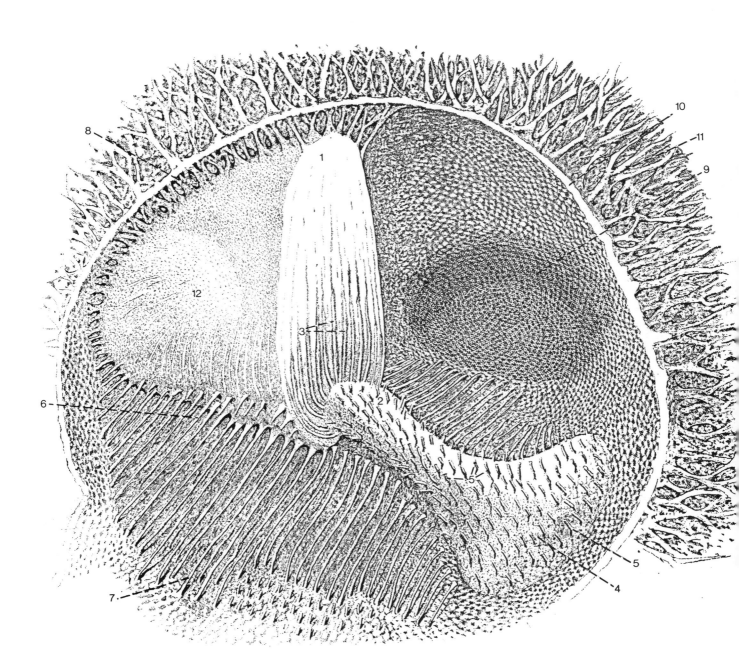

The macula of the utricle (After Hillman)

Both the utricle and the saccule of the inner ear contain receptors that are sensitive to tilting the head and to moving and stopping in a linear direction. These receptors are flattened areas called maculae (Latin, *macula,* spot) on the walls of the utricle and saccule. The two maculae are essentially clusters of receptor hair cells, each of which is covered by an overlying gelatinous otolithic membrane. The macula of the utricle lies in a horizontal plane, and that of the saccule in a vertical plane. The otolithic membrane tends to slide whenever the head moves and stimulates the hair cells by bending their cilia.

Color and label

1. **Otolithic membrane** (Greek, *otos,* ear; *lithos,* stone). This gelatinous structure overlies the receptor cells and supporting cells to which it is attached by a meshwork of fine fibers called the filamentous base.

2. **Pores in otolithic membrane.** These tiny holes overlie each receptor hair cell.

3. **Otoliths.** These small concretions of calcium carbonate lie upon the otolithic membrane. Because of their greater density, they cause the otolithic membrane to slide back when the head moves forward (inertia in response to linear acceleration) and slide forward when the movement stops (momentum in response to linear deceleration). Tilting the head will likewise cause the otolithic membrane to move in the direction of the tilt.

4. **Kinocilium.** Note its expanded terminal bulb that is attached to the otolithic membrane at the edge of the pore above it. Movement in the direction of the open arrow bends the kinocilium away from the stereocilia and excites the hair cell by depolarizing it which fires off its afferent nerve fibers. Movement in the direction of the shaded arrow silences the receptor cell by hyperpolarizing it.

5. **Stereocilia.** These are arranged in a pipe-organ configuration, with the tallest next to the kinocilium.

6. **Receptor (or sensory) hair cell.** Type I. These have a bottle shape and are enclosed by a chalice-shaped nerve ending that almost entirely encloses it.

7. **Receptor hair cell.** Type II. These are thinner than type I and are innervated by several smaller nerve endings.

8. **Chalice nerve ending**

9. **Nerve terminals on type II receptor hair cell.** The asterisk (*) marks one that has been cut open.

10. **Nerve fibers (axons).** These are both afferent and efferent. The latter presumably have an inhibitory function.

11. **Cuticular plate.** This is a rigid supportive plate in the apical cytoplasm of the hair cell and serves as a support for the stereocilia. The kinocilium is not connected to the cuticular plate.

12. **Microvilli on supporting cells**

13. **Filamentous base.** This is a meshwork of fine fibers that extends from the surface of the hair cells and supporting cells to the undersurface of the otolithic membrane.

14. **Supporting cell**

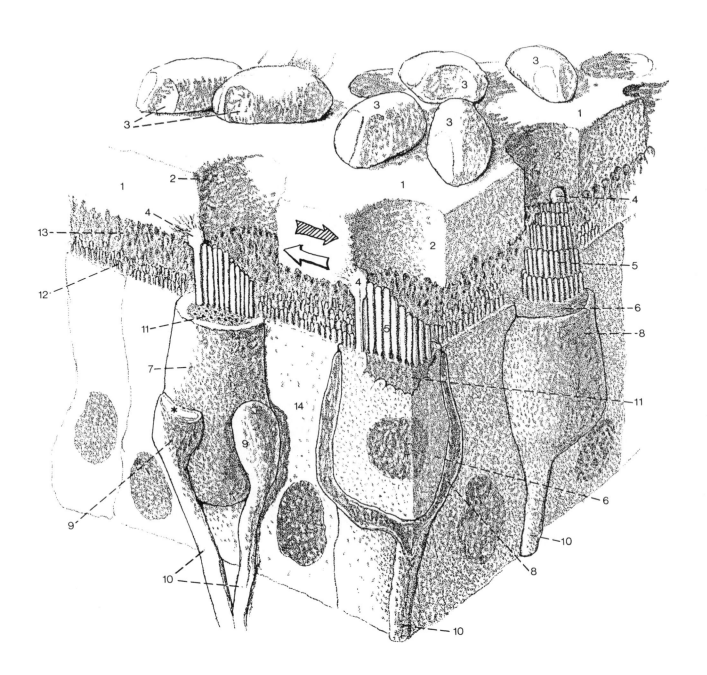

The vestibular portion of the vestibulocochlear nerve (N VIII) consists of the central processes of bipolar vestibular ganglion neurons (1). The peripheral processes of the bipolar cells begin as synapses at five different sites: three on the hair cells in the three ampullary crests and two on the hair cells on the two maculae. They are labelled on the opposite page as follows: crest of superior semicircular duct (2); crest of lateral duct (3); crest of posterior duct (4); macula of the utricle (5); and macula of the saccule (6). Fibers (7) that arise from the two maculae divide upon entering the brain stem into an ascending branch ending in the lateral vestibular nucleus (8) and a descending branch ending in the medial vestibular nucleus (9). Fibers that arise from the three ampullary crests (10) also divide, with one branch ending in the superior vestibular nucleus (11) and another in the rostral portion of the medial vestibular nucleus.* The ascending portion of the **medial longitudinal fasciculus** (MLF) arises from both the superior and medial vestibular nuclei, but not from the other two nuclei. The fibers that arise from the superior vestibular nucleus (12) remain essentially homolateral and supply the motor nuclei of nerves III and IV. In addition, they supply the contralateral nuclei III and IV by means of collaterals that cross the midline. (Figure A). The superior vestibular nucleus may also send a minor contribution to the homolateral nucleus VI. Some fibers ascend to end in the homolateral interstitial nucleus of Cajal (13).

The rostral portion of the medial vestibular nucleus gives rise to MLF fibers that cross the midline and ascend on the opposite side. One set of fibers (14) crosses the midline and ascends on the opposite side where it bypasses nuclei VI and IV, and supplies only nucleus III, where it supplies both sides. It then continues to the interstitial nucleus of Cajal. Another set of fibers (15) also crosses the midline and supplies only the contralateral nuclei VI and IV. Both sets of contralateral MLF fibers that are derived from the medial vestibular nucleus are shown more fully in Figure B (lower right). The MLF also descends into the spinal cord as far as the upper thoracic segments, where it is also called the **medial vestibulospinal tract.** These descending MLF fibers arise mainly from the medial vestibular nucleus and descend on both sides of the spinal cord, contralateral (16) and homolateral (17). The **lateral vestibulospinal tract** (18), which is much larger and much longer than the medial vestibulospinal tract, extending the full length of the cord, originates from neurons in the lateral vestibular nucleus. Unlike the medial vestibulospinal tract the lateral vestibulospinal tract remains strictly homolateral. It projects to all levels of the spinal cord and ends mainly on interneurons, and has facilitatory action on extensor motor neurons, both alpha and gamma. This tract helps us catch our balance when we feel ourselves falling.

The three ampullary crests (also called canal receptors) respond to turning the head (angular acceleration). The four vestibular nuclei are connected to the eye muscle nuclei by the MLF and coordinate eye movement with turning the head, thus allowing one's eyes to remain fixed upon a stationary object even as the head turns from side to side. Damage to the inner ear, particularly to the semicircular canals, may result in **nystagmus,** which is an involuntary oscillatory movement of the eyeballs.

Abbreviations: MLF, medial longitudinal fasciculus; III, oculomotor nucleus; IV, trochlear nucleus; VI, abducent nucleus; ml, midline.

Directions: Color and label the three ampullary crests 2,3,4. Color and label the two maculae 5 and 6. Starting with fiber (7), trace the course of the vestibular fibers (7, 10) centrally to their endings in the lateral, medial, and superior vestibular nuclei. Then trace the ascending MLF fibers, using one color for homolateral fibers (12) and another for the contralateral fibers (14 and 15). Do the same for the medial and lateral vestibulospinal tracts (16, 17, 18).

---

*Only two central processes (7, 10) and two vestibular ganglion neurons (both marked 1) are shown in the diagram. Naturally each fiber has its own cell body and several axons do not arise from one cell body as the peripheral processes appear to do in this drawing.

Brodal A: Neurological Anatomy. New York, Oxford University Press, 1981.
Tarlov E: Organization of vestibulo-oculomotor projections in the cat. Brain Research 20: 159-179, 1970.

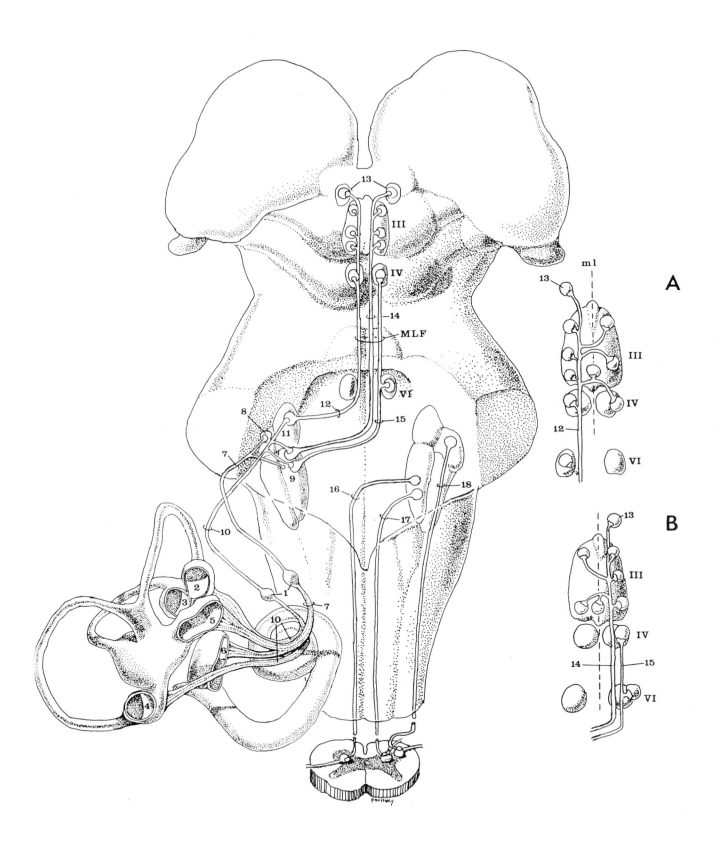

A

B

m l

13

III

IV

12

VI

13

III

IV

14   15

VI

13

III

IV

14

MLF

VI

12

8

11

7

9

15

16

18

17

10

7

1

2

3

5

10

6

7

4

poritsky

Color and label

1   Facial motor nucleus. This is the largest of the cranial nerve motor nuclei, with approximately 10,000 neurons.

2   Facial nerve fibers arising from facial motor nucleus. These innervate the muscles of facial expression.

3   Genu of facial nerve around abducent nucleus (after Brodal, 1981)

4   Perikaryon of facial motor fiber. These alpha motor neurons are special visceral efferent (SVE) fibers because they supply muscles derived from branchial arch 2.

5   SVE fiber within facial nerve. These number about 7,000.

6   Parasympathetic perikarya within superior salivatory ganglion.

7   Parasympathetic fibers (preganglionic) within nervus intermedius, which is part of the facial nerve. These fibers are general visceral efferent (GVE). They end as synapses in the pterygopalatine ganglion and submandibular ganglion.

8   Taste neuron perikaryon in geniculate ganglion.

9   Taste fiber. Distally it contacts taste buds in the tongue and palate. Taste fibers are SVA (special visceral afferent). The taste fiber central process ends in the solitary nucleus (18).

10   Perikaryon of GSA (general somatic afferent) fiber.

11   GSA fiber carrying pain, touch, and temperature from ear canal. It enters spinal tract of V (16) and ends in spinal nucleus of V (17).

12   Abducent nucleus

13   Abducent nerve (N VI)

14   Perikaryon of abducent motor neuron

15   General somatic efferent (GSE) fiber in abducent nerve (VI). It supplies the lateral rectus muscle of eye. Extraocular eye muscles arise from somites.

16   Trigeminal spinal tract (seen inside brain stem on right side)

17   Trigeminal spinal nucleus (seen inside brain stem on right side)

18   Solitary nucleus (inside brain stem)

19   Geniculate ganglion. Note efferent fibers GVE and SVE pass through geniculate ganglion, which contains cell bodies for afferent fibers GSA and SVA (taste). SVA, GVA, and GVE fibers compose the nervus intermedius of the facial nerve.

20   Fourth ventricle.

Figure in upper right shows plane of cross-section.

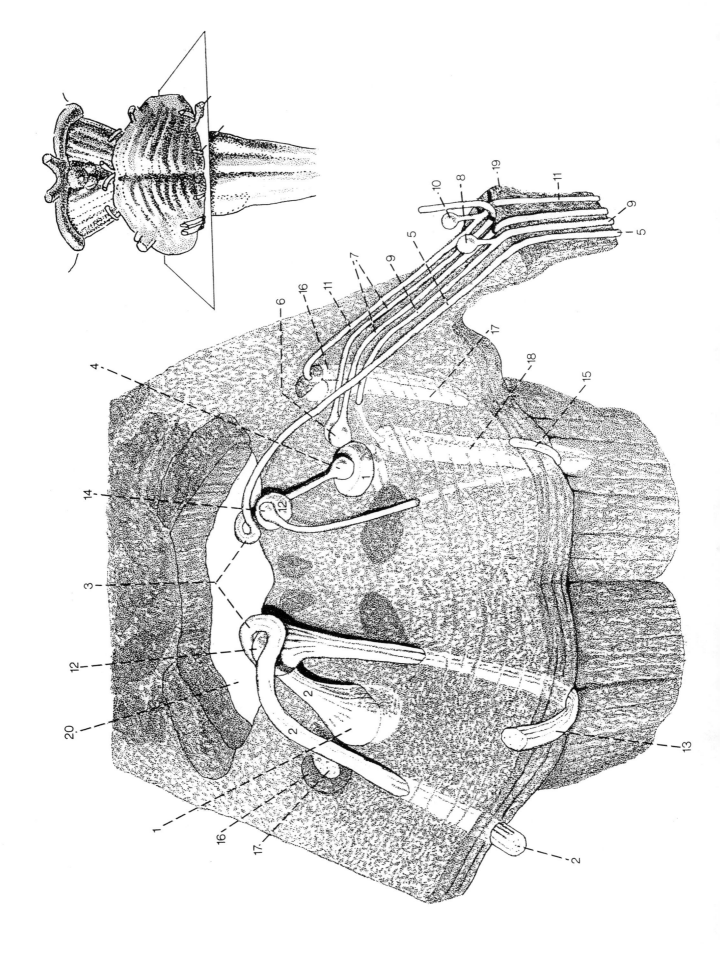

Etymological cartoon: Latin, *pes anserinus,* goose's foot

There are two goose feet, or *pes anserini,* in the body. One is on the face and is formed by the branches of the facial nerve. As the branches of the facial nerve spread out on the side of the face, they are connected to one another by connecting links of nerve fibers that loop from one branch to another. With a little bit of imagination, they resemble a goose's webbed foot.

The other *pes anserinus* is on the knee and is formed by the tendons of three muscles as they insert on the medial surface of the tibia. These are the tendons of the gracilis, sartorius, and semitendinosus muscles, which insert in a web-like formation. Thus the pes anserinus in the face is made by nerve fibers and that on the knee is made by tendons.

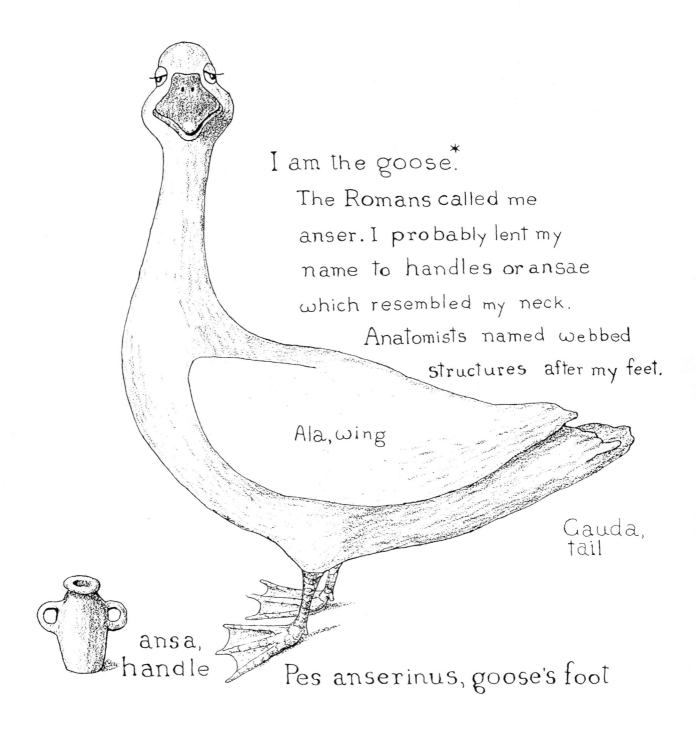

I am the goose.*

The Romans called me anser. I probably lent my name to handles or ansae which resembled my neck.

Anatomists named webbed structures after my feet.

Ala, wing

Cauda, tail

ansa, handle

Pes anserinus, goose's foot

*Occasionally I am a verb transitive; to startle someone by poking in a posterior sensitive part.

Facial nerve motor fibers arise from cell bodies in the facial motor nucleus (1). Notice that fibers that innervate the upper facial muscles (2) such as the frontalis muscle (3) arise from somata (4) that receive ipsilateral corticonuclear (corticobulbar) fibers (5) as well as contralateral corticonuclear fibers (6). Facial motor fibers (7) that innervate the lower facial muscles, however, such as the buccinator muscle (8), receive only contralateral corticonuclear fibers (9). Therefore a lesion such as a cerebral hemorrhage in the internal capsule (10) could possibly destroy all corticospinal and corticonuclear fibers (the great majority of which end in the opposite side of the brain stem and spinal cord), thus paralyzing the opposite side of the body. Following such an accident, fibers innervating the upper facial muscles (2) would still function because they continue to receive some motor commands from the undamaged ipsilateral corticonuclear fibers. Thus the eye could still be closed. However, motor neurons that give rise to fibers (7) innervating the lower facial muscles would receive no conscious motor control, since their corticonuclear fibers were destroyed in the capsular hemorrhage and these muscles would remain paralyzed.

Damage to the facial motor nucleus or to the facial nerve itself (13), such as occurs in Bell's palsy, would result in paralysis of all the ipsilateral muscles of facial expression, both upper as well as lower facial muscles. Because the facial motor neurons are alpha motor neurons and because their axons directly innervate voluntary muscle, their destruction results in instant flaccid paralysis. If regeneration does not occur, eventual atrophy of the muscles of facial expression will happen. There is an additional "emotional pathway" from undetermined centers in the brain that supplies the facial motor nucleus with "emotional motor commands" (as opposed to the voluntary motor commands from the cerebral cortex). These "emotional pathways" are believed to arise either from the globus pallidus (11) or from the hypothalamus (12). Paradoxically in the case of destruction of corticonuclear fibers and the resultant paralysis of the contralateral lower facial muscles, genuine emotions such as laughter and sorrow are surprisingly expressed in the afflicted muscles, even though these same muscles remain unresponsive to conscious controls. In fact, the extent of the smile is greater, occurs earlier, and lasts longer on the affected side. This observation, plus the loss of facial expression in diseases such as Parkinson's, suggest a dual control of the facial motor nucleus by higher motor centers, a voluntary one from the cerebral cortex and an "emotional" one arising from subcortical structures, such as the globus pallidus or hypothalamus.

Directions: Using a different color for each of the following, color and trace the course of the facial nerve motor fibers (2 and 7), the homolateral corticonuclear fibers (5), the contralateral corticonuclear fibers (6 and 9), and the hypothetical "emotional" pathway originating from either the globus pallidus (11) or hypothalamus (12).

Label

1	Facial motor nucleus
3	Frontalis muscle
5	Ipsilateral corticonuclear fibers
6	Contralateral corticonuclear fibers
8	Buccinator muscle
10	Cerebral hemorrhage in internal capsule
11	Globus pallidus
12	Hypothalamus
13	Indication of nerve damage

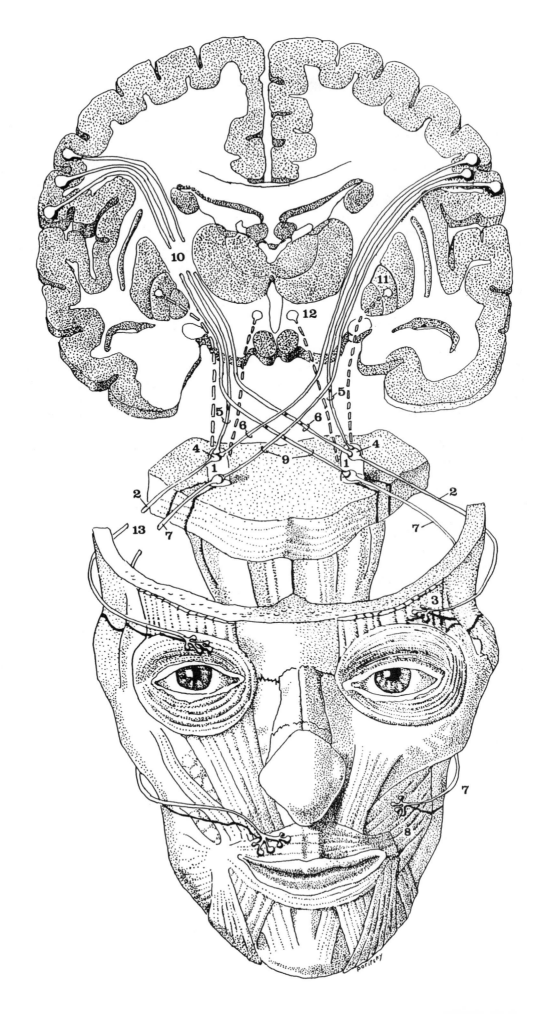

76 Facial nerve and its branches

Color and label

1 Facial nerve
2 Geniculate ganglion
3 Greater petrosal nerve
4 Chorda tympani nerve
5 Nerve to stapedius muscle
6 Lingual nerve (cut; part of mandibular nerve)
7 Deep petrosal nerve
8 Nerve of pterygoid canal
9 Pterygopalatine ganglion
10 Internal carotid plexus (sympathetic fibers)
11 Submandibular ganglion
12 Maxillary nerve (cut; part of trigeminal nerve)
13 Infraorbital nerve
14 Posterior superior alveolar nerve
15 Palatine nerves
16 Pterygopalatine nerves
17 Middle superior alveolar nerve
18 Zygomatic nerve
19 Communicating branch to lacrimal nerve
20 Lacrimal nerve (branch of ophthalmic nerve)
21 Internal carotid artery
22 Mastoid process
23 Styloid process
24 Eardrum and malleus
25 Stylomastoid foramen
26 Facial canal
27 Carotid canal
28 Foramen lacerum
29 Medial pterygoid plate
30 Canal and groove for greater petrosal nerve
31 Orbit
32 Internal auditory meatus (roof removed)

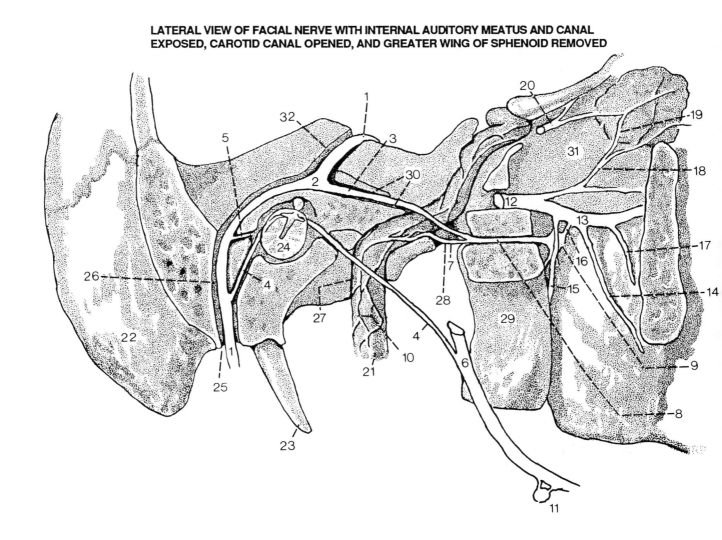

Color and label these nerve fibers and their brainstem nuclei

1   Motor neuron to muscles of facial expression
2   Facial motor nucleus
3   Parasympathetic neuron to submandibular ganglion
4   Parasympathetic neuron to pterygopalatine ganglion
5   Superior salivatory nucleus
6   Cell body of taste neuron carrying taste from the tongue via the chorda tympani nerve
7   Cell body of taste neuron carrying taste from the palate via the greater petrosal nerve
8   Neuron in solitary nucleus (second order; relays taste from tongue)
9   Neuron in solitary nucleus (second order; relays taste from palate)
10   Nucleus of solitary tract
11   Parasympathetic neuron (postganglionic) in pterygopalatine ganglion supplying lacrimal gland
12   Parasympathetic neuron (postganglionic) to nasal glands
13   Pterygopalatine ganglion
14   Parasympathetic neuron (postganglionic) in submandibular ganglion supplying submandibular gland
15   Parasympathetic neuron (postganglionic) supplying sublingual gland
16   Sympathetic neuron (preganglionic) in spinal cord
17   Sympathetic neurons (postganglionic)
18   Superior cervical ganglion
19   Internal carotid plexus
20   Geniculate ganglion
21   Greater petrosal nerve (taste and parasympathetic fibers)
22   Deep petrosal nerve (sympathetic fibers)
23   Nerve of pterygoid canal
24   Nerve to stapedius
25   Chorda tympani nerve (taste and parasympathetic fibers)
26   Facial canal
27   Stylomastoid foramen
28   Maxillary nerve in foramen rotundum
29   Lacrimal nerve
30   Zygomatic nerve
31   Zygomaticotemporal nerve
32   Communicating branch between zygomaticotemporal nerve and lacrimal nerve
33   Facial nerve (VII) exiting stylomastoid foramen
34   Genu of facial nerve (intrapontine)

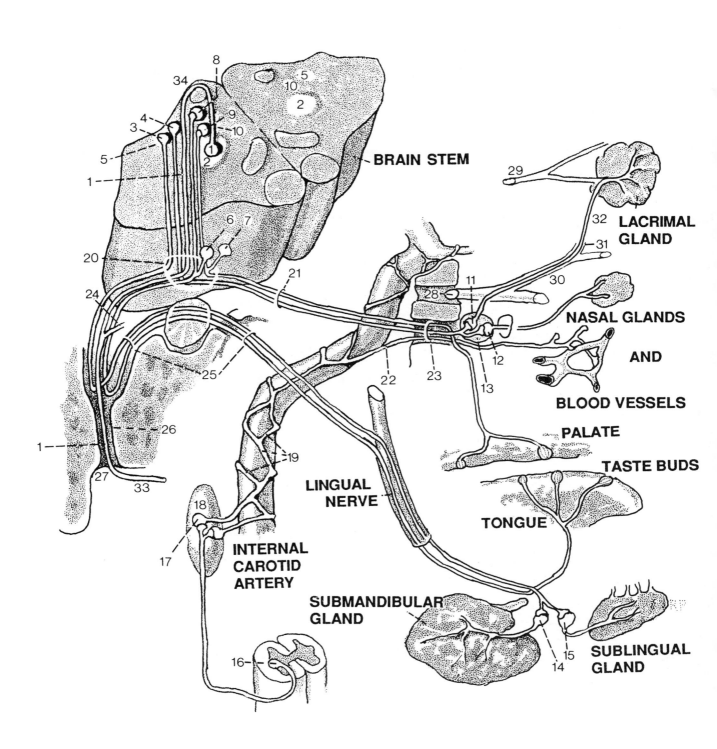

BRAIN STEM

LACRIMAL
GLAND

NASAL GLANDS

AND

BLOOD VESSELS

PALATE

TASTE BUDS

TONGUE

LINGUAL
NERVE

INTERNAL
CAROTID
ARTERY

SUBMANDIBULAR
GLAND

SUBLINGUAL
GLAND

The most common disorder of the facial nerve is peripheral facial nerve paralysis or Bell's palsy. This idiopathic (meaning of unknown cause; originally the term meant a disease arising by itself–having its own origin, without any external cause) disorder is presumably due to some kind of inflammation or compression of the facial nerve in its course through the facial canal before its exit from the stylomastoid foramen. The causative agent has been attributed to viruses, or to vascular impingement against the nerve, or to abnormal bone growth compressing the nerve within the facial canal. Approximately 1 in 60 persons in a lifetime will suffer this affliction.

The affected muscles are all the muscles of the facial expression (or mimetic muscles) on the same side as the affected nerve plus the posterior belly of the digastric and the stylohyoid. The stapedius muscle of the middle ear receives a small branch from the facial nerve in the upper part of the facial canal and is spared if the nerve blockage is below the origin of its nerve.

If the paralysis is complete, all movement of the muscles of the facial expression is lost on the same side. The face is asymmetrical because the muscles on the normal side pull on the affected side. The surface of the affected side is smooth, and common facial features such as the nasolabial fold are lost. The patient is unable to frown or to close the eye due to paralysis of the orbicularis oculi. Moreover, the area of the open eye will be even greater than normal. This is due to the unopposed action of the levator palpebrae muscle, which is supplied by nerve III. The cornea may be in danger of drying and ulceration.

The mouth cannot be closed properly, The affected corner of the mouth (oral angle) is lower than normal, with saliva sometimes drooling from it.

Since this is a type of peripheral or lower motor neuron paralysis, the affected facial muscles will be flabby and, if regeneration of the facial nerve does not occur, the paralyzed muscles will atrophy (waste away).

The affected muscles will not partake in any of the normal facial movements such as speaking, weeping, or eating, and food will tend to accumulate between the teeth and the paralyzed buccinator muscle. Taste sensation will be lost on the affected side if the chorda tympani branch of the facial nerve is also affected.

The onset of Bell's palsy is usually sudden. The paralysis may only last for a few hours and then disappear. Eighty percent of the patients tend to recover within a few weeks.

Unlike supranuclear facial palsy, in which the upper facial muscles such as the orbicularis oculi and frontalis retain their function, peripheral facial nerve paralysis involves all the ipsilateral mimetic muscles.

BELL'S PALSY

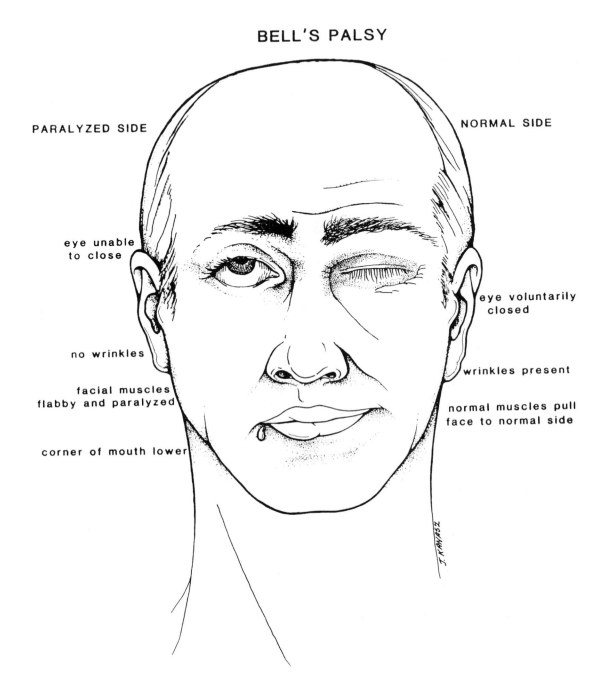

PARALYZED SIDE

NORMAL SIDE

eye unable
to close

eye voluntarily
closed

no wrinkles

wrinkles present

facial muscles
flabby and paralyzed

normal muscles pull
face to normal side

corner of mouth lower

Color and label

1	Trigeminal ganglion (semilunar ganglion)
V_1	Ophthalmic division of trigeminal nerve
V_2	Maxillary division of trigeminal nerve
V_3	Mandibular division of trigeminal nerve
2	Trigeminal spinal nucleus
3	Trigeminal pontine nucleus (new name; old name is "main sensory nucleus")
4	Trigeminal mesencephalic nucleus
5	Trigeminal motor nucleus
6	Oral nucleus (upper third of trigeminal spinal nucleus)
7	Interpolar nucleus (middle third of trigeminal spinal nucleus)
8	Caudal nucleus (lower third of trigeminal spinal nucleus)
9	Trigeminal spinal tract
10	Root of trigeminal nerve
11	Trigeminal mesencephalic tract
12	Ventral trigeminothalamic tract (trigeminal lemniscus)
13	Dorsal trigeminothalamic tract
14	Reticular formation fibers
15	Posterior thalamic nucleus
16	Projection of centromedian fibers
17	Thalamocortical fibers
VII	Facial nerve fibers entering trigeminal spinal tract
IX	Glossopharyngeal nerve fibers entering trigeminal spinal tract
X	Vagus nerve fibers entering trigeminal spinal tract

The trigeminal nerve (cranial nerve V) carries pain, touch, temperature, and proprioception from the face, eyes, teeth, jaws, and mucosa (mucous membrane) of the nose, mouth, and anterior two-thirds of the tongue. The trigeminal nerve contains about 140,000 sensory fibers and about 8,100 motor fibers. Most of the sensory fibers have cell bodies in the trigeminal ganglion (semilunar ganglion) (1). Somewhat surprisingly, sensory fibers conveying proprioception from the jaw muscles and from receptors around the teeth, which signal the force of the bite, have cell bodies in the slender trigeminal mesencephalic nucleus. Motor fibers in the trigeminal nerve arise from cell bodies in the trigeminal motor nucleus (5) and supply the powerful muscles of the jaw (muscles of mastication) plus a few more.

The sensory fibers in the trigeminal nerve end either in the trigeminal spinal nucleus (2) or in the trigeminal pontine nucleus (3) (formerly the main or principal trigeminal sensory nucleus). The trigeminal spinal nucleus (2) and trigeminal pontine nucleus (3) both project sensory data to the thalamus by the crossed ventral trigeminothalamic tract (12) (trigeminal lemniscus) and by the uncrossed dorsal trigeminothalamic tract (13). The ventral trigeminothalamic tract ascends close to the medial lemniscus and terminates in the ventral posterior medial (VPM) nucleus of the thalamus. Thalamocortical fibers then relay this information to the face region of the cerebral cortex. The uncrossed dorsal trigeminothalamic tract (13) arises from the trigeminal pontine nucleus and ends on the VPM nucleus of the thalamus.

Traveling with the dorsal trigeminothalamic fibers are pain-carrying reticular formation fibers (14). These carry pain from the trigeminal spinal nucleus (7,8), ascend on both sides, and form a diffuse multisynaptic pathway. The combined fibers of the dorsal trigeminothalamic tract and reticular fibers end not only in the VPM nucleus, but also in the centromedianum (CM) nucleus and posterior thalamic nuclei (15) as well. The CM nucleus projects to wide areas of the frontal cortex and parietal cortex (16). The posterior thalamic nuclei (15) are also involved in pain perception.

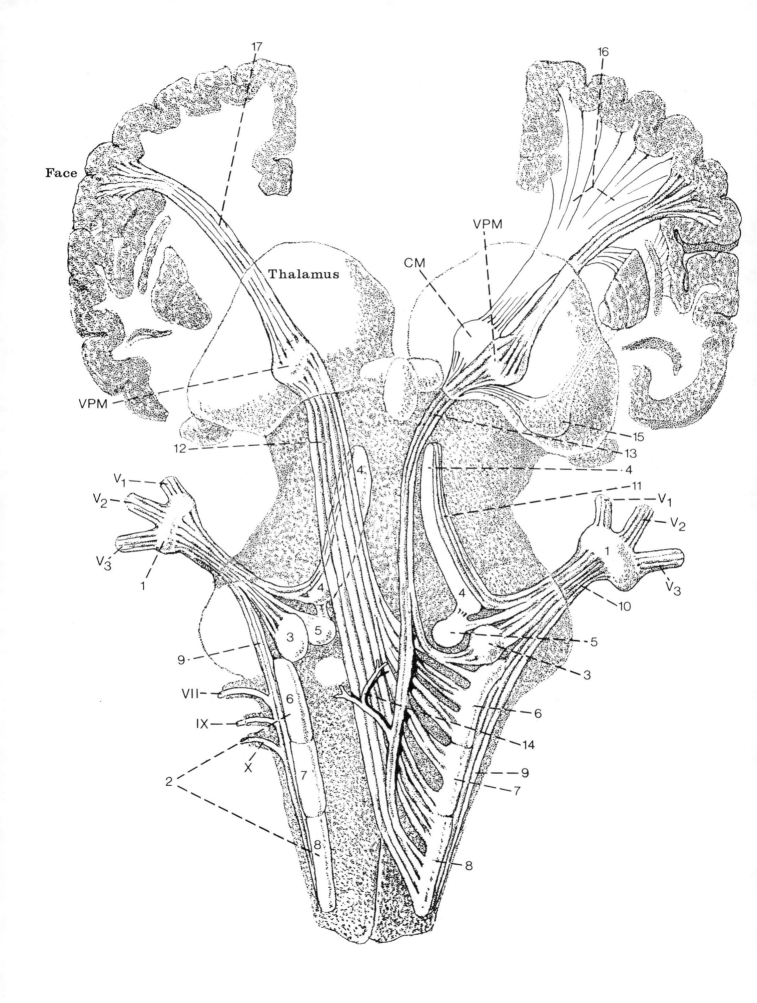

Face

Thalamus

VPM

CM

VPM

17

16

15

13

12

4

11

4

V₁

V₂

V₃

1

V₁

V₂

V₃

10

3

5

9

3

5

VII

6

6

IX

14

X

9

2

7

7

8

8

The trigeminal nerve is named the **triplet nerve** because it divides into three large branches, the ophthalmic, the maxillary, and mandibular. *Trigeminus* in Latin means triplet.

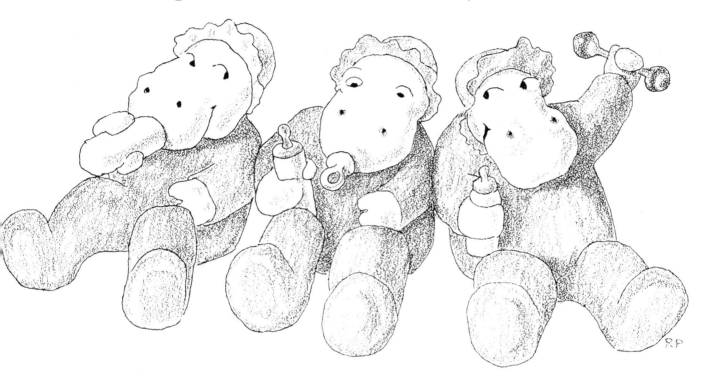

Trigemini, Latin, triplets

The trigeminal nerve has three large branches (Latin, *trigeminus,* three-fold or triplet). The ophthalmic (V_1), the maxillary (V_2), and the mandibular (V_3).

Locate fiber number 1, which is a large-diameter afferent fiber carrying discriminative touch or proprioceptive information from the mouth, tongue, or lips. Its unipolar perikaryon lies in the trigeminal ganglion and its central process terminates upon neuron 2 in the pontine nucleus, which gives rise to an ascending fiber that crosses the midline and joins the ventral trigeminothalamic tract (V trig tr). The fiber then ascends to the ventral posterior medial (VPM) nucleus of the thalamus, where neuron 3 relays the impulse to the "face" region of the somatosensory cortex.

The pontine nucleus also gives rise to another ascending bundle of fibers, the dorsal trigeminothalamic tract (d trig tr). This tract (4), unlike the ventral trigeminal tract, remains entirely ipsilateral. Its function is not understood. It arises from a part of the main sensory nucleus that is concerned with the mouth and terminates in its own region of nucleus VPM (5). It may possibly be involved in taste or intraoral sensation.

Locate fiber 6, which is a pain fiber traveling with the mandibular nerve and carrying pain from one of the teeth in the lower jaw. Its unipolar perikaryon is in the semilunar ganglion and its central process turns caudally and descends within a bundle of fibers, the spinal trigeminal tract (sp tr V). It descends to the lowest of the three nuclei that comprise the spinal trigeminal nucleus, the caudal nucleus (caud), where it ends by synapsing upon second-order neuron 7, which projects its fiber across the midline and joins the ventral trigeminal tract to the opposite VPM nucleus. Third-order neuron 8 in the VPM then projects this information to the somatosensory "face" cortex.

The nucleus caudalis appears to process pain and temperature data from the face, mouth, and nose. It resembles the dorsal horn of the spinal cord, with which it blends at about the third cervical level. The spinal tract of V likewise blends with the dorsolateral fasciculus (tract of Lissauer), which carries pain and temperature fibers from the rest of the body. There is another pathway through which pain from the face reaches the thalamus; this is a multineural network within the reticular formation (9). It has been proposed that the ventral trigeminal tract carries the sharp, well-defined pain similar to that carried in the lateral spinothalamic tract, whereas the reticular formation carries the dull, diffuse, aching pain similar to that carried by the spinoreticular tract in the spinal cord.

Return to the right side and locate fiber 10, which carries light touch. Note that it bifurcates upon entering the brain stem, with one branch going to the pontine nucleus (TPN) and the other to the nucleus oralis. Second-order neuron 11 relays this tactile information via the ventral trigeminothalamic tract to the opposite VPM nucleus. Nerves VII, IX and X also contribute fibers to the spinal trigeminal tract. These three nerves carry general sensibilities from the external and middle ear. Their central processes descend in the spinal trigeminal tract and end in the spinal nucleus of V.

Locate fiber 12 in both mandibular nerves. It is a first-order sensory fiber (or primary afferent), but it is unique because its cell body is not in a ganglion, but rather in the trigeminal mesencephalic nucleus (mes nuc V). This is the only case of a first-order sensory perikaryon lying within the CNS instead of within a ganglion. These fibers form a small but well-defined tract, the trigeminal mesencephalic tract (mes tr V), which lies directly lateral to the mesencephalic nucleus of V. The mesencephalic nucleus of V is believed to process proprioceptive information that controls the force of the bite. The fibers within the mesencephalic tract of V arise from proprioceptors in the jaw muscles, the temporomandibular joint, and the periodontal membrane of the teeth. Collaterals from the afferent fibers in the mesencephalic tract of V project to the trigeminal motor nucleus (mot nuc V) where they synapse directly upon motor neurons 13 within this nucleus. Axons arising from these motor neurons (13) form the motor component of the V nerve. They travel with the mandibular nerve and supply motor control to the jaw muscles.

Neuron 14 is a mesencephalic neuron whose collateral projects to the cerebellum (cut in drawing). On the left, fiber 15 carries touch from the conjunctiva of the eye. Its central process enters the spinal tract of V and ends upon a second-order neuron in the nucleus oralis which relays this to motor neurons 16 in both facial motor nuclei (nuc VII) which in turn reflexly send motor commands, via nerve VII, to both orbicularis oculi muscles to blink. Fiber 17 on the left represents a pain fiber from the eye.

Directions: *Color* the listed nerve fibers using a different color for each functional group.

Color and label

TG	Trigeminal ganglion
TPN	Trigeminal pontine nucleus (former name, main sensory nucleus of V)
sp tr V	Trigeminal spinal tract
sp nuc V	Trigeminal spinal nucleus
oral	Oral nucleus
inter	Interpolar nucleus
caud	Caudal nucleus
mot nuc V	Trigeminal motor nucleus
mes tr V	Trigeminal mesencephalic tract
mes nuc V	Trigeminal mesencephalic nucleus
v trig tr	Ventral trigeminothalamic tract
d trig tr	Dorsal trigeminothalamic tract
nuc VII	Facial motor nucleus
VPM	Ventral posterior medial nucleus of thalamus
face	Face region of somatosensory cortex

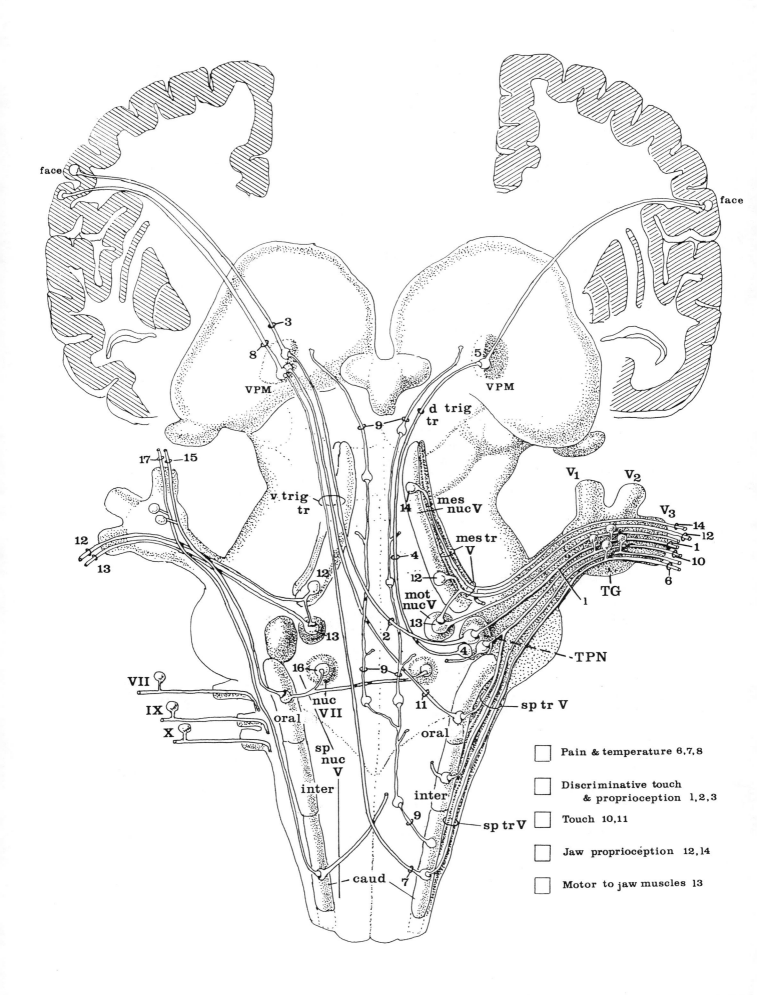

face

face

3

8

VPM

5

VPM

d trig
tr

9

17 15

v. trig
tr

V₁ V₂

V₃

14
mes
nuc V

12

14
12
1
10

12

mes tr
V

6

13

4

l2

1

TG

12

mot
nuc V

13

1

2

13

4

TPN

16

9

nuc
VII

11

sp tr V

VII

oral

IX

oral

sp
nuc
V

X

inter

inter

9

sp tr V

caud 7

Pain & temperature 6,7,8

Discriminative touch
& proprioception 1,2,3

Touch 10,11

Jaw proprioception 12,14

Motor to jaw muscles 13

Figure A shows a human embryo at 32 days, at which time four branchial (Greek, *branchia,* gill) arches appear on the sides of the head and neck. The numbers 1, 2, 3, 4 indicate the four arches and the Roman numerals V, VII, IX, X are the four cranial nerves that supply motor innervation to the muscles that develop in each of the four arches. Actually, there are six arches; but arch five rapidly disappears leaving no derivatives, and arch six does not form a definitive arch that is visible externally. However, arch six gives rise to most of the muscles of the larynx. **Color and label** nerves V, VII, IX, X in Figure A.

Figure B shows a horizontal section through the branchial arches, each with its own cranial nerve. **Color and label** each of these cranial nerves (V, VII, IX, X).

Figure C shows a portion of the developing brain with the motor nuclei that contain the motor neuron cell bodies that supply the branchial muscles. Branchial **arch one** is the **mandibular arch**. It is supplied by the **trigeminal nerve (V)**. The motor neuron perikarya lie in the **motor nucleus of V** and supply all the muscles that come from this arch; these are the muscles of mastication, which include the masseter, temporalis, medial pterygoid, and lateral pterygoid. Also derived from the first arch and supplied by the V nerve are the mylohyoid, anterior belly of the digastric, tensor veli palatini, and tensor tympani muscles.

Figure D shows the temporalis and masseter muscles. **Color** nerve V starting with its perikaryon in motor nucleus of V (also called trigeminal motor nucleus). The **second arch** is the **hyoid arch** and is supplied by the **facial nerve (VII)**. Starting with the motor nucleus of VII (or the facial motor nucleus), color the course of a motor neuron of nerve VII. Note that it makes a loop before leaving the brain. The second branchial arch gives rise to all the **muscles of facial expression**. These are relatively small muscles that often insert into the skin. Some are essential, such as the orbicularis oculi that protects the eye. The orbicularis oris and buccinator are used in normal chewing and sucking. In addition to supplying motor control to the muscles of facial expression, the facial nerve also supplies the posterior belly of the digastric, the stylohyoid, and the stapedius.

The **third arch** gives rise to the upper pharynx, and its nerve is the glossopharyngeal (IX). Nerve IX carries sensation from the posterior tongue and upper pharynx, and one would expect that the muscles of the upper pharynx, such as the superior constrictor and muscles of the soft palate, would also be supplied by IX. But the only muscle supplied solely by IX is the stylopharyngeus (asterisk in Figure F). **Color** and trace the course of nerve IX. Its soma lies in the rostral part of the nucleus ambiguus and also takes a curved course in the brain stem.

The **fourth arch** develops into the muscles of the lower pharynx, which are supplied by the vagus nerve (Figure G). The muscles of the larynx actually develop from the sixth arch (not shown) and are supplied by the **recurrent laryngeal** branch of nerve X. **Trace** the course of nerve X and note that its cell body lies in the caudal portion of the nucleus ambiguus.

The muscles that are derived from the branchial arches are called **branchiomeric** muscles. These muscles are striated and voluntary, and histologically identical to muscles that develop from somites (somatic or myomeric muscles). The only apparent difference is their embryonic origin. The nerves that supply these branchiomeric muscles are called **special visceral efferent** or simply **SVE**. Each of these four cranial nerves has one or two ganglia that contain the sensory cell bodies of its sensory fibers, which may greatly outnumber the motor fibers. These ganglia (Figure C) are the **semilunar** ganglion (gg V) for nerve V, the **geniculate** ganglion (gg VII) for nerve VII, the **superior** and **inferior** ganglion (gg IX) for nerve IX, and the **superior** and **inferior** ganglion (gg X) for nerve S. The motor fibers in these four cranial nerves pass through these ganglia with no interruption. In fact, none of the ganglia contains any synapses, only unipolar perikarya of sensory fibers. **Color and label** the four sets of ganglia.

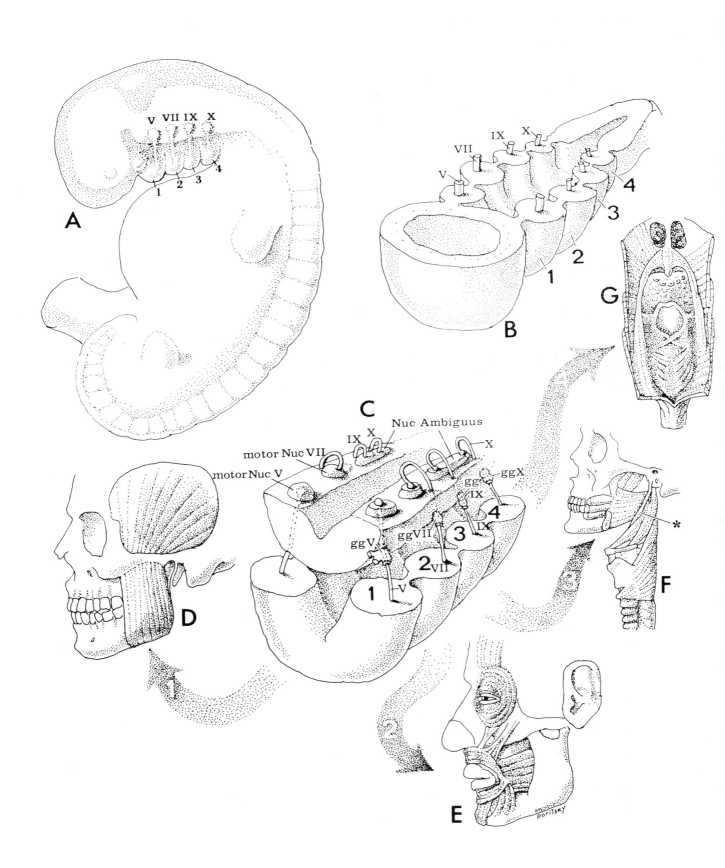

A

V VII IX X

1 2 3 4

B

VII

V

IX X

4

3

2

1

G

C

Nuc Ambiguus

motor Nuc VII

IX X

X

motor Nuc V

ggX

gg
IX

ggVII

4

ggV

3 IX

2 VII

1 V

D

E

F

*

poritsky

Color and label

1 **Sclera.** The white of the eye; a major part of outer fibrous coat.
2 **Choroid.** Major part of middle vascular coat.
3 **Retina: inner coat of eye with neural layers.** Photoreceptive part of eye.
4 **Retina: pigment layer.** Non-nervous part of retina.
5 **Ciliary body.** Thickened portion of middle coat. It forms a muscular ring around the lens.
6 **Cornea.** The anterior transparent part of the outer fibrous coat.
7 **Lens.** The biconvex lens inverts the incoming light rays and focuses them upside down on the posterior retina.
8 **Iris.** This is the anterior colored part of the vascular coat. The iris has a central hole, the pupil (asterisk), which it can either enlarge or constrict, like the diaphragm in a camera. The pigmentation of iris determines whether the eyes are brown, blue, green or hazel.
9 **Anterior chamber.** This space lies behind the cornea and in front of the lens and iris. It is filled with a clear liquid, the **aqueous humor.**
10 **Posterior chamber.** This narrow space lies behind the iris and in front of the peripheral part of the lens and the zonule fibers. It also contains aqueous humor.
11 **Zonule fibers.** Collectively these form the suspensory ligament of the lens. They extend from the ciliary processes to the lens.
12 **Canal of Schlemm** (new name: **scleral venous sinus**). This drains the aqueous humor from the anterior chamber.
13 **Vitreous body.** This is a clear gel that is 99% water. A network of fine filaments runs through it.
14 **Fovea centralis.** This small crater-like depression in the retina contains only small, tightly packed cones, thus giving the fovea the greatest power of visual resolution and acuity.
15 **External sheath of optic nerve**
16 **Optic nerve.** Cranial nerve II. Contains about 1,200,00 myelinated fibers.
17 **Central retinal artery and vein.** The artery is a branch of the ophthalmic artery.
18 **Pupil** (Latin, doll, girl, or puppet; asterisk). It was so named because one can see one's reflection in another person's pupil when close by.
19 **Equator of the lens**
20 **Optic disk.** This is the blind spot due to the absence of rods and cones.
21 **Lamina cribrosa of the sclera.** This portion of the sclera contains holes for the passage of bundles of optic nerve fibers.
22 **Hyaloid canal.** In the embryo this transmitted the hyaloid artery, which disappears in the ninth month. The artery and canal are straight in the embryo; however, the residual canal becomes wavy in the adult.

Axes of rotation and planes of right eye

Color and label

1 **Anterior-posterior axis**
2 **Transverse axis**
3 **Vertical axis**
4 **Intorsion.** An inward rotation of the upper iris (and eye) about the anterior-posterior axis. Indicative of malfunction of one or more extraocular muscles.
5 **Extorsion.** An outward rotation of the upper iris (and eye) about the anterior-posterior axis. Intorsion and extorsion will cause the visual field to abnormally tilt away from the horizontal. Intorsion and extorsion should normally never occur, and, if present, are indicative of malfunctioning extrabulbar muscles.
6 **Elevation.** Gaze directed up.
7 **Depression.** Gaze directed down.
8 **Abduction.** Lateral rotation. Gaze directed laterally.
9 **Adduction.** Medial rotation. Gaze directed medially.
10 **Equator of eye.** Divides eyeball into anterior and posterior hemispheres.
11 **Horizontal meridian of eye.** Divides eyeball into superior and inferior hemispheres.
12 **Anterior pole of eye.** Center of cornea.

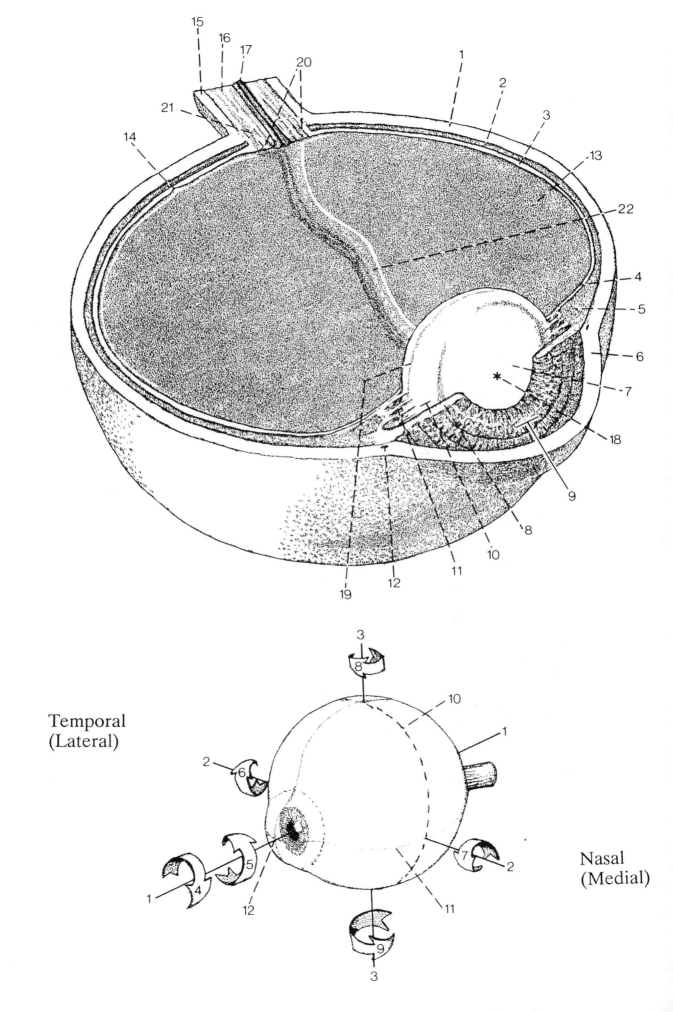

Temporal
(Lateral)

Nasal
(Medial)

Upper figure is an enlarged segment of area marked by dashed lines in lower figure.

Color and label

1   **Cornea**
2   **Iris**
3   **Anterior chamber.** Filled with aqueous humor
4   **Posterior chamber.** Filled with aqueous humor
5   **Lens.** The lens is held in its flat biconvex shape by the radial pull of the zonule fibers that extend from the surrounding ciliary processes to the lens. Because the natural tendency of the lens is to assume a more round or globular shape, constriction of the circular ciliary muscle relaxes the peripheral outward pull by the zonule fibers and allows the lens to increase its curvature and thus focus light from near objects (accommodation). In its flatter shape the lens focuses light from far objects.
6   **Ciliary processes.** There are about 70 of these tiny, radial-arranged, wrinkled folds. They lie in the pars plicata or a folded part of the ciliary body (also called the ciliary crown).
7   **Ciliary body** (muscular part). This completely encircles the lens and consists of smooth muscle that controls the curvature of the lens (the muscle of accommodation).
8   **Anterior zonule fibers.** These pass to the front of the lens where they fuse with the lens capsule.
9   **Posterior zonule fibers.** These pass to the back of the lens where they fuse with the lens capsule.
10 **Trabecular meshwork.** An irregular network of tiny beams (trabeculae) at the periphery of the anterior chamber where the iris joins the the cornea. The convoluted passages between the trabeculae contain aqueous humor, which slowly flows outward eventually to be absorbed by the scleral venous sinus (canal of Schlemm).
11 **Scleral venous sinus** (canal of Schlemm). This varicose vein encircles the inner part of the corneoscleral junction (limbus). It drains the aqueous humor from the anterior chamber.
12 **Limbus.** The corneoscleral junction
13 **Conjunctiva.** The transparent mucous membrane on the sclera (bulbar conjunctiva). It is also reflected onto the inner surface of the eyelid (palpebral conjunctiva).
14 **Sclera**
15 **Choroid**
16 **Retina**
17 **Fovea centralis**
18 **Outer dural sheath of optic nerve**
19 **Central artery and vein of retina**
20 **Optic nerve**
21 **Ciliary body.** Pars plana (smooth part); also called the ciliary ring. Covered internally by the non-nervous part of the retina.

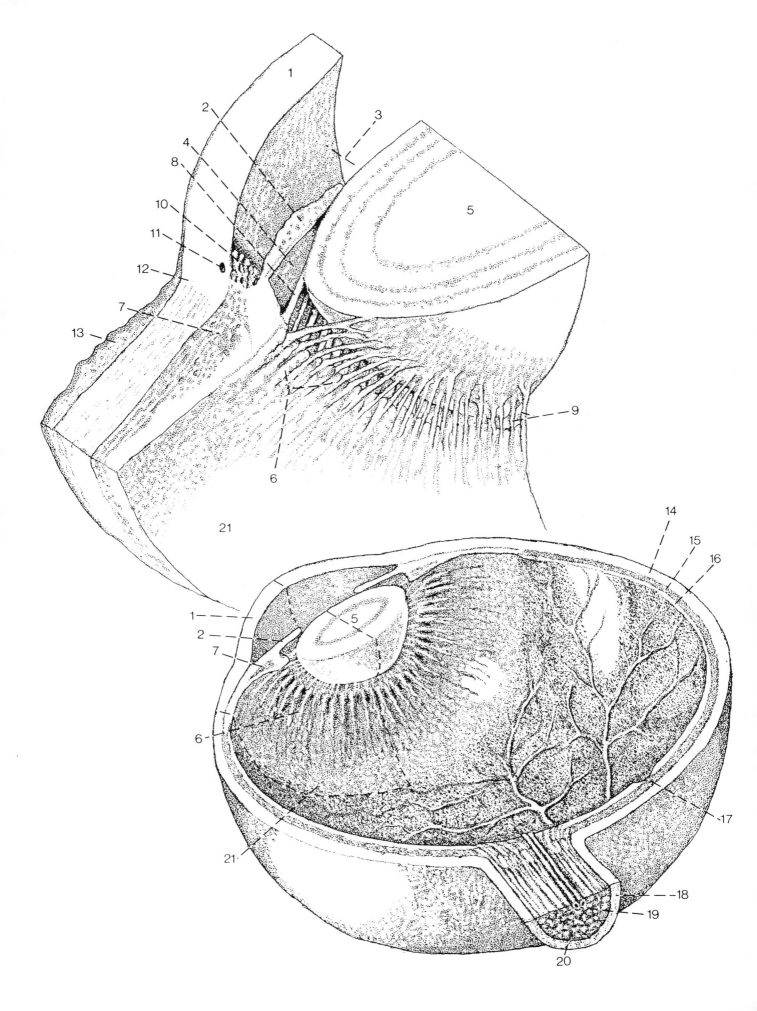

Arrow L indicates direction of light.

Figure A. Upper left: cone and rod

Color and label (these labels also apply to Figure B)

1   Cone outer segment
2   Cone inner segment
3   Cone outer fiber. This is present only in the longer cones. See Figure C.
4   Zonula adherens. Adhering junction between the cone and the surrounding Müller cell. Until the electron microscope revealed this to be a specialized junction between cells, it was mistakenly identified as a membrane. Even though it is not a membrane, it is still called the external limiting membrane.
5   Cone cell body with its nucleus
6   Cone inner fiber
7   Cone pedicle: cone synaptic ending. This synapses with both bipolar cells and horizontal cells.
8   Rod outer segment
9   Rod inner segment
10   Zonula adherens (outer limiting membrane)
11   Outer rod fiber
12   Rod cell body with nucleus
13   Inner rod fiber
14   Rod spherule: rod synaptic ending
15   Microvilli projecting from outer surface of Müller cell
16   Concavities in Müller cells formed by rod and cone cell bodies

Figure B.   Label the 10 layers of the retina (large numbers 1-10)

1   Pigment epithelium (PE)
2   Layer of rods (R) and cones (C): inner and outer segments
3   Outer limiting "membrane": adhering zones between photoreceptors and Müller cells.
4   Outer nuclear layer: nuclei of rods and cones. There are about 120 million rods and about 7 million cones.
5   Outer plexiform layer. Synaptic region where rods and cones synapse with bipolar cells (BP) and horizontal cells (H).
6   Inner nuclear layer: nuclei of bipolar cells (BP), horizontal cells (H), amacrine cells (A), and Müller cells.
7   Inner plexiform layer: region of synaptic contact between bipolar cells (BP), ganglion cells (G), and amacrine cells (A).
8   Ganglion cell layer. The ganglion cells give rise to the optic nerve fibers.
9   Nerve fiber layer. The optic nerve fibers are ensheathed by Müller cell end feet as they converge toward the optic disk.
10   Inner limiting membrane: basal laminae of Müller cells

Color and label rods (R), cone (C), bipolar cell (BP), horizontal cell (H), and amacrine cell (A), and notice the extent of the Müller cells (M) stretching from layer 3 to layer 10. Note also the hollows and concavities on the Müller cell surface where its membrane enfolds the various other cells in the retina and fills up all the intercellular space.

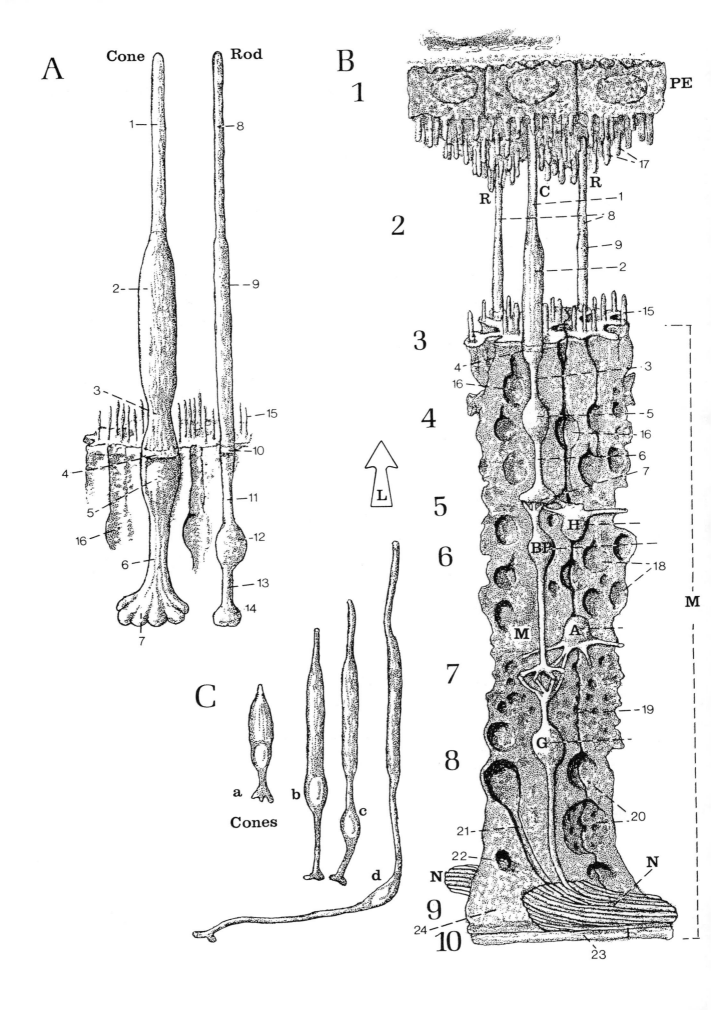

A

Cone   Rod

1
8
2
9
3
15
4
10
5
11
16
12
6
13
7
14

B
1
2
3
4
5
6
7
8
9
10

L

C
a   b   c   d
Cones

PE
17
R   C   R
1
8
9
2
15
4
3
16
5
16
6
7
H
BP
18
M   A
19
G
20
21
22
N   N
24
23
M

85 The retina: Rods, cones, and Müller cells
(Continued)

Arrow L indicates direction of light.

Color and label

17 Microvilli of pigment epithelium
18 Concavities for bipolar cells, horizontal cells, and amacrine cells
19 Border between two Müller cells
20 Concavities for ganglion cells
21 Groove for optic nerve fiber
22 Hole in Müller cell for passage of bundles of optic nerve fibers
23 Basal lamina of Müller cell (inner limiting membrane)
24 Müller cells end feet

Figure C. Bottom center

Cones from different areas of the retina: **a,** from the periphery of the retina (note that only these peripheral cones have the classic cone shape); **b,** from the edge of the macula lutea; **c,** from the macula lutea; **d,** from the fovea centralis. (After Greeff, cited in Copenhaver, 1978.)

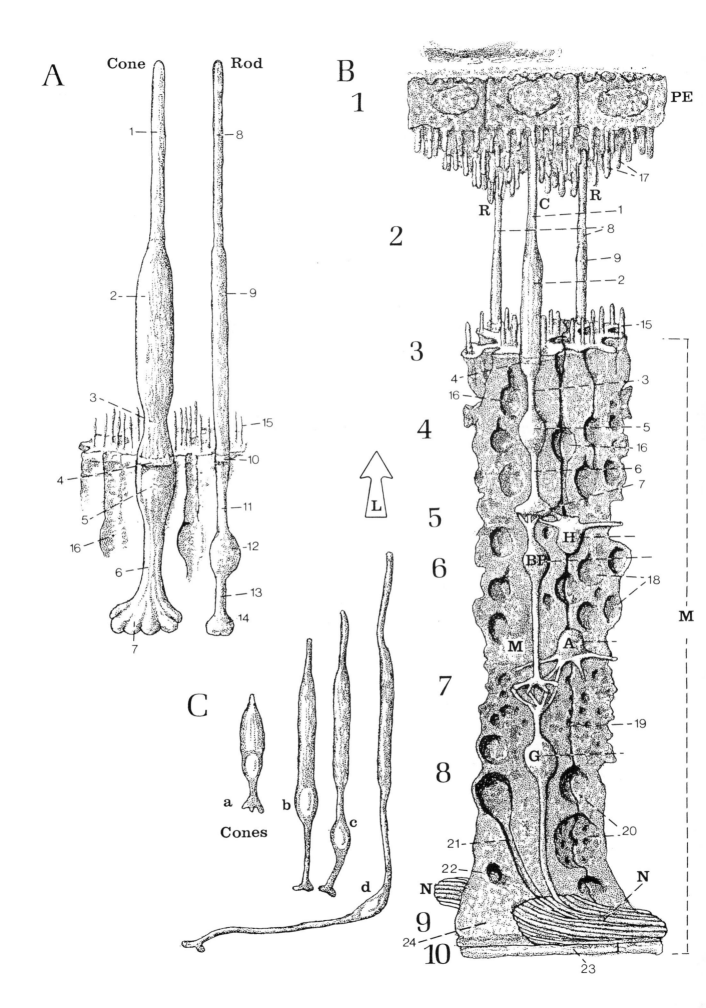

A

Cone Rod

1
8

2
9

3
15

4
10
5
11
16
12
6
13
7
14

C

a
b
c
d

Cones

L

B

1 PE
R C R
17

2
1
8
9
2

3
15
4
3
16
5
16
6
7

4

5
H
BP
18

6
M A

7
19

G

8
20

21
22
N N
9
24
10 23

M

Figure A. Cells

Color and label   *Label*

C   Cone cell   COS   Cone outer segment
R   Rod Cell   CIS   Cone inner segment
BP   Bipolar cell   Cped   Cone pedicle
H   Horizontal cell   nf   Optic nerve fibers
A   Amacrine cell
G   Ganglion cell

Figure B. Enlargement of junction of cone cell outer and inner segments

Color and label

ms   Membranous sac. These sacs contain visual pigment. There are 3 different pigments
      in cone cells, each of which responds maximally to either red, green, or blue light.
st   Connecting stalk. This is a modified flagellum.
mt   Microtubules. There are 9 pairs of microtubules.
bb   Basal body

Note that the membranous sacs in cones are continuous with the cell membrane of the outer
segment (double arrows).

Figure C. Cone pedicle.   Encircled area is enlarged below as D.

Hp   Horizontal cell process
BPd   Bipolar cell dendrite

Figure D. Enlargement of cone pedicle indented with processes of bipolar and horizontal cells

Cped   Cone pedicle
BPd   Bipolar cell dendrite
Hp   Horizontal cell process
sv   Synaptic vesicles
sr   Synaptic ribbon

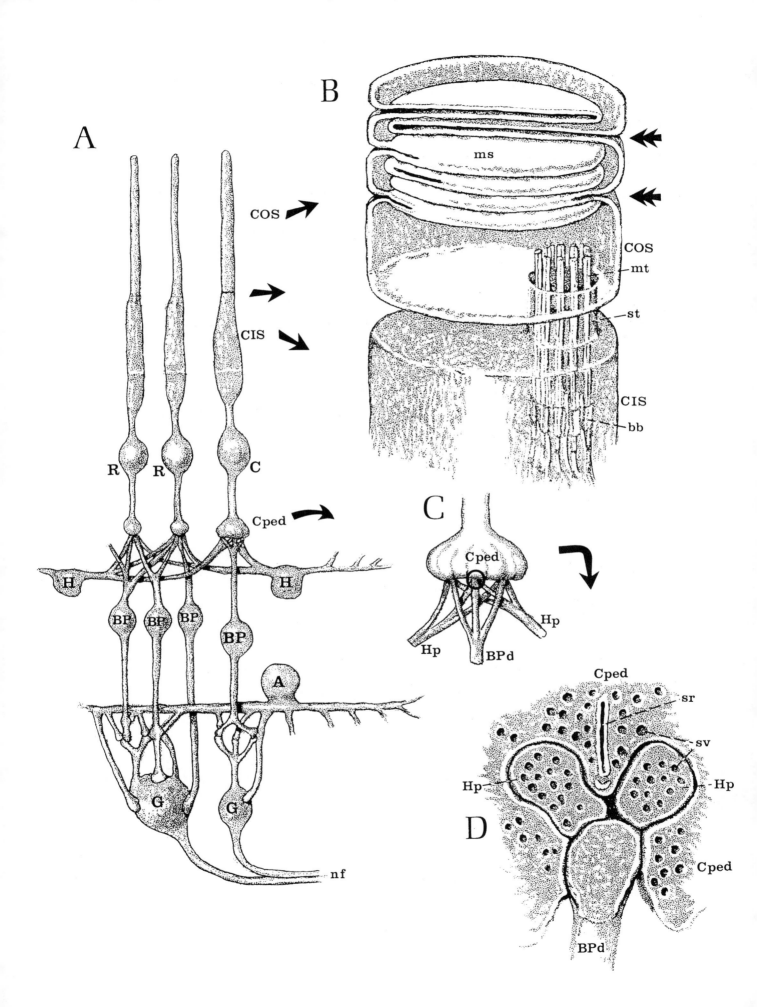

A

COS

CIS

R R C

Cped

H H

BP BP BP BP

A

G G

nf

B

ms

COS
mt

st

CIS
bb

C

Cped

Hp
Hp
BPd

D

Cped
sr

sv

Hp
Hp

Cped

BPd

RIGHT EYE, LOWER HALF

Color and label

1 **Optic disk.** Blind spot. It is pink or white and much paler than surrounding retina. Contains no rods or cones.

2 **Macula lutea** (Latin, yellow spot). Lies about 3 mm lateral to the optic disk. It is a yellowish circular depression with sloping sides.

3 **Fovea centralis** (Latin, central pit). This central depressed area of the macula lutea contains only tightly packed narrow cones that give this small area of the retina the greatest visual activity (sharp vision). At the fovea centralis the cones are exposed directly to the incoming light because the overlying layers of cells lie off to the sides of the fovea. Also there are no overlying retinal blood vessels in front of the cones at the fovea centralis as there are in the rest of the retina. The peripheral clivus does, however, contain blood vessels.

4 **Sclera.** Fibrous outer tunic. The anterior part of the sclera is the white of eye visible beneath the transparent conjunctiva. The sclera protects the eye and maintains its shape. Posteriorly the sclera fuses with the three meninges that surround the optic nerve.

5 **Choroid.** This is the thin, highly vascular, and highly pigmented middle layer that lies between the outer sclera and the inner retina. Its blood vessels supply the outer layers of the retina including the rods and cones.

6 **Pigment layer of the retina.** This is the outermost layer (layer 1); it absorbs light and prevents reflection.

7 **Outer nuclear layer of retina.** Nuclei of rods and cones

8 **Inner nuclear layer.** Nuclei of bipolar cells, horizontal cells, and amacrine cells

9 **Ganglion cell layer.** Note the relative thickness of the three nuclear layers in the retina. There are about 130 million rods and cones, which are indicated by the thick outer nuclear layer. There are considerably fewer bipolar horizontal cells and amacrine cells, as indicated in the thinner inner nuclear layer. There are only about one million ganglion cells and their layer is the thinnest of the three.

10 **Lamina cribrosa of the sclera.** This is the weakest part of the sclera because it is full of holes for the passage of optic nerve fibers. Consequently, it may bulge outward in the case of increased intraocular pressure, as in glaucoma, or bulge inward in the case of increased intracranial pressure.

11 **Arachnoid sheath** (arachnoid mater) and **subarachnoid space.** The optic nerve is the only nerve that is enveloped by the three meninges as well as the subarachnoid space filled with cerebrospinal fluid.

12 **Dural sheath** (dura mater) of optic nerve

13 **Central vein of retina.** Note that the central vein lies lateral to the artery at the optic disk and that the branches of the central artery lie in front of (actually more internal than) the tributaries of the central vein.

14 **Central artery of the retina.** This is the first branch of the ophthalmic artery. It pierces the optic nerve about 12 mm behind the eyeball, travels in its center, and enters the eye at the middle of the optic disk. Its branches spread out on the inner surface of the retina just behind (peripheral to) the delicate basal lamina of the Müller cells. Thus the retinal blood vessels are easily seen with an ophthalmoscope. The central artery supplies the inner (vitreal) layers of the retina.

15 **Circle of Zinn.** This is an arterial circle within the sclera that surrounds the optic nerve at its junction with the eye. It supplies that part of the optic nerve and the adjacent retina.

16 **Optic nerve.** The axons of the optic nerve arise from the ganglion cells in the retina. They are unmyelinated as they course across the inner surface of the retina where they comprise layer 9. They converge on the optic disk, and once they pass through the lamina cribrosa of the sclera and enter the optic nerve, they become myelinated. Because the retina develops as an outgrowth of the brain, the optic nerve should really be called the optic tract. However, the first part up to the chiasm has been designated **optic nerve**, and the second part, from chiasm to lateral geniculate body, has been designated **optic tract**.

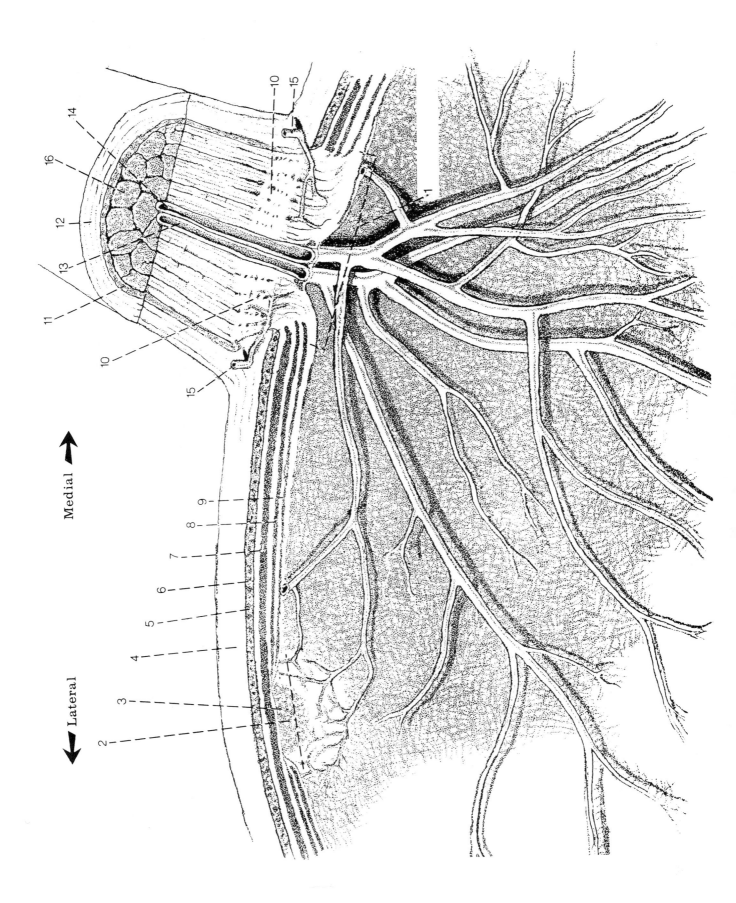

Lateral ← → Medial

Color and label

1   Superior rectus muscle
2   Lateral rectus muscle
3   Medial rectus muscle
4   Inferior rectus muscle
5   Superior oblique muscle
6   Inferior oblique muscle
7   Levator palpebrae muscle (*cut*)
8   Anulus tendineus communis (common tendinous ring)
9   Trochlea
10   Optic nerve
11   Conjunctiva (tunica conjunctiva)
       (cut edge)
12   Frontal sinus
13   Maxillary sinus
14   Pterygopalatine fossa
15   Sphenopalatine foramen

After Wolf-Heidegger.

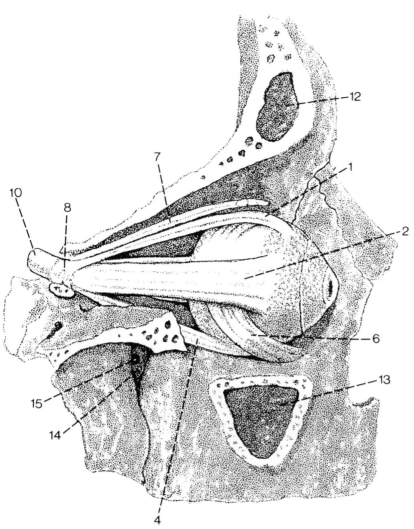

**LATERAL VIEW OF RIGHT EYE (ABOVE)
WITH LATERAL WALL REMOVED**

**SUPERIOR VIEW OF RIGHT EYE (BELOW)
WITH ROOF OF ORBIT REMOVED**

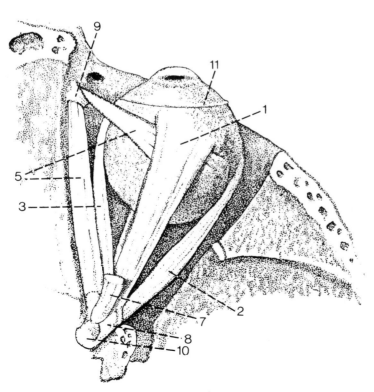

Cranial nerves VI, IV, and III

Six extrinsic ocular muscles move the eye and determine the direction of gaze: the superior rectus, lateral rectus, medial rectus, inferior rectus, superior oblique, and inferior oblique. A seventh muscle, the levator palpebrae, raises the eyelid. These seven muscles are supplied by three cranial nerves, the abducent (VI), trochlear (IV), and oculomotor (III) nerves.

The abducent nerve contains approximately 6,600 fibers, the trochlear approximately 3,400, and the oculomotor approximately 24,000. The abducent nerve (N VI) arises from a cluster of motor somata that comprise the abducent nucleus (Nuc N VI) in the medial dorsal pons, just under the floor of the IV ventricle. Neuron 1 is a motor neuron in the abducent nucleus. Its axon enters the orbit through the superior orbital fissure (not shown), passes through the anulus tendineus, which is a ring of fibrous tissue at the back of the orbit from which the four recti muscles arise, and supplies a single muscle, the lateral rectus (LR). The action of the lateral rectus muscle is abduction of the eye, that is, turning the eye outward or laterally. Damage to the abducent nerve or lateral rectus muscle will result in an inability of the eye to gaze laterally, plus an inward turning of the eye when staring straight ahead due to the unopposed action of the antagonist medial rectus muscle.

The trochlear nerve (N IV), like the abducent nerve, also innervates only one muscle, the superior oblique. The trochlear nerve is unique among the cranial nerves in two respects: First, it is the only cranial nerve that completely decussates, thus innervating a structure on the opposite side; and, second, it is the only cranial nerve that emerges from the dorsal surface of the brain. The axon of neuron 2 in the left trochlear nucleus (Nuc N IV) *crosses* the midline and ends upon the right superior oblique muscle (SO). Like the abducent nerve and oculomotor nerve, the trochlear nerve passes through the superior orbital fissure, but unlike nerves VI and III, which pass *through* the anulus tendineus, the trochlear nerve passes *above* the anulus. Paralysis of the superior oblique will be most apparent when an attempt is made to direct the eye down and to the front, as in walking down stairs.

The remaining five muscles are all innervated by the oculomotor nerve (N III), which arises from motor neurons in the oculomotor nucleus. This nerve also contains a contingent of preganglionic parasympathetic neurons in its visceral efferent nucleus of Edinger-Westphal (now called accessory oculomotor nucleus). These preganglionic parasympathetic fibers leave the brain stem as part of the oculomotor nerve. Both the oculomotor nucleus (Nuc N III) and trochlear nucleus (Nuc N IV) lie in the mesencephalon near the midline, somewhat ventral to the cerebral aqueduct. The trochlear nucleus lies beneath the inferior colliculus and the oculomotor nucleus beneath the superior colliculus. The oculomotor nucleus is partly paired and partly unpaired; the unpaired portion lies in the midsagittal plane and unites the two paired portions.

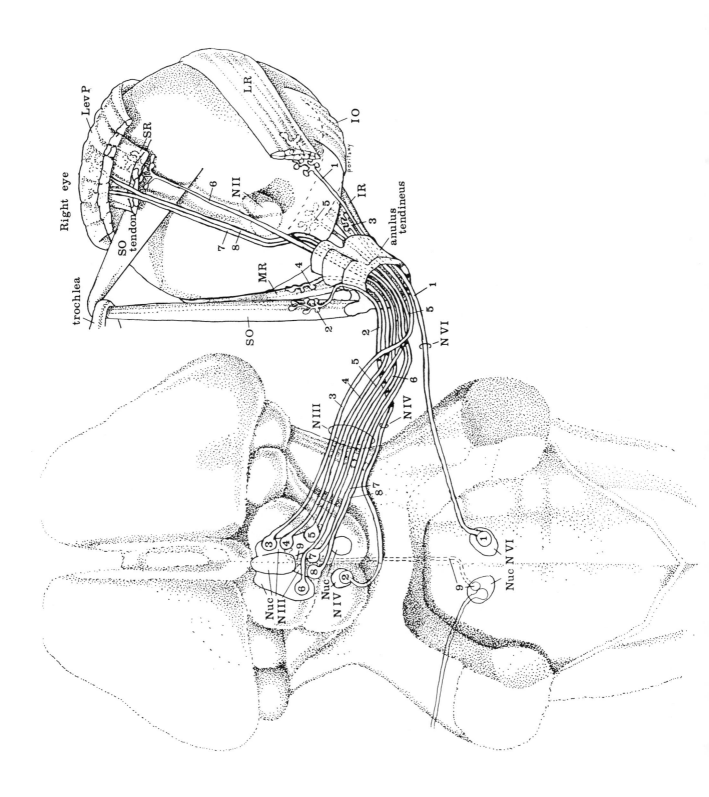

Although the majority of fibers within the oculomotor nerve remain uncrossed and supply muscles on the same side, some fibers arise from somata in the opposite side of the nucleus. Neurons 3 through 8 represent groups of motor neurons within the oculomotor nucleus, each of which supplies one of five muscles. Their positions within the nucleus indicate the relative front-to-back localization of these neuronal groups. Neuron 3 supplies the inferior rectus (IR), neuron 4 supplies the medial rectus (MR), and neuron 5 innervates the inferior oblique (IO). Neuron 6 on the *left* side is exceptional because its axon crosses the midline to supply the *right* superior rectus. Hence, the superior rectus muscle is supplied by crossed fibers. Neurons 7 and 8 both supply the levator palpebrae. Note that 7 is homolateral and 8 is on the opposite side. Thus the levator palpebrae receives both crossed and uncrossed fibers, which may account for the fact that both eyelids are raised (and blinked) simultaneously.

Severance of the oculomotor nerve would result in paralysis of four extrinsic ocular muscles and the levator palpebrae. Hence, the eyelid could not be raised due to paralysis of the levator palpebrae. Drooping of the eyelid is called ptosis ("a falling," from the Greek, *ptoma*, to fall). If the trochlear and abducent nerve were still functioning, the superior oblique muscle (N IV) would turn down the eye, and the lateral rectus (N VI) would abduct it; thus with exclusive nerve III damage, the eye would be somewhat depressed and abducted. The pupil constriction reflex in response to light would also be lost due to interruption of the parasympathetic fibers within the oculomotor nerve destined for the sphincter muscle in the iris. Recent work has demonstrated the existence of **internuclear cells** within these three nuclei. The axons of these cells run from the one nucleus to another. Neuron 9 is one such internuclear neuron; it lies in the left abducent nucleus and its axon ends in the right oculomotor nucleus upon a motor neuron that supplies the right medial rectus muscle. Internuclear neurons are probably responsible for coordinating **conjugate** eye movements, that is, movements in which both eyes move in the same direction. In order to turn both eyes to the left, the left lateral rectus and right medial rectus work together. Conversely, antagonist muscle must be inhibited; contraction of the right lateral rectus muscle must be accompanied by reciprocal inhibition of the right medial rectus. Thus there must be inhibitory and excitatory internuclear connections.

Color and label the muscles and the nerves that supply them.

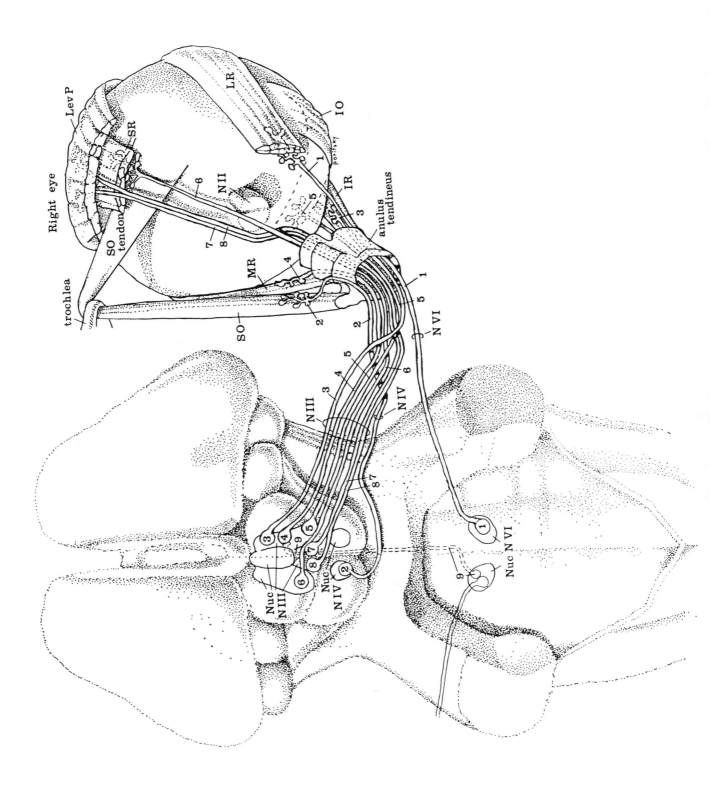

If you were to encounter a penguin holding a sign "**penguin**" and standing in front of another sign that said "**up**," the penguin and signs would constitute your **visual field**–that is, your **visual field** is what you **see**. By staring at the penguin's perplexed expression, you would cause its face to be projected upon the central portion of your retina, the macula lutea or "yellow spot." The macular portion of your visual field is indicated by the lighter area that encompasses the penguin's face. The biconvex lens in each eye would focus the image of the penguin upside-down on the retina in the back of each eye. The center of your visual field, in this case the penguin's face, would fall upon the macula lutea. Hence, the retinal fields in each eye would be an upside-down penguin. The retinal field is an inverted visual field. Ganglion cells in the retina give rise to the axons that comprise the optic nerve (N II) and convey visual impulses centrally to a nuclear mass in the back of the thalamus, the **lateral geniculate body**.

Each eye is drawn so that only its bottom half is shown. The two inverted penguins are the retinal fields. The enlarged inserts behind each eye show that the penguin's eyes and beak fall in the macular field, one eye in each of the two lower quadrants and half of the beak in each of the two upper quadrants of the macula. Note that the optic nerve only extends to the chiasma; beyond the chiasma it is called optic tract.

Four ganglion cells (1, 2, 3, 4) are shown. Note that the two ganglion cells that arise from the **lateral** or **temporal retinal fields** (1, 4) have axons that project to the lateral geniculate bodies on the **same side**, that is, they do not cross but remain **ipsilateral**. The fibers that arise from ganglion cells in the **medial** or **nasal retinal fields** (2, 3) cross at the chiasma and project to the **opposite** or **contralateral** lateral geniculate body. Neurons within the lateral geniculate body give rise to axons that compromise the **optic radiation** or **geniculocalcarine tract**, which is a large, curved bundle of fibers that arises in the lateral geniculate body and ends mainly in the medial surface of the occipital lobe of the cerebral hemispheres.

The lateral geniculate body is divided into six layers, or laminae, of which layers 2, 3, 5 receive **uncrossed** fibers from the **lateral** half of the ipsilateral retina and layers 1, 4, 6 receive fibers from the **medial** half of the contralateral retina. Thus ganglion cells 1 and 3, which both lie in the **left** half of each retina, project to the **left** lateral geniculate body, and ganglion cells 2 and 4, which lie in the **right** half of each retina, project to the **right** lateral geniculate body. Because of this arrangement the same half of the penguin will be projected to each lateral geniculate body. The macular projection occupies the wedge-shaped posterior central region of the lateral geniculate body and peripheral retinal fields occupy the remaining medial and lateral parts.

The drawing shows an image of each half of the penguin occurring twice in each lateral geniculate body. The macular projection, which is half of the penguin's beak and one eye, is disproportionately large. It occupies layers 5 and 6 with corresponding parts lying side by side but in separate layers. The rest of the penguin is shown in layers 3 and 4. It is probable that each half of the retinal field is represented not twice, but four or even six times, once in each layer of the lateral geniculate body. In the visual cortex the macular representation is exceedingly large and located most posteriorly. In the drawing each cortical macula is represented as a greatly enlarged upside-down eye and half a beak. The rest of the penguin that falls within the peripheral fields is located more anterior and is quite small, especially when compared with the large size of the peripheral visual field and peripheral retinal field. In terms of what you look at, the world about you is projected onto your visual cortex upside-down, with the **right half** of the **visual field** ending in the **left half** of the brain, and the **left visual field** ending in the **right half** of the brian. Note that the sign "up" is now **down** and entirely within the **right** lateral geniculate body and **right** visual cortex because in the visual field it lies in the **left** half.

Directions: Use one color for ganglion cells 1, 3 and the left optic radiation, and another for ganglion cells 2, 4 and the right optic radiation.

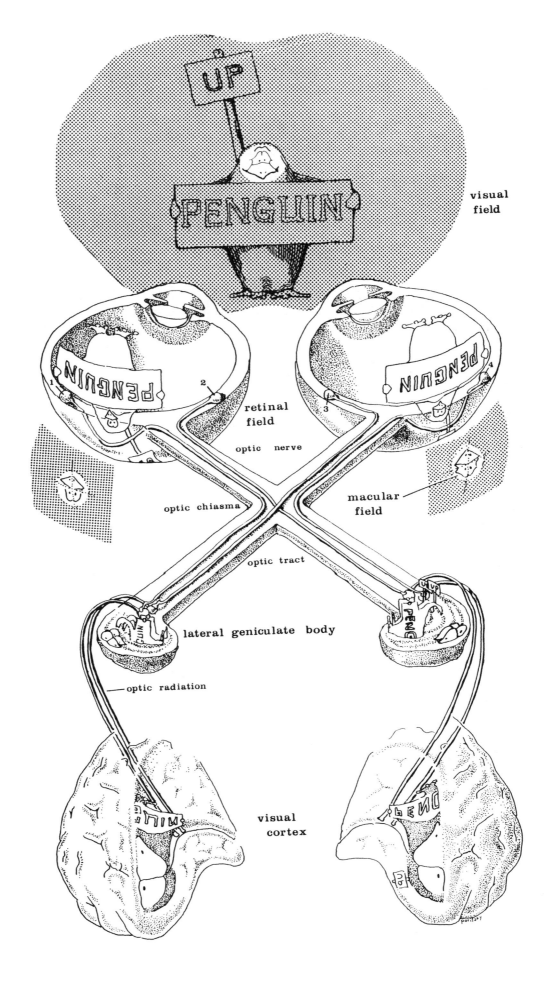

visual
field

retinal
field

optic nerve

optic chiasma

macular
field

optic tract

lateral geniculate body

optic radiation

visual
cortex

Top figure from right side
Bottom figure from left, above, and in front

Color and label the visual pathways

1	Eye
2	Optic nerve
3	Optic chiasma (or chiasm)
4	Optic tract
5	Lateral geniculate body
6	Optic radiation (geniculocalcarine tract)
7	Temporal genu of optic radiation (Meyer's loop)*
8	Primary visual cortex. Mainly on medial surface of occipital cortex.
9	Frontal horn of lateral ventricle
10	Thalamus
11	Inferior (temporal) horn of lateral ventricle

_____

*Damage to the temporal lobe can interrupt fibers in the **lower half** of the optic radiation. This results in a loss of vision in the **upper quadrant** on the **opposite side** of both visual fields.

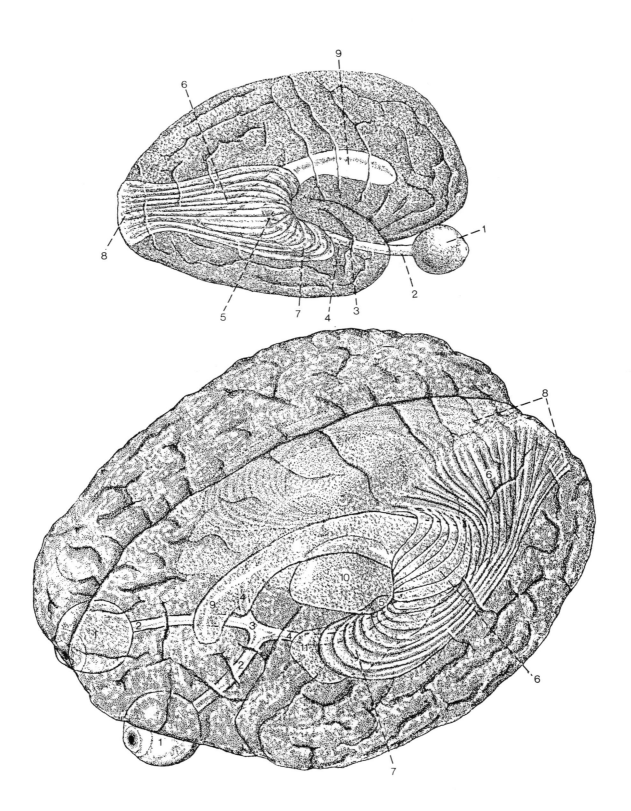

(After Wolf-Heidegger)

Color and label

1   Olfactory bulb
2   Olfactory tract
3   Optic nerve
4   Optic chiasm (Latin, chiasma opticum)
5   Optic tract
6   Temporal genu (bend) of optic radiation (Meyer's loop)
7   Medial root of optic nerve
8   Lateral geniculate body
9   Pulvinar of thalamus
10 Superior colliculus (cut)
11 Optic radiation (geniculocalcarine tract)
12 Pineal body
13 Lateral ventricle (roof of posterior horn)
14 Splenium of corpus callosum
15 Primary visual cortex (area 17 of Brodmann; also called striate cortex because of the prominent striation in layer 4, the line of Gennari, or Gennari's band)
16 Cerebral aqueduct (new name, mesencephalic aqueduct; old name, aqueduct of Sylvius) and cut surface of midbrain (mesencephalon)
17 Medial geniculate body
18 Mamillary body and posterior perforated substance
19 Tuber cinereum and infundibulum
20 Putamen (cut surface)
21 Anterior commissure
22 Anterior perforated substance
23 Olfactory trigone

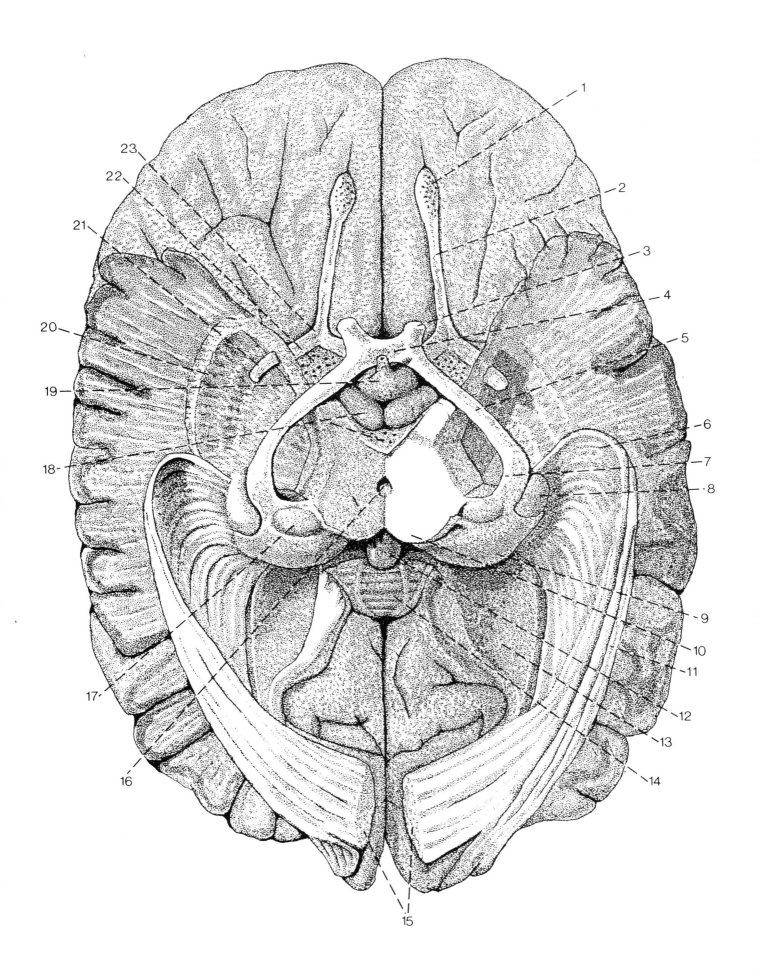

93 Left homonymous hemianopsia

The visual deficit or loss is always described in terms of what the patient sees or does not see. In this case, the patient has lost vision in the left half of both visual fields. The patient has a **left homonymous hemianopsia** (Greek, *homos,* same; *onyma,* name) (Greek, *hemi,* half; *an,* not; *opsis,* vision [no half vision]). Such a visual deficit is caused by a lesion in the right optic tract, which contains axons from the **right** halves of both retinas, or in the **right** optic radiatiion. An extensive lesion in the right visual cortex would have a similar effect.

Color the functional visual pathways one color and the nonfnctional (blind) visual pathways another color.

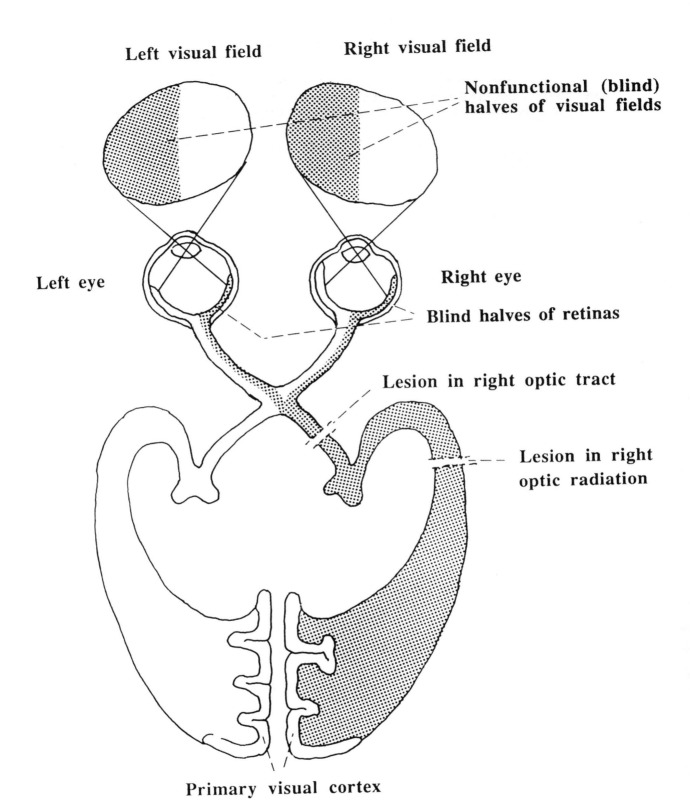

Left visual field

Right visual field

Nonfunctional (blind) halves of visual fields

Left eye

Right eye

Blind halves of retinas

Lesion in right optic tract

Lesion in right optic radiation

Primary visual cortex

A lesion in the optic chiasm such as a tumor of the pituitary gland, would interrupt fibers that **cross** at the chiasm. Crossing fibers arise from the **medial** (or nasal) halves of both retinas. Since the medial halves of the retinas receive light from the **lateral** (or temporal) halves of the visual fields, the patient will have a loss of vision in both of the **lateral** visual fields, or a **bitemporal hemianopsia**.

Color the functional visual pathways (empty) one color and the nonfunctional (blind or shaded) visual pathways another.

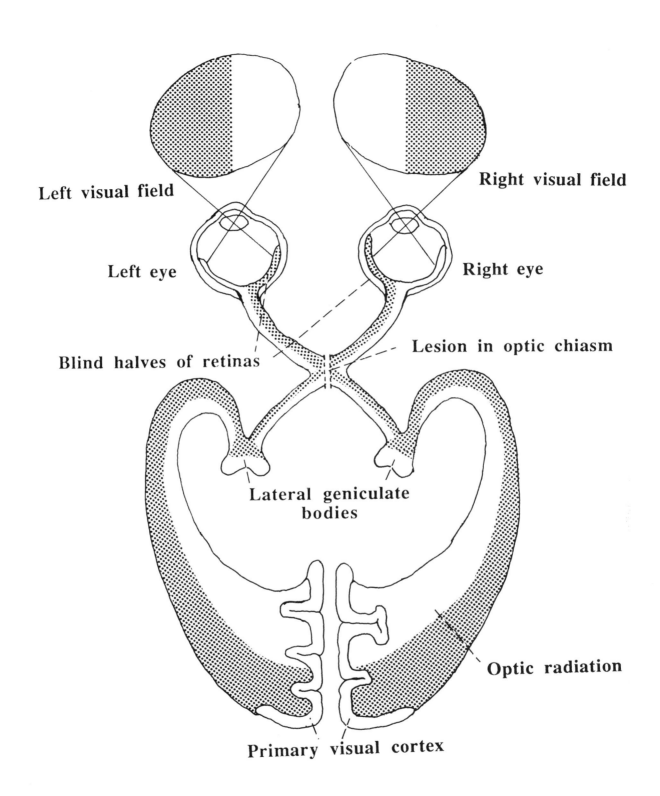

Left visual field

Right visual field

Left eye

Right eye

Blind halves of retinas

Lesion in optic chiasm

Lateral geniculate
bodies

Optic radiation

Primary visual cortex

95   Etymological Cartoon: Hemianopsia
      (Greek, *hemi*, half; *an*, not; *opsis*, vision)
      = One half not seeing

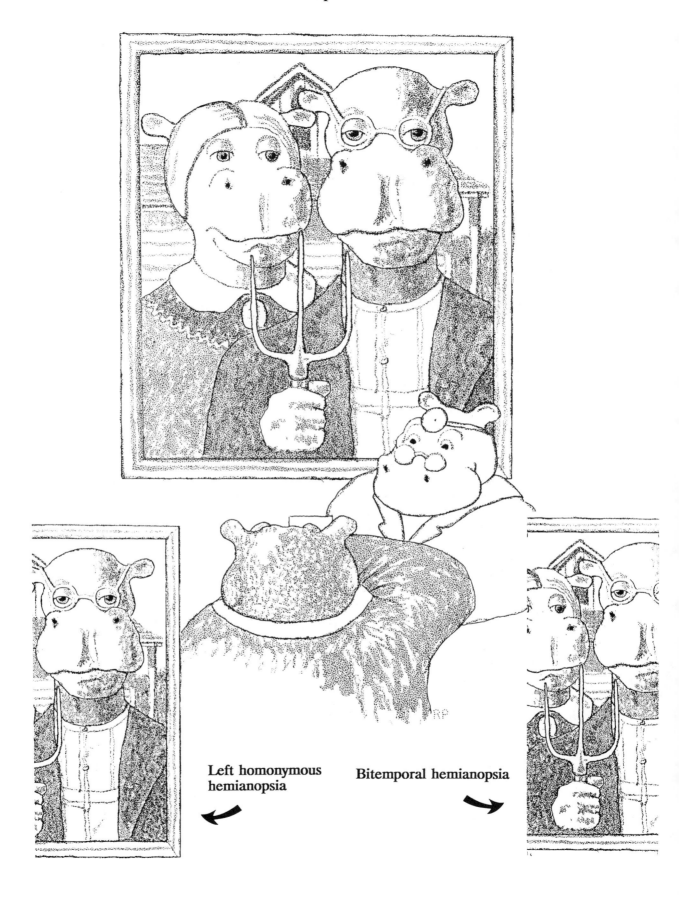

Left homonymous
hemianopsia

Bitemporal hemianopsia

(After Wolf-Heidegger)

Upper figure: from above and behind

Color and label

CH	Cerebellar hemispheres
V	Vermis (Latin, worm)
1	Primary fissure. Divides the cerebellum into an anterior (actually superior) lobe and a much larger posterior (actually inferior) lobe.
AL	Anterior lobe
PL	Posterior lobe
2	Horizontal fissure. Runs roughly along border between the superior surface and inferior surface.
3	Posterior superior fissure

Lower figure: from the front

Color and label

V	Vermis
2	Horizontal fissure
4	Nodulus (part of both vermis and flocculonodular lobe)
5	Flocculus. The nodulus and two flocculi comprise the flocculonodular lobe (also called the archicerebellum), which functions with the vestibular system to regulate balance and equilibrium.
6	Middle cerebellar peduncle (cut). Formerly called brachium pontis (Latin, arm of the pons).
7	Inferior cerebellar peduncle (cut). Formerly called restiform body (Latin, rope-like body).
8	Superior cerebellar peduncle (cut). Formerly called brachium conjunctivum (Latin, arm that is joined).
9	Anterior (superior) medullary velum. This forms the superior roof of the fourth ventricle.
10	Nervus intermedius: part of the facial nerve
11	Facial nerve (N VII)
12	Vestibulocochlear nerve (N VIII)
13	Choroid plexus of ventricle IV
14	Lateral aperture of ventricle IV (foramen of Luschka)

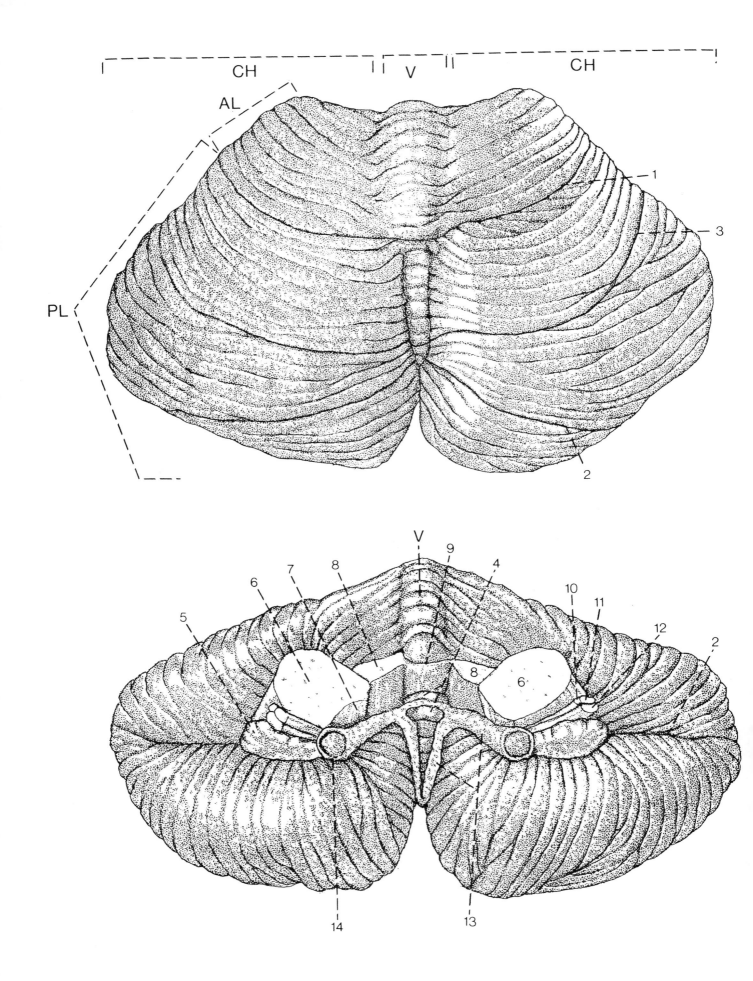

Figure A.   Dorsal aspect of cerebellum

This a simplified view of the dorsal aspect of the cerebellum showing the three lobes: the anterior lobe (ant lobe), the posterior lobe (post lobe), and the small flocculonodular lobe (fl-nod-fl). The flocculonodular lobe is actually situated beneath (in front of) the posterior lobe and not inferior as indicated in the picture. The cerebellar cortex is divided into three longitudinal zones: a central **vermis** (Latin, worm); two intermediate zones (**int**) on either side of the vermis; and the much larger lateral zones (**lat**) that cover the bulk of the cerebellar hemispheres. Note that the nodulus is part of both the vermis and the flocculonode. In terms of its function and its connections, the cerebellum is divided into three parts: the vestibulocerebellum, which occupies the flocculonodular lobe; the spinocerebellum, which consists of most of the anterior lobe (indicated by "LEG" and "ARM") and a portion of the posterior lobe (also indicated by "ARM" and "LEG"); and the neocerebellum, which comprises the greater part of the human cerebellum, encompassing the large hemispheres of the posterior lobe and the vermis between them. The terms archicerebellum, paleocerebellum, and neocerebellum are often used synonymously for vestibulocerebellum, spinocerebellum, and pontocerebellum, respectively.

Color and label flocculonodular lobe, spinocerebellum ("ARM," "LEG"), and pontocerebellum (lat).

Figure B. Purkinje neurons and outflow from the cerebellum.

Neurons 1, 2, 3, and 4 are Purkinje neurons in the cerebellar cortex. There are an estimated 15 million Purkinje neurons in the cerebellar cortex. The axons of the Purkinje neurons run centrally to the interior of the cerebellum, where they end upon neurons in one of the four cerebellar nuclei. **Color and label** these nuclei: the dentate (Den), emboliform (Emb), globose (Glob), and fastigial (Fast). Notice that the Purkinje cells in the cerebellar hemispheres project to the dentate nucleus (1). Those in the intermediate zone project to the emboliform nucleus and globose nucleus (2, 3), and those in the vermis project to the fastigial nucleus (4). Purkinje neurons in the flocculonodulae lobe project to the fastigial nucleus (5) and also directly to the vestibular nuclei (6) in the medulla and pons. **Color Purkinje neurons 1–6.** Neurons in the dentate nucleus (7) and in the emboliform nucleus (8) and globose nucleus send their axons into the superior cerebellar peduncle. Dentate nucleus neurons (7) project mainly to the ventral lateral nucleus (VL) in the thalamus, which in turn projects to the motor cortex. Axons arising from neurons in the emboliform nucleus (8) and globose nuclei end in the red nucleus (RN). Neuron 9 in the red nucleus gives rise to either a rubro-olivary (not shown) fiber or a rubrospinal fiber (not shown). Neuron 10 gives rise to a thalamocortical fiber. **Color neurons 7, 8, 9, and 10.**

Color and label

Cereb Hemis	Cerebellar hemispheres	Decuss	Decussation of superior cerebellar
Int Z	Intermediate zone (paravermal zones)		peduncle
V	Vermis	RN	Red nucleus
Vent IV	Fourth ventricle	Midbr	Midbrain (or mesencephalon)
Floc	Flocculus	Vest N	Vestibular nuclei
Nod	Nodulus	Thal	Thalamus
Sup Cereb Ped	Superior cerebellar peduncle	VL	Ventral lateral nucleus of thalamus

Figure C.   Cerebellar peduncles

The cerebellum is attached to the brain stem by three peduncles (Latin, a little foot or stalk) on each side. The three **left** peduncles are superimpose on the **right** cerebellum (CBL).

Color and label: sup, superior cerebellar peduncle; mid, middle cerebellar peduncle; inf, inferior cerebellar peduncle; den, dentate nucleus.

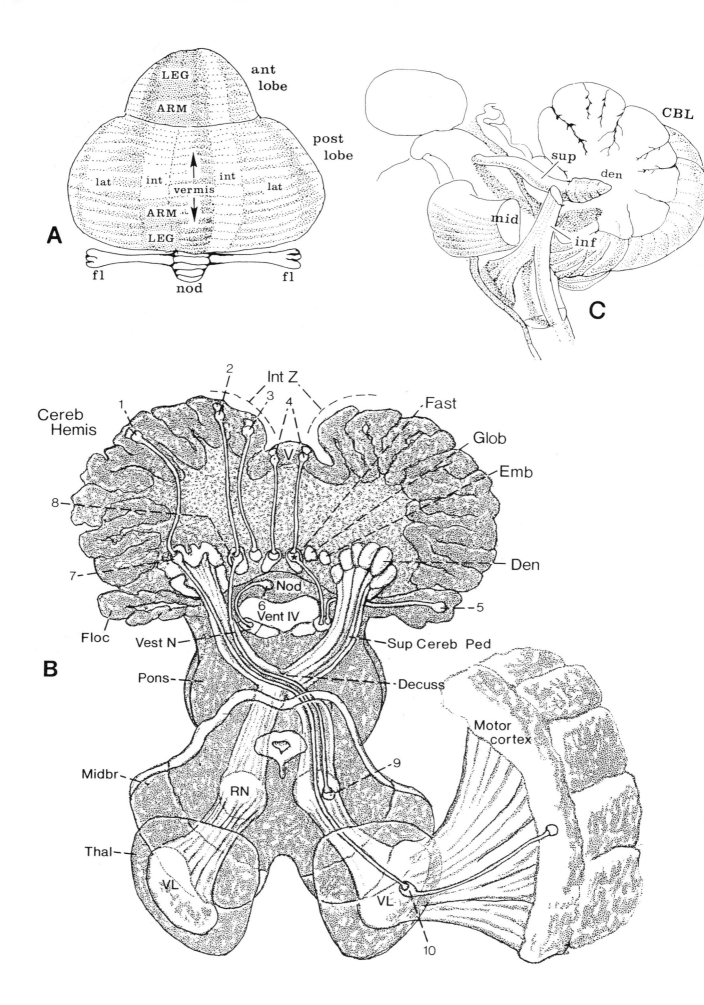

Color and label the four cerebellar nuclei deep within the cerebellum.

D   Dentate nucleus
E   Emboliform nucleus
G   Globose nucleus
F   Fastigial nucleus

The only fibers that leave the cerebellar cortex are the axons of Purkinje neurons. Purkinje neurons (1, 2, and 3) in the cortex of the cerebellar hemispheres project axons centrally to end upon neurons (4) in the dentate nucleus. Dentate neurons (4) send axons rostrally to end upon neurons (5) in the ventral lateral (VL) nucleus of the thalamus. Thalamic VL neurons then project axons to the motor cortex. Purkinje neuron 6 in the intermediate zone projects its fiber to the emboliform nucleus, where it ends upon neuron 7. Neuron 7 projects to the red nucleus where it ends upon red nucleus neuron 8. Red nucleus neuron 8 projects to the inferior olive. Inferior olive neuron 9 projects to the opposite cerebellar cortex. Purkinje neurons 10 in the vermal cortex project to the fastigial nucleus. Color neurons 1-10.

Color and label

V	Vermis of cerebellum
Inf Olive	Inferior olivary nucleus
CH	Cerebellar hemisphere
RN	Red nucleus
Dec sup cbl ped	Decussation of the superior cerebellar peduncle (hence its former name, Latin, *brachium conjunctivum,* the arm that is joined)
Thal	Thalamus
VL	Ventral lateral nucleus of thalamus
11	Dentatothalamic fibers
12	Emboliform to red nucleus fiber
13	Rubro-olivary fiber. Formerly, central tegmental tract
14	Olivocerebellar fibers. These enter the cerebellum via the inferior cerebellar peduncle
15	Climbing fibers. These climb like vines and make numerous synapses upon Purkinje neurons. Climbing fibers arise exclusively from the opposite inferior olivary complex (inferior olivary nucleus, medial accessory olivary nucleus, dorsal accessory olivary nucleus).
16	Thalamocortical fibers

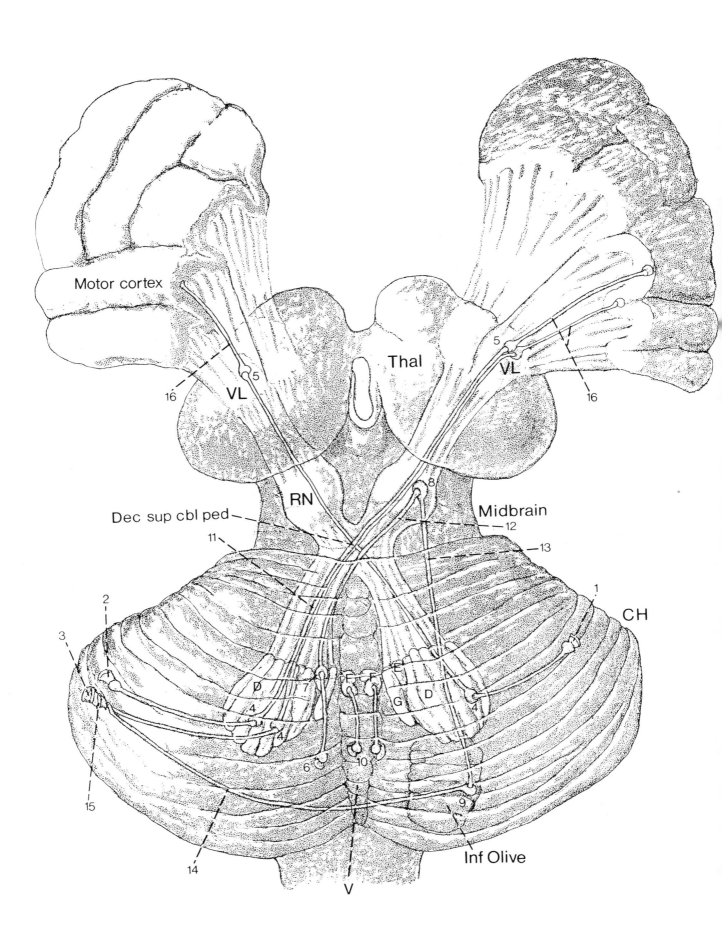

Motor cortex

VL

16

5

Thal

RN

VL

5

16

Dec sup cbl ped

Midbrain

8

12

11

13

2

1

CH

3

D

7

F F F

E

G

D

4

4

15

6

10

9

14

Inf Olive

V

Color and label

PN	Pontine nuclei. Partially dissected (in pons ventral to cerebellum)
Inf O	Inferior olivary nucleus: partially dissected (in medulla)
Med acc O	Medial accessory olivary nucleus
D	Dentate nucleus
E	Emboliform nucleus
G	Globose nucleus
F	Fastigial nucleus
ECN	External cuneate nucleus (in medulla)
DSCT	Dorsal spinocerebellar tract
VSCT	Ventral spinocerebellar tract

The **dorsal spinocerebellar tract** (DSCT) carries touch, temperature, and proprioception from the leg and lower trunk to the two spinal regions of the cerebellar cortex . Neurons 1 and 2 are the cells of origin of the DSCT. They lie in the nucleus dorsalis (Clark's column). Their axons group together ascend as the dorsal spinocerebellar tract, and then enter the cerebellum by way of the inferior cerebellar peduncle. The dorsal spinocerebellar tract projects to the "leg" region of both homolateral spinocerebellar cortices. Neuron 1 projects to the anterior spinocerebellar cortex and neuron 2 projects to the posterior spinocerebellar cortex. Each spinocerebellar cortex receives a complete projection of the same half of the body. **Color** neurons 1 and 2.

The **cuneocerebellar tract** is the arm and upper trunk equivalent of the dorsal spinocerebellar tract. It carries proprioception, touch, and temperature from the arm and upper trunk to the corresponding cortical regions of the spinocerebellar cortex. Its cells of origin (7 and 8) lie in the **external cuneate nucleus** (ECN), which is the cervical equivalent of the nucleus dorsalis. Its fibers also enter the cerebellum by way of the inferior cerebellar peduncle. **Color** neurons 7 and 8.

The **ventral spinocerebellar tract** (VSCT) crosses the midline and is largely a crossed tract that ascends on the opposite side of the spinal cord. It enters the cerebellum via the superior cerebellar peduncle. However, it crosses the midline again and ends in the "leg" and "lower trunk" region of homolateral spinocerebellar cortex. The VSCT carries proprioception from the leg and lower trunk. **Color** neurons 5 and 6.

The **rostral spinocerebellar tract** (RSCT) is the arm and upper trunk equivalent of the ventral spinocerebellar tract. Its cells of origin (3, 4) lie in the gray matter of the cervical spinal cord. Its fibers end in the "arm" and "upper trunk" region of both spinocerebellar cortices. **Color** neuron 3 and 4.

Neurons 9 and 10 in the inferior olivary nucleus (Inf O) and neuron 11 in the medial accessory olivary nucleus (Med acc O) project by way of olivocerebellar fibers to the opposite cerebellar cortex, where specific cortical strips (indicated by arrows) are supplied by specific regions of the inferior olivary nucleus. **Color** neurons 9, 10, and 11.

The pontocerebellar fibers arise from neuron cell bodies in the pontine nuclei (12, 13, and 14) and make up the largest input into the cerebellum (approximately 20 million fibers). Pontocerebellar fibers cross the midline, group together as the middle cerebellar peduncle (brachium pontis), and project to the entire cerebellar cortex with the exception of the nodulus. Pontocerebellar fibers end as mossy fibers in the cerebellar cortex, as do the four spinocerebellar tracts. Olivocerebellar fibers, on the other hand, end as climbing fibers. Pontocerebellar fibers from particular parts of the pontine nucleus end in the opposite cortex in the small circular zone indicated by PC. **Color** neurons 12, 13, and 14.

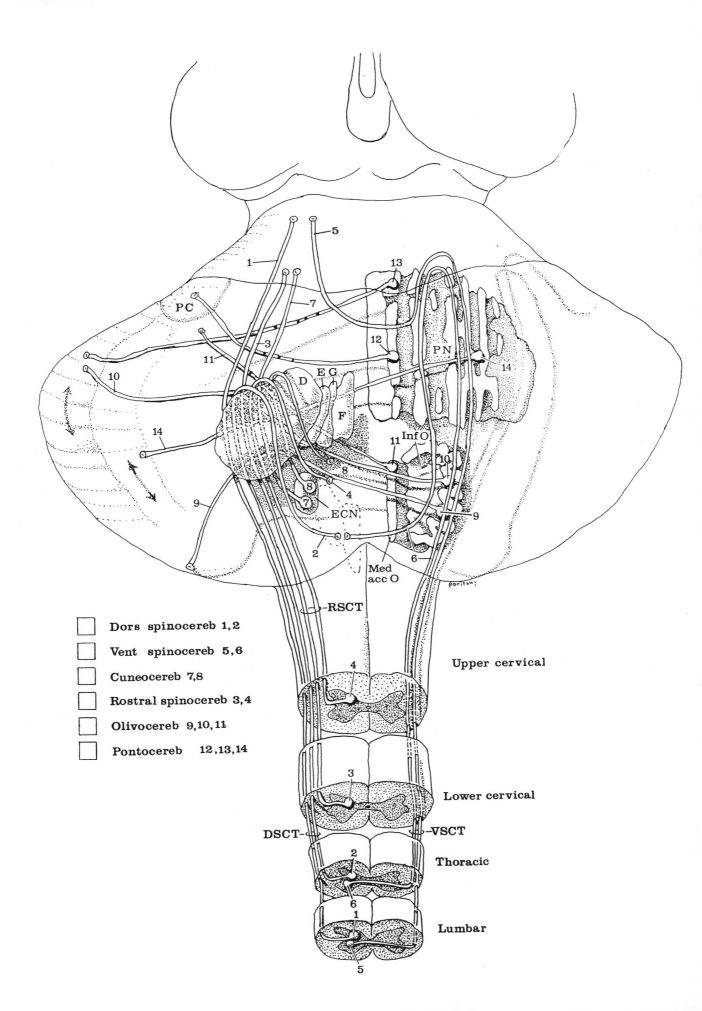

Dors spinocereb 1,2
Vent spinocereb 5,6
Cuneocereb 7,8
Rostral spinocereb 3,4
Olivocereb 9,10,11
Pontocereb 12,13,14

Upper cervical

Lower cervical

Thoracic

Lumbar

PC
13
1
5
7
12
PN
3
11
D
E G
14
10
F
14
InfO
11
8
10
8
9
7
4
ECN
9
2
6
Med
acc O
RSCT
4
3
DSCT
VSCT
2
6
1
5

Neuron 1 in the motor cortex projects its **corticopontine** axon to the pons where it synapses upon pontine neuron 2. Pontine neuron 2 sends a pontocerebellar fiber to the opposite cerebellar cortex where it becomes a **mossy fiber** and synapses with granule cell 3. The axon of granule cell 3 divides like a T into a **parallel fiber** (pf) that makes synaptic contact with the dendritic tree of Purkinje neurons 4 and 5. Purkinje neurons 4, 5, and 6 project their axons centrally to the **dentate nucleus** (D) where they contact dentate nucleus neurons 7, 8, and 9. Neuron 7 gives off a **nucleocortical** collateral fiber (ncf) that extends back to the cerebellar cortex. The main axon of neuron 7 joins fibers 8 and 9 and together form the **brachium conjunctivum** (bc, superior cerebellar peduncle). These fibers cross the midline (decussate) and enter the opposite red nucleus where fiber 7 gives off a collateral to neuron 12. Fibers 7 and 8 continue rostrally to the ventral lateral thalamic nucleus (VL) where they end with synaptic terminals upon neurons 10 and 11. The latter two then project up to the motor cortex.

The loop of neurons is believed to function as a feedback mechanism by which motor commands issuing from the cerebral cortex are sent to the cerebellar cortex where they are compared with all ongoing muscle activity. The cerebellum appears to correct and modify these muscle commands by its projection back to the motor region of the cerebral cortex. Another probable feedback loop involves the red nucleus. Neuron 12 in the red nucleus projects caudally to the inferior olive where it synapses upon neuron 13. Neuron 13 in the inferior olive sends its olivocerebellar fiber to the opposite cerebellar cortex where it ends as a climbing fiber (cf) upon Purkinje neuron 6. The loop is completed by the neuron 6 projection to 7, which projects back to 12.

Purkinje neuron 14 (left center) projects to neuron 15 in the **emboliform nucleus** (E), which sends its axon via the brachium conjunctivum to the opposite red nucleus where it synapses upon neuron 25. Neuron 25 gives rise to the **rubrospinal** fiber, which crosses the midline and descends in the lateral funiculus of the spinal cord (RST). Purkinje neuron 16 in the posterior vermis projects to the **fastigial nucleus** (F) where it contacts fastigial neuron 17. Note that fastigial neurons 17 and 18, which lie in the posterior part of the fastigial nucleus, both send their axon across the midline, **through** the opposite fastigial nucleus to the opposite medial (M) and inferior (I) vestibular nuclei. Purkinje neuron 19 projects to fastigial neuron 20 which, together with fastigial neuron 21, projects to the ipsilateral vestibular nuclei, neuron 20 to the superior vestibular nucleus (S), and 21 to the medial vestibular nucleus (M). Purkinje neurons 22 and 23, both in the vermis of the anterior lobe, project to the lateral vestibular nucleus (L). Note that 22, which is anterior (leg), projects to the posterior part of the lateral vestibular nucleus, whereas posterior 23 (arm) projects to the anterior part. Neuron 24 in the flocculus projects directly to the superior vestibular nucleus (S).

Abbreviations

BC	Brachium conjunctivum (superior cerebellar peduncle)	L	Lateral vestibular nucleus
		I	Inferior vestibular nucleus
D	Dentate nucleus	RST	Rubrospinal tract
E	Emboliform nucleus	RN	Red nucleus
G	Globose nucleus	VL	Ventral lateral nucleus of the thalamus
F	Fastigial nucleus	mf	Mossy fiber
Inf O	Inferior olivary nucleus	pf	Parallel fiber
S	Superior vestibular nucleus	cf	Climbing fiber
M	Medial vestibular nucleus	ncf	Nucleocortical fiber

Color and label

1	Corticopontine fiber	9	Dentatorubro fiber
2	Pontocerebellar fiber	10,11	Thalamocortical fibers
3	Granule cell	12	Rubro-olivary fiber
4,5,6	Purkinje neurons	13	Olivocerebellar fiber
7,8	Dentatothalamic fibers		

Trace and color the course of neurons 14-25.

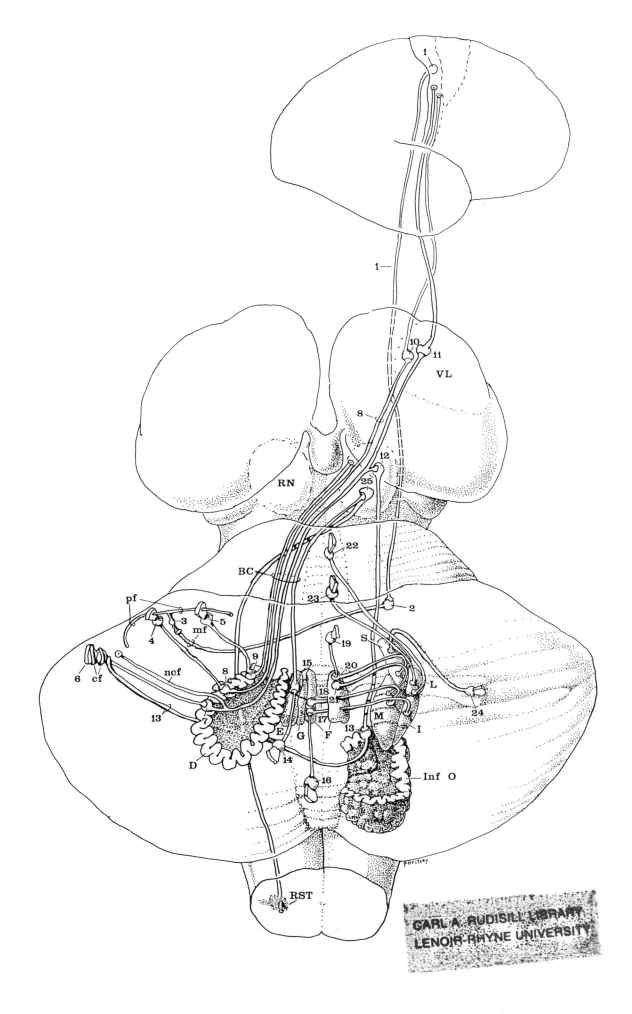

Figure A. Sagittal view of the cerebellum and brain stem

The cerebellar cortex consists of narrow leaf-like gyri or folds, each of which is called a folium, which means leaf in Latin (plural, folia). Only about 15% of the cerebellar cortex is visible. The remaining 85% lies hidden in deep folds and subfolds. Beneath the cortex lies the white matter, consisting of myelinated fibers running to and from the cortex. Earlier anatomists likened the cerebellar white matter to a tree and called it the *arbor vitae* (Latin, the tree of life). The encircled area is enlarged in Figure B. **Label the following:** (1) nodulus, (2) fourth ventricle. (3) pons, (4) medulla, (5) pineal gland, (6) spinal cord, and (7) cerebral aqueduct.

Figure B. Simplified view of the cerebellar cortex

Unlike the cerebral cortex, which varies in cell types from one region to another, the cerebellar cortex is remarkably uniform and has the same neuronal cells throughout its entire extent. This view shows the three cortical layers: the outer molecular layer (mol), the intermediate Purkinje layer (Pur), and the inner granule layer (gr). Note the arrangement of the Purkinje cell dendrites (p den), which lie in a plane that is transverse to the folds or folia of the cortex. **Color and label** the Purkinje neurons (p), their dendritic trees shown in fan-like planes (p den), and their axons running into the white matter.

Figure C. Cerebellar cortical neurons and interneuron connections

Incoming impulses reach the cerebellar cortex by only two kinds of fibers, mossy fibers and climbing fibers. **Locate mossy fiber 1 and follow it as it ascends.** Note that it gives off a collateral fiber to cerebellar nucleus neuron 13 that lies in one of the four cerebellar nuclei. **Color and label** mossy fiber 1 and cerebellar nucleus neuron 13. Note that mossy fiber 1 divides into several terminal branches, each of which makes synaptic contact with the dendrite of a granule neuron (2). Each mossy fiber-to-granule cell dendrite synapse also involves the terminal of a Golgi cell axon (8). These three elements form a cerebellar rosette (**Figure D**). The axon (3) of granule cell 2 extends to the molecular layer where it divides like a T and forms parallel fiber 4. Fiber 9 is a parallel fiber from another granule cell. Parallel fibers run along the axis of the folium, where a single parallel fiber will synapse upon Golgi cell dendrites (5), Purkinje cell dendrites (6), stellate cell dendrites (10), and basket cell dendrites (15). **Color and label** the granule cell, its axon, and its parallel fiber (2,3,4,9).

The total length of a parallel fiber probably exceeds 3 mm (3,000 μm) and one parallel fiber may act upon 450 Purkinje neurons. A single Purkinje neuron may have as many as 400,000 parallel fibers passing through its dendritic tree and hence be affected by a tremendous number of granule cells. The Golgi cell is an inhibitory neuron, and its axonal branches form inhibitory terminals on the mossy fiber axon endings. **Color Golgi 7, its dendrites (5), and its axonal branches (8). Color stellate neurons 10 and 11**, which make inhibitory synapses on Purkinje cell bodies. **Color basket neuron 14 and its axon**, which make basket-like endings (18) on Purkinje cell bodies. **Color the course of climbing fiber 12.** Note that, like the mossy fiber, it gives off a collateral fiber to cerebellar nuclear neuron 13. It also sends fibers to basket cell 14 and stellate cell 15. Its main axon (12) is directed to Purkinje cell 16 and its dendrites, which it entwines and climbs upon like ivy tendrils on a tree (17). Of the five cell types in the cerebellar cortex, *four are inhibitory neurons* and only *one is excitatory*. The granule cell is excitatory. The other four are inhibitory. **Color the Purkinje cells (16) and the basket cell (14).** The squares in the lower right may be used as color keys.

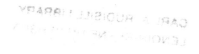

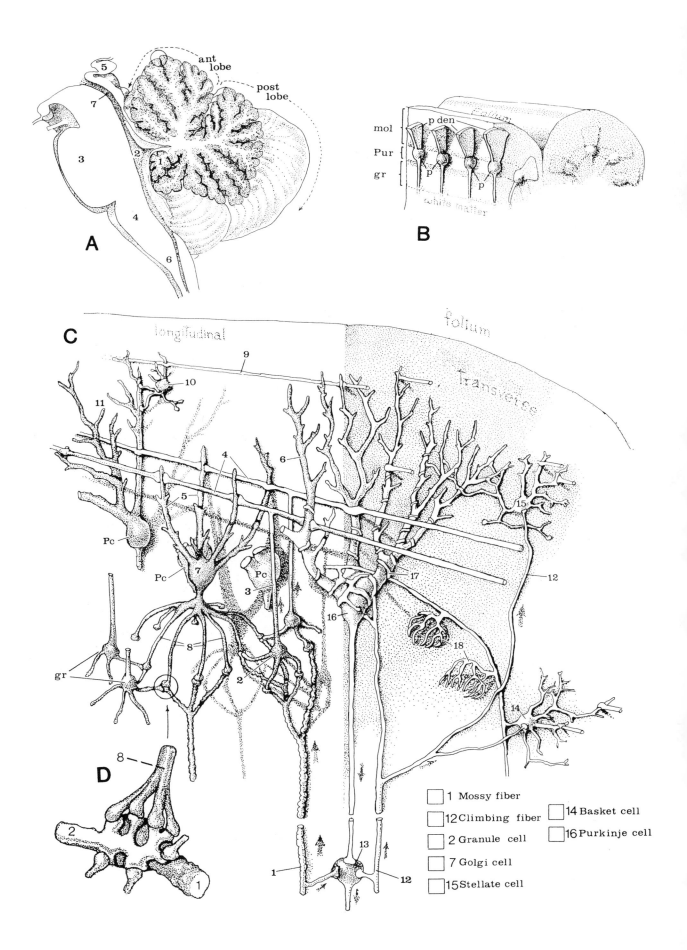

A

ant lobe
post lobe
5
7
3
2
1
4
6

B

mol
Pur
gr
p den
p
p
folium
white matter

C

longitudinal
folium
transverse
9
10
11
4
6
5
Pc
Pc
7
3
Pc
8
gr
2
17
16
18
12
15
14
13
1
12

D

8
2
1

1 Mossy fiber	14 Basket cell
12 Climbing fiber	16 Purkinje cell
2 Granule cell	
7 Golgi cell	
15 Stellate cell	

Cerebellar dysfunction is most marked if either the superior cerebellar peduncle or dentate nucleus is damaged. If either of these structures is affected, the following symptoms are likely to occur and will be on the same side as the cerebellar damage.

Figure A.   Dysmetria

The inability to correctly judge distance and direction when performing a movement. It is seen particularly when the patient tries to touch his nose or the examiner's finger. The hand overshoots its mark (hypermetria) or veers to the side.

Figure B.   Loss of the check reflex

The inability to stop a movement against resistance if the examiner suddenly removes his restraining hand from the patient's limb (Holmes rebound phenomenon).

Figure C.   Jerky conjugate gaze

Movement of the eyes is jerky rather than smooth. Nystagmus may or may not be present. Nystagmus is a spontaneous, rapid, rhythmic movement of the eyes. It can occur either when the eyes are moving or when the eyes are fixed on a stationary object. Nystagmus can be indicative of damage to a number of sites such as the cerebellum, the vestibular part of the inner ear, or the nuclei of nerves III, IV and VI.

Figure D.   Adiadochokinesia

A clumsiness in performing rapid alternating movements such as pronation and supination of the hands and forearms.

Figure E.   Intention tremor (or action tremor)

This occurs only during movement and becomes worse at the end of the movement.

Figure F.   Hypotonia (decrease in muscle tone).   Muscles feel flabby when

examined and there is a marked lessening of resistance to passive movement.

Ataxia. Unsteadiness and incoordination of movement. Tendency to deviate to the affected side on walking. Gait is wide-based, unsteady, and irregular. The patient may lurch from side to side.

Dysarthria. A slowness of speech. Words are not pronounced correctly, and the syllables of each word are unnaturally separated (scanning). Some words may be uttered with excessive force (explosive speech) and others lack sufficient breath to be heard.

Figures A, B, C, D, and F drawn by Janice Lalikos.

SYMPTOMS OF CEREBELLAR DISEASE

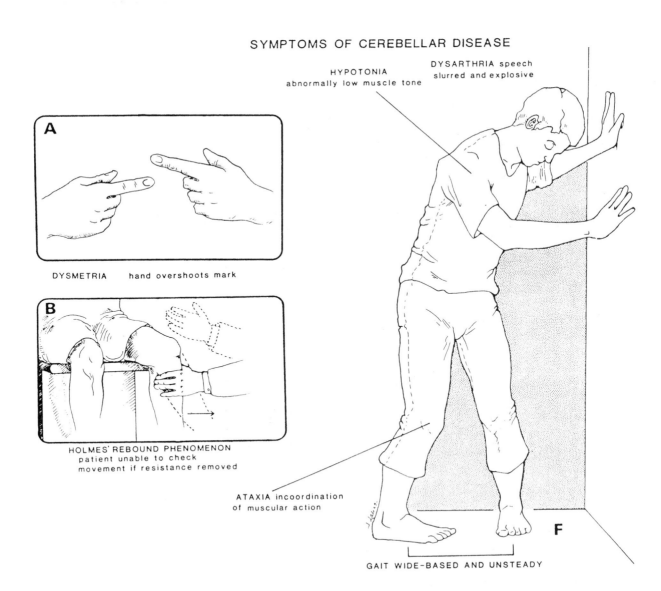

HYPOTONIA
abnormally low muscle tone

DYSARTHRIA speech
slurred and explosive

A

DYSMETRIA   hand overshoots mark

B

HOLMES' REBOUND PHENOMENON
patient unable to check
movement if resistance removed

ATAXIA incoordination
of muscular action

F

GAIT WIDE-BASED AND UNSTEADY

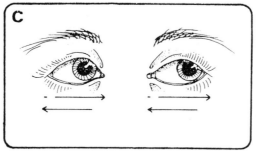

C

CONJUGATE GAZE IS JERKY

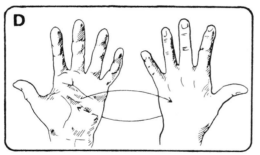

D

ADIADOCHOKINESIA   difficulty in performing
rapid alternating movements

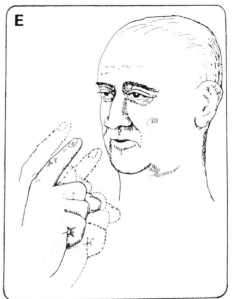

E

INTENTION TREMOR worst at end of movement

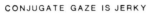

The main outflow from the corpus striatum is by two fiber tracts that arise in the medial segment of the globus pallidus and end in the thalamus. Thus, in terms of their origin and ending, they are **pallidothalamic** tracts (or fasciculi). These two tracts are the **fasciculus lenticularis** and the **ansa lenticularis.**

Fasciculus lenticulus. The fibers of the fasciculus lenticularis begin in the dorsal part of the medial pallidal segment (1,2), emerge from its dorsal medial segment, and penetrate the internal capsule in little bundles (fasc lent). The fibers continue posteriorly and converge in the space between the subthalamic nucleus below and the zona incerta above. This region is **field (or area) H2 of Forel.** They then proceed posteriorly and medially to the region in front of the red nucleus. This region is **field (or area) H of Forel,** or the prerubral field. Most of the fibers then turn superiorly and laterally to join the **thalamic fasciculus,** which ascends between the zona incerta and the thalamus. The fibers of the fasciculus lenticulus end in thalamic nuclei VL (ventral lateral) (5) and ventral anterior (VA) (not shown in drawing).The thalamic fasciculus itself constitutes **field (or area) H1 of Forel.** The drawing shows the thalamus as hollow with only its border, which is partly cut away.

Ansa lenticularis. The fibers that make up the **ansa lenticularis** (Latin, *ansa,* curved handle) begin with cell bodies (3,4) that lie in the medial pallidal segment. They sweep rostrally and medially and make a loop (or ansa) around the internal capsule, thus forming the ansa lenticularis (ansa lent). Continuing posteriorly they join fibers from the fasciculus lenticularis in the prerubral field H and ascend with them as part of the **thalamic fasciculus.** Fibers in the ansa lenticulus end on neurons (5) in the VL thalamic nucleus, whereas those in the fasciculus lenticulus end in both the VL thalamic nucleus (5) as well as the more rostral VA thalamic nucleus. Fibers arising from neurons (5) in the VA/VL complex then project to the motor cortex.

Neurons 8 and 9 indicate an efferent pathway from the **corpus striatum** (caudate nucleus and lentiform nucleus) to the **substantia nigra.** Hence, it is a **striatonigral** pathway. Two fibers arise from neuron 8 in the putamen and the other from neuron 9 in the caudate nucleus. Both fibers labelled 8 pass through the globus pallidus where they give off collaterals to neurons 3 and 4. The main axons of 8 continue caudally and obliquely through the internal capsule to the substantia nigra to end upon nigral neurons 13. Caudate nucleus neuron 9 also gives rise to striatonigral fiber that passes through the globus pallidus where it too gives off a collateral fiber to pallidal neuron 1, and eventually ends on another nigral neuron 13.

Fibers 10, 11, 12 represent **corticostriatal** fibers that project from the cerebral cortex to the caudate nucleus and putamen. Thus there is a neuronal loop formed by fibers from cerebral cortex to striatum, which projects to the globus pallidus, which projects to the thalamus, which then projects back to the cerebral cortex.

Fibers 6 and 7 represent the anterior and posterior limbs of the internal capsule, respectively.

Directions: use one color for neurons 3 and 4 and label them **ansa lenticularis;** use another for neurons 1 and 2 and label them **fasciculus lenticularis;** and use a third color for neurons 8 and 9 and label them **striatopallidonigral** fibers.

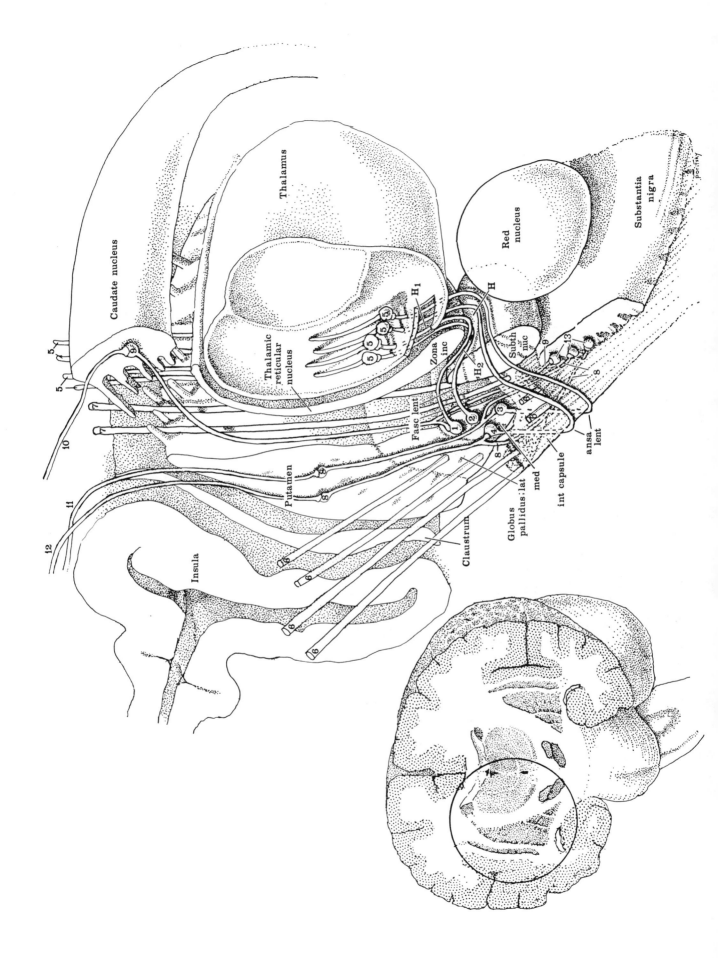

Caudate nucleus

Thalamus

Thalamic
reticular
nucleus

Red
nucleus

Substantia
nigra

H₁

H

Zona
inc

Subth
nuc

Fasc lent

H₂

Putamen

Globus
pallidus : lat
med

ansa
lent

int capsule

Claustrum

Insula

porttky

Neuron 1 in the head of the caudate nucleus gives rise to **striatonigral fiber** that sends a collateral to a pallidal neuron as it passes through the globus pallidus. The caudate nucleus and putamen are the *striatum*; *nigro* stands for the substantia nigra. Thus fiber 1 is a **striatonigral fiber**. **Neuron 2** in the dorsal **pars compacta** of the substantia nigra gives rise to **nigrostriatal fiber** 1 that ends upon a neuron in the head of the caudate. Fibers 3 and 5 are also nigrostriatal fibers that start in the substantia nigra, but these end in the putamen. Nigrostriatal fibers such as 2, 3, and 5 use **dopamine** as their neurotransmitter. Thus these fibers function as **dopaminergic** fibers, that is, they release dopamine at their synaptic endings (Greek, *ergon*, work). The loss of these cells in the substantia nigra and the degeneration of their dopaminergic fibers appear to be the cause of Parkinson's disease. Neuron 4 in the substantia sends a **nigrothalamic** fiber to the ventral lateral (VL) thalamic nucleus.

Color and label

Fiber 1	Striatonigral fiber
Fibers 2,3,5	Nigrostriatal fibers
Fiber 4	Nigrothalamic fiber

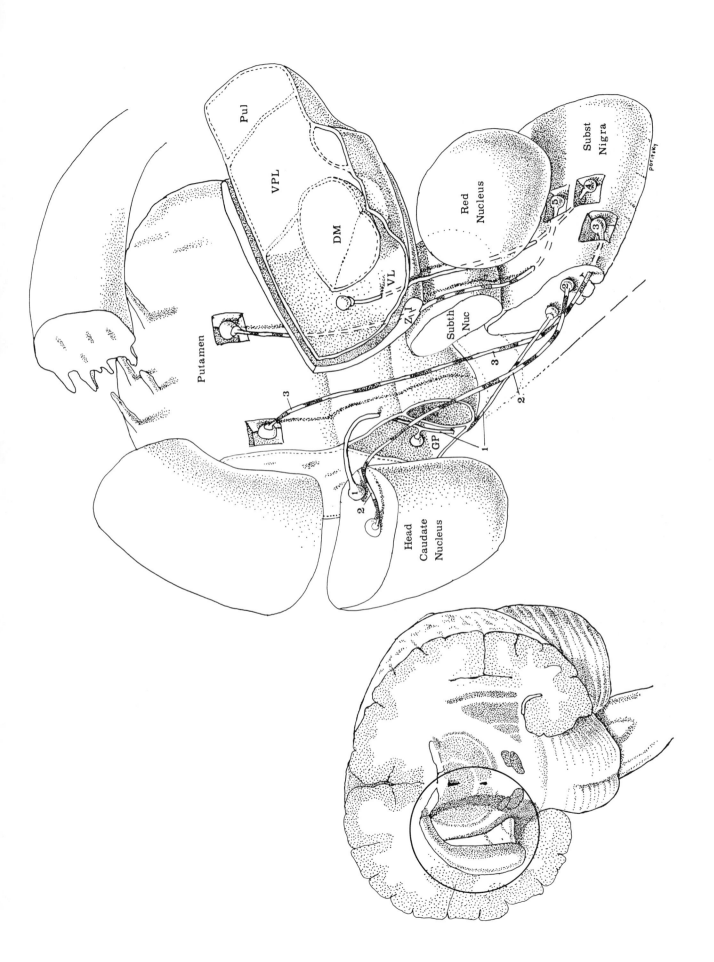

Parkinson's disease, first described by James Parkinson in 1817, is caused by the destruction of pigmented cells in the substantia nigra and in other pigmented nuclei such as the locus ceruleus. These pigmented cells release dopamine at their terminals, and their degeneration results in a depletion of dopamine in both the putamen and caudate nucleus. The term **parkinsonism** refers to a group of symptoms that characterize this disease.

Symptoms of Parkinson's Disease

An **expressionless, mask-like face** that conveys no emotion. Extra wide, unblinking eyes impart a blank staring appearance, the reptilian stare.

A **cogwheel rigidity** is felt when the examiner moves a limb. As the limb is passively moved and the muscles stretched, the examiner feels the muscles alternately relax, then briefly contract, then further relax. This alternate relaxing and contracting feels, to the examiner, like the limb is being pulled over the teeth of a cogwheel.

A **poverty and slowness of all voluntary movement**. This includes an absence of swinging the arms in walking, a slowness in chewing, and an absence of adjustment movements in both sitting and standing. It may take an hour to eat a meal. Handwriting becomes cramped and small (micrographia). The voice weakens until it is only a whisper and conveys practically no emotion.

Shuffling gait. Walking is reduced to a shuffle, with the patient frequently losing his balance. Walking turns into a rapid, stiff shuffle as the patient chases his center of gravity. This ever-accelerating gait is the festinating gait (Latin, *festinare,* to hasten).

Resting tremor. The disease usually begins as a slight tremor of one hand, arm, or leg. This usually takes the form of a four-per-second "pill-rolling" tremor that affects the thumb and fingers. It is a "resting" tremor because it occurs only in the absence of movement. It disappears during voluntary movement only to reappear when the movement ceases. It is not uncommon to see a patient who has been trembling violently raise a full glass of water to his lips and drain its contents without spilling a drop.

Intellectual decline. Intellectual deterioration does not occur until late in the disease, with dementia eventually affecting one-third of patients. The symptoms are aggravated by stress and anxiety, but alleviated by relaxation and encouragement. Depression is common. However, exercise and special home aids can improve both the sufferer's mobility and morale. Drugs, particularly levodopa, which the body converts to dopamine, have proved somewhat effective in reducing the symptoms, but they cannot halt the degeneration of brain cells. Moreover, the beneficial effects of levodopa may suddenly stop, necessitating that another drug or combination of drugs be given.

Adams R, Victor M (eds): Principles of Neurology, 4th ed. New York, McGraw-Hill, 1989.

Clayman, CB (ed): The American Medical Association Encyclopedia of Medicine. New York, Random House, 1989: p. 772.

Drawn by Joseph Kanasz.

PARKINSON'S DISEASE

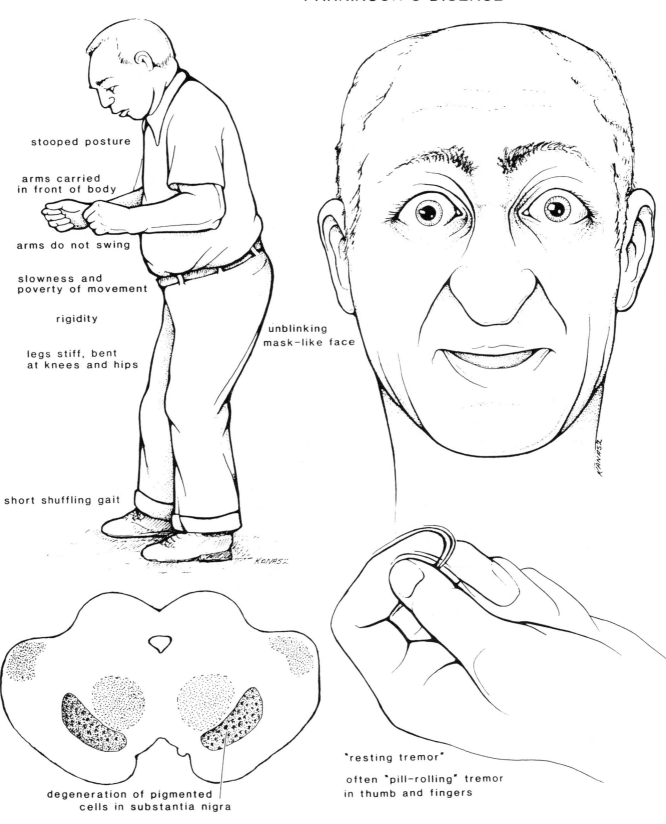

stooped posture

arms carried
in front of body

arms do not swing

slowness and
poverty of movement

rigidity

legs stiff, bent
at knees and hips

short shuffling gait

unblinking
mask-like face

degeneration of pigmented
cells in substantia nigra

'resting tremor'

often 'pill-rolling' tremor
in thumb and fingers

Chorea is the name given to certain convulsive movements of a forcible and rapid nature that resemble a sort of dance. (*Chorea* means dance in Greek.) It is caused by the degeneration of neurons in the caudate nucleus and putamen.

Huntington's chorea is a progressive neurological disorder characterized by mental deterioration and choreiform (dance-like) movements. It is a hereditary disease that usually first appears between 35 and 45 years of age, although in rare instances it shows up in early childhood. It is transmitted from parent to offspring as a dominant genetic factor, the faulty gene located on the terminal segment of the short arm of chromosome 4. Children of one parent with Huntington's chorea have a 50% chance of inheriting the disease. The choreiform movements are sudden, purposeless, and jerky, and usually affect the muscles of the trunk, shoulders, and hips. Facial grimacing is common in the early stages of the disease. As the disease progresses, the simple act of walking is compounded by sudden twisting movements of the trunk and forward tipping of the pelvis, so the individual's gait appears to be part walking and part prancing. These abnormal movements are exacerbated by emotional stress; however, they disappear during sleep. Memory impairment is progressive and is accompanied by a failing intellect, a disregard for personal cleanliness, and general apathy . There may be fits of depression, irritability, impulsive behavior, and even outbursts of violence. Eventually the irreversible mental deterioration and bizarre emotional behavior necessitate that the patient be institutionalized. There is no cure for the disease, which is progressive. It ends in death about 15 years from the time of its first appearance, not from the disease itself but usually from an acquired infection. Suicide is not uncommon.

Sydenham's chorea (also called Saint Vitus' dance, rheumatic chorea, chorea minor) is a CNS disorder that is also characterized by chorea or sudden, aimless, spasmodic movements. It is rarely fatal, with the patient usually recovering in one to four months. However, the affliction usually results in a loss of neurons in the corpus striatum. The disease is apparently caused by the same streptococcal bacillus that causes rheumatic fever, in which case it follows the infection by several months after all other symptoms have disappeared. Once inside the brain, these same bacilli affect neurons in the caudate nucleus and subthalamic nucleus. The choreiform movements are sudden, jerking, and flinging, and affect the face, tongue, and limbs. It most often affects children, adolescents, and young adults. In addition to the choreic movements, the victim will display emotional lability . Following recovery, the emotional lability may persist for a considerable period and relapses may follow upper respiratory infection. Rheumatic heart disease is an occasional sequel.

Drawn by Joseph Kanasz.

CHOREA

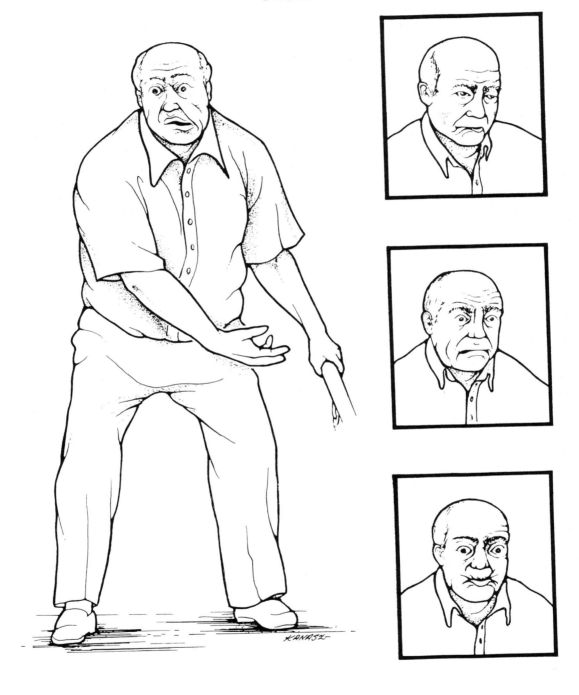

Athetosis (Greek, not stable; *a*, not; *theto*, put or fixed). This is a peculiar type of dyskinesia (abnormal movement) characterized by continuous, slow, twisting, writhing, worm-like movements usually involving the hands and feet. The affected individual is unable to sustain any group of muscles in one position. The disease results from damage to the corpus striatum. Emotional stimulation intensifies the movements, whereas they improve with rest and disappear during sleep. A typical athetoid movement is shown on the opposite page, in which the forearm and hand continually alternate between flexion/supination and extension/pronation. Athetoid movement is slower than that seen in chorea.

Hemiballism (Greek, a half throwing; *hemi*, half; *ballo*, to throw). It is so named because of the violent flinging of the arm and/or leg confined to one side of the body. The muscles of the shoulders and/or hips undergo sudden and forceful rotary contractions that result in the limbs being thrown about aimlessly. The movements are continuous but cease during sleep. In the past the thrashing about often resulted in death from exhaustion. It can now be treated with tranquilizing drugs and stereotactic surgery. This affliction is the result of an infarction (tissue death from occluded blood flow) in the opposite subthalamic nucleus.

Drawn by Joseph Kanasz.

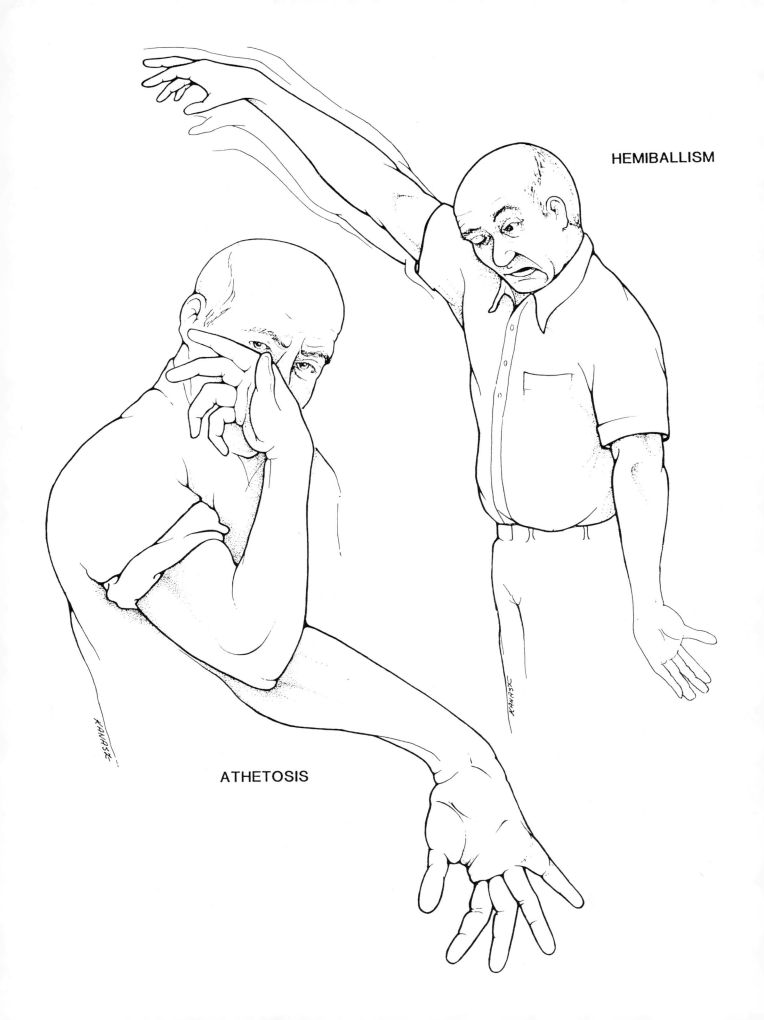

HEMIBALLISM

ATHETOSIS

Amygdala, stria terminalis, and ventral amygdalofugal pathway

The amygdala (amygdaloid body or complex) is an almond-shaped mass of nerve cells just beneath the medial surface of the temporal lobe (Greek, *amygdale*, almond). It is usually divided into corticomedial and basolateral cell groups. The figures below show two of its main efferent pathways in highly simplified form.

The stria terminalis is a bundle of fibers that arises from neurons in the corticomedial part of the amygdala and ends mainly in the hypothalamus. The stria terminalis curves in an arc along the medial surface of the tail of the caudate nucleus, beginning at the amygdala and ending just above the anterior commissure (ac).

Figure A shows the **left amygdala and left stria terminalis** superimposed upon the **right half** of the brain. Figures B and C have a similar orientation. Figure E is a frontal section of the right amygdala in the plane indicated by X-X in Figure A and by plane Y-Y in Figure D. The fibers in the stria terminalis fall into three groups:

Commissural fibers (1,12), which **cross** via the anterior commissure to the opposite side and end in the opposite amygdala.

Precommissural fibers (2,6,8,10), which pass in **front** of the anterior commissure and end in the hypothalamus.

Postcommissural fibers (3,13,14), which pass **behind** the anterior commissure and end in the hypothalamus.

Commissural fiber 1 originates with neuron 1 in Figure A, which lies in the corticomedial part of the amygdala. Fiber 1 travels within the stria terminalis until it reaches the anterior commissure. It enters the anterior commissure, crosses to the opposite side, travels backwards in the opposite stria terminalis, and finally ends in the opposite amygdala.

Precommissural fiber 2 originates with neuron 2 in the corticomedial nuclear group, travels in the stria terminalis, and passes in front of the anterior commissure. It then proceeds downwards and backwards to end in the medial preoptic hypothalamic nucleus (4).

Postcommissural fiber 3 originates with neuron 3 in the basolateral nuclear group. It enters the stria terminalis, passes behind the anterior commissure, and ends in either the anterior hypothalamic nucleus (5) or in the bed nucleus of the stria terminalis, which is collections of neurons lying adjacent to the stria terminalis (Figure C).

Figure B shows the path of three precommissural fibers. Amygdala neuron 6 projects to the medial hypothalamic nucleus (7). Amygdala neuron 8 projects to the anterior hypothalamic nucleus (9). Amygdala neuron 10 projects to the ventromedial hypothalamic nucleus (11).

Figure C shows the trajectory of two postcommissural fibers. Neuron 13 projects to the bed nucleus of the stria terminalis. Neuron 14 projects to the anterior hypothalamic nucleus by passing posterior to the anterior commissure. Commissural neuron 12 in the cortical amygdaloid nucleus projects via anterior commissure to the opposite cortical amygdaloid nucleus.

The **ventral amygdalofugal pathway** refers to a large assortment of fibers that leaves the amygdala in a medial direction and passes along the base of the brain to widely diverse sites.

Figures D and E show three amygdalofugal neurons. Neuron 15 projects to the dorsomedial thalamic nucleus (16). Neuron 17 projects to the lateral preoptic nucleus (18), and neuron 19 (cut) projects to the medial frontal cerebral cortex. Disruption of the ventral amygdalofugal pathway abolishes the defensive reactions in experimental animals.

Directions: Color each of these fiber groups a different color: commissural fibers (1 and 12); precommissural fibers (2,6,8, and 10); postcommissural fibers (3,13, and 14); and ventral amygdalofugal fibers (15,17, and 19).

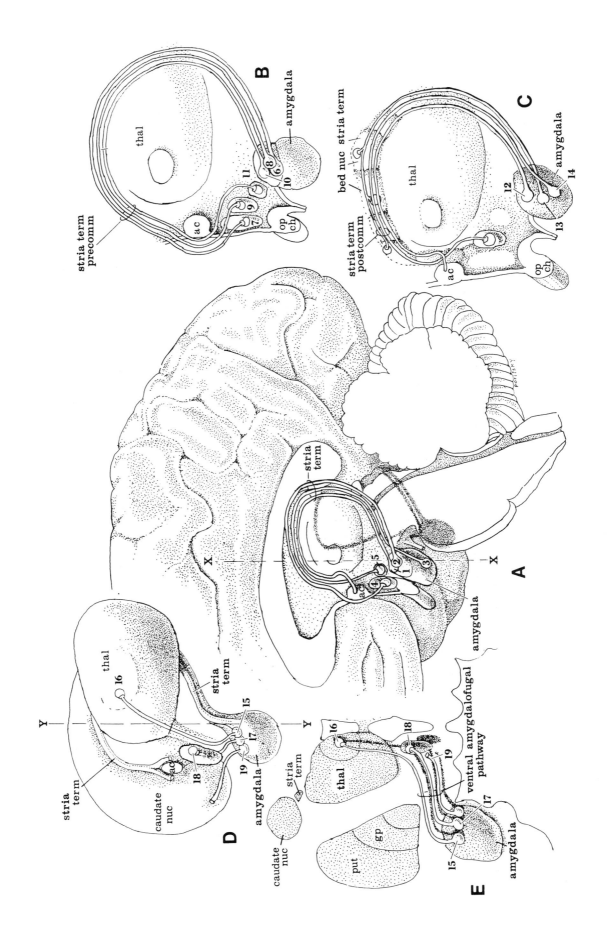

B

stria term
precomm

thal

amygdala

ac

op
ch

11

8
6
10

9
7

C

bed nuc   stria term

stria term
postcomm

thal

amygdala

ac

op
ch

12

14

13

A

stria
term

amygdala

X

X

ac

1
2
5
3
4

D

thal

stria
term

stria
term

caudate
nuc

amygdala

ac

16

15

17

18

19

E

Y

Y

caudate
nuc

thal

stria
term

ventral amygdalofugal
pathway

amygdala

amygdala

gp

put

16

18

19

17

15

The amygdala receives afferents from widely diverse sites in the brain. Some of these afferents are shown on the opposite page in highly simplified form.

Figure A (central figure) shows the lateral view of the left amygdaloid body cut at plane X to reveal its component nuclei. The **cortical nucleus** (cort) and **medial nucleus** (med) are small in humans, receive afferents from the olfactory bulb (1) and the anterior olfactory nucleus (2), and most likely have an olfactory function. The **basal nuclear group** (b) and **lateral nucleus** (lat) are large in humans and probably function in rage and defensive reactions.

Figure B shows the left amygdala and some afferents superimposed on the right half of the brain.

Color and trace amygdala afferent neurons 1–11:
Neuron 1 in the olfactory bulb projects to the corticomedial nuclear group.
Neuron 2 in the anterior olfactory nucleus also projects to the corticomedial group.
Neuron 3 in the primary olfactory cortex projects to the basolateral group.
Neuron 4 in the anterior cingulate gyrus also projects to the basolateral group.
Neuron 5 in the medial frontal cortex projects to the basal, lateral, and central amygdaloid nuclei by entering the stria terminalis, traveling backwards, leaving the stria at the midthalamic level, descending through both the internal capsule and globus pallidus, and ending extensively in the amygdala.
Neuron 6 in the inferior temporal gyrus projects to the basolateral group.
Neuron 7 in the dorsomedial thalamic nucleus projects to the basolateral group.
Neuron 8 in the ventromedial hypothalamic nucleus projects to the central amygdaloid nucleus.
Neuron 9 in the dorsal raphe nucleus projects to the central amygdaloid nucleus.
Neuron 10 in the locus ceruleus projects to the central amygdaloid nucleus.
Neuron 11 in the lateral preoptic hypothalamic nucleus projects to most of the amygdaloid nuclei by way of the stria terminalis.

Uncinate epileptic seizures. The uncus is the hook-shaped rostral end of the parahippocampal gyrus on the medial surface of the temporal lobe directly overlying the amygdala. Uncinate seizures, which have their focus in or near the uncus, often evoke olfactory or gustatory hallucinations, occasionally with chewing movement. In addition there may be emotional hallucinations in which the patient experiences overpowering feelings of dread.

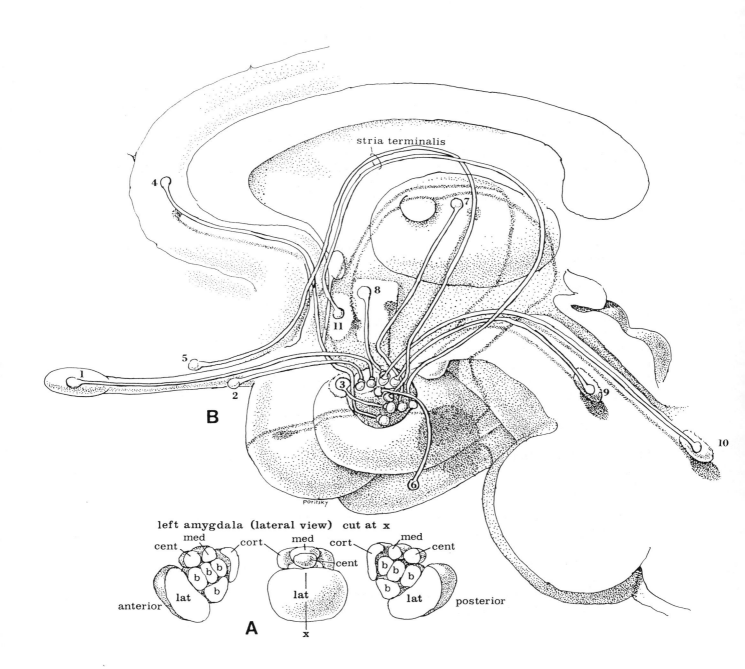

stria terminalis

4

7

8

11

5

1

2

3

9

B

6

10

Poritsky

left amygdala (lateral view) cut at x

cent   med   cort   med   cort   med   cent
                                                       cent
         b b   b   b
      b   b   b   b   b
         b   b
anterior   lat   lat   lat   posterior
                                 x

A

The hippocampal formation (Greek, sea horse) is the ancient three-layered (archicortex) part of the cerebral cortex rolled up inside the temporal lobe of the the brain. It cannot be seen from the outside. It can only be seen if the medial surface of the temporal lobe is pulled apart, exposing the lateral ventricle where the hippocampus forms an arched elevation in the floor of the inferior horn of the lateral ventricle. The **hippocampal formation** consists of two gyri, the **dentate** (Latin, toothed) **gyrus** and the **hippocampus proper** (also **Ammon's horn** or *cornu Ammonis**).The main afferents to the hippocampal formation originate in the entorhinal cortex of the parahippocampal gyrus. Its main outflow is by the fornix, which contains about 1,200,000 fibers and projects to the mamillary nuclei, septal nuclei, and anterior nuclei of the thalamus.

Figure A shows the left hippocampal formation, left fornix (Latin, arch), and left mamillary (breast-like) body superimposed upon the right half of the brain.

Color the hippocampal formation, the fornix, and mamillary body.

Figure B shows some of the hippocampal neural connections.

Trace and color the following:

Neuron 1 in the parahippocampal gyrus (entorhinal cortex; area of the cortex medial to the rhinal fissure; also area 28 of Brodmann) projects to dentate gyrus neuron 2.

Neuron 2 in the dentate gyrus projects to Ammon's horn.

Neuron 3 in Ammon's horn projects to the subiculum (Latin, a small underlying or supporting structure). The subiculum is the superior part of the parahippocampal gyrus, beneath the hippocampus (Ammon's horn).

Neuron 4 in the subiculum gives rise to a fiber that enters the arched fornix and ends in the mamillary body.

Neuron 5 in Ammon's horn sends its fiber into the fornix and ends in septal nucleus neuron 8.

Neuron 6 in the parasubiculum (parahippocampal cortex medial to the subiculum) projects by way of the fornix to the neuron 9 in the anterior thalamus.

Neuron 7 in the cingulate gyrus projects by way of the cingulum (Latin, belt or girdle) in a sweeping arch backward to end in the subiculum.

Neurons destined for the mamillary body originate in the subiculum and not in Ammon's horn, as previously believed. The pyramidal cells in Ammon's horn project largely to the septal nuclei, which are located in front of the columns of the fornix.

* Named for the horns of the ancient Egyptian deity Ammon or Amun, who had the head of a ram and the body of a human.

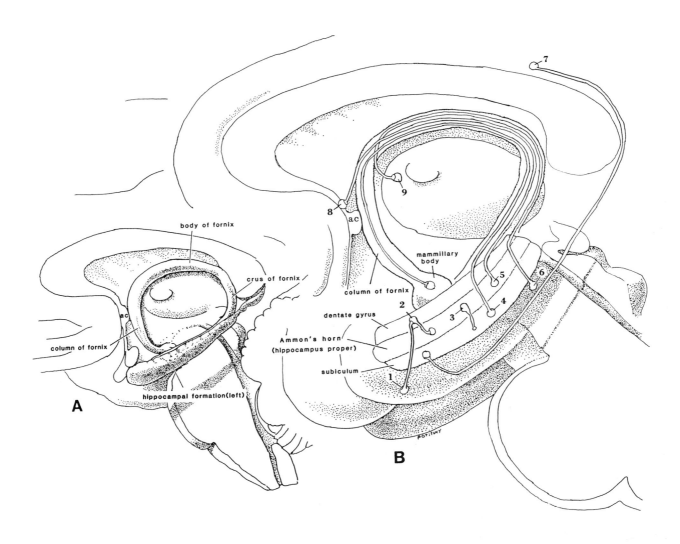

body of fornix

crus of fornix

ac

column of fornix

hippocampal formation(left)

A

column of fornix

mammillary body

dentate gyrus

Ammon's horn (hippocampus proper)

subiculum

ac

8

9

7

5

6

2

3

4

1

B

BOTITSKY

Etymological cartoon: Hippo campus

Color and label

BHOC Big hippo on campus
EH   Englebert Hippodink
AH   Albert Hippostein. Note his familiar baggy sweater,
      pipe, and shock of white hair.
HPF   Hippo playing Frisbee (after Mother Frisbie's pie tins,
      originally used by students at Yale for playing the game)
HRB(PA) Hippo riding bicycle (posterior aspect)
H   Sea horse hippocampus

The hippocampus was probably so named because it resembles the small sea horse, hippocampus. In Greek mythology the *hippocampus* was a beast with a horse's head and a serpent's tail that pulled Neptune (Poseidon) in his large conch across the sea. *Hippos* is Greek for horse and *kampos* is sea monster. Hippopotamus means river horse: *hippos*, horse; *potamos*, river. Hippology is the study of horses. The name Phillip means "love of horses" and even Hippocrates (460-377 B.C.), the "Father of Medicine," whose oath, or a variation thereof, all physicians must take before they can practice medicine, had a horse in his name: Hippocrates is derived from *hippos*, (horse) and *kratos*, (power) hence, rule by horses or horsepower.

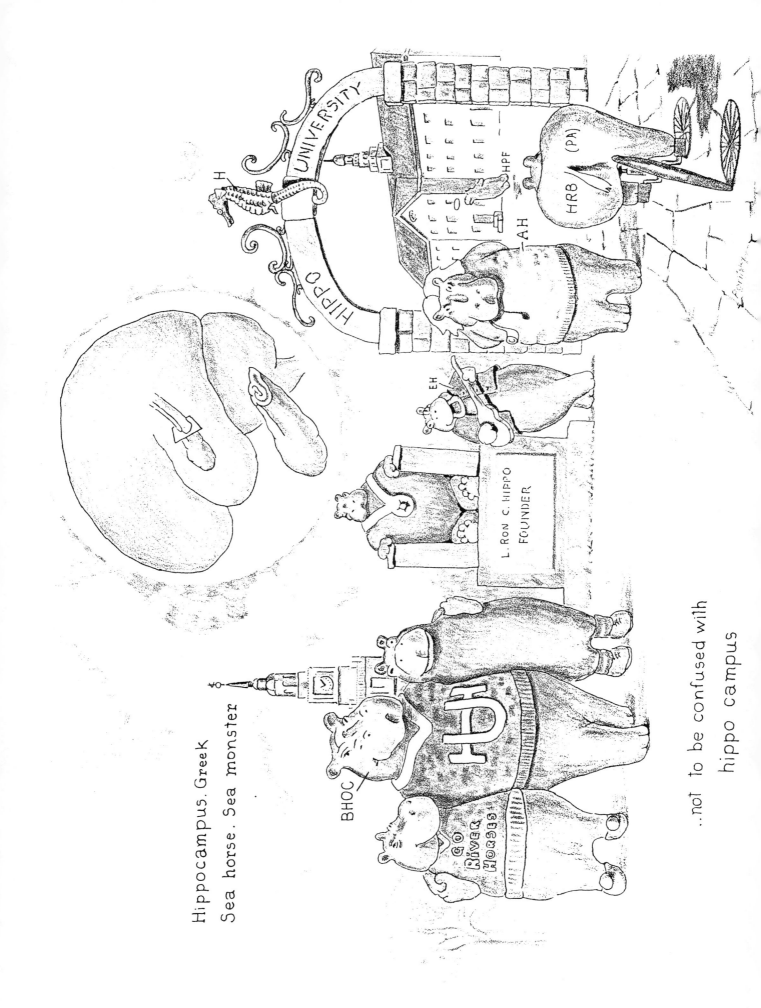

Hippocampus. Greek
Sea horse. Sea monster

..not to be confused with
hippo campus

Figure A is a frontal view of a dissected brain with the right hippocampal formation, fornix, and mamillary body exposed.

Figure B is a medial view of the same structures.

Color the hippocampal formation, fornix, and mamillary body in both Figures A and B.

Figure C shows both hippocampal formations, fornices, and mamillary bodies in frontal view. The left hippocampus (viewer's right) has been cut to reveal some of the internal structure.

Trace and color neurons 1, 2, 3, and 4.

Neuron 1 in the subiculum sends its axon into a curved bundle of axons called the **alveus** (Latin, a hollow container). The alveus consists of efferent myelinated fibers forming a layer of white matter external to the hippocampal gyri. This is the reverse of the usual pattern in the cerebral cortex, in which the white matter lies beneath the gray matter. As the fibers of the alveus travel backward, they converge and form a narrow band of white matter, the **fimbria** (Latin, fringe) of the hippocampus. The fibers of the fimbria then form the **crus** (Latin, leg) of the **fornix**. As the arched **fornix** curves upward and forward, its name changes to **body of the fornix**, which in turn becomes the **column of the fornix** as the fibers turn downward and finally backward in their course to the mamillary body. Fiber 1 ends on neuron 2 in the mamillary body.

Neuron 3 is a pyramidal neuron in Ammon's horn and its fiber ends upon a septal nucleus neuron 4.

Figure D shows a disassembled hippocampal formation. Note that the fimbria is made up of myelinated axons that course on the ventricular surface of the hippocampus proper as the alveus. Note how the hippocampus proper (Ammon's horn) and the dentate gyrus have the shape of two interlocking Cs. Only the hippocampus proper has the pyramidal cells, and the dentate gyrus has the granule cells. The subiculum, presubiculum, and parasubiculum are all parts of the parahippocampal gyrus.

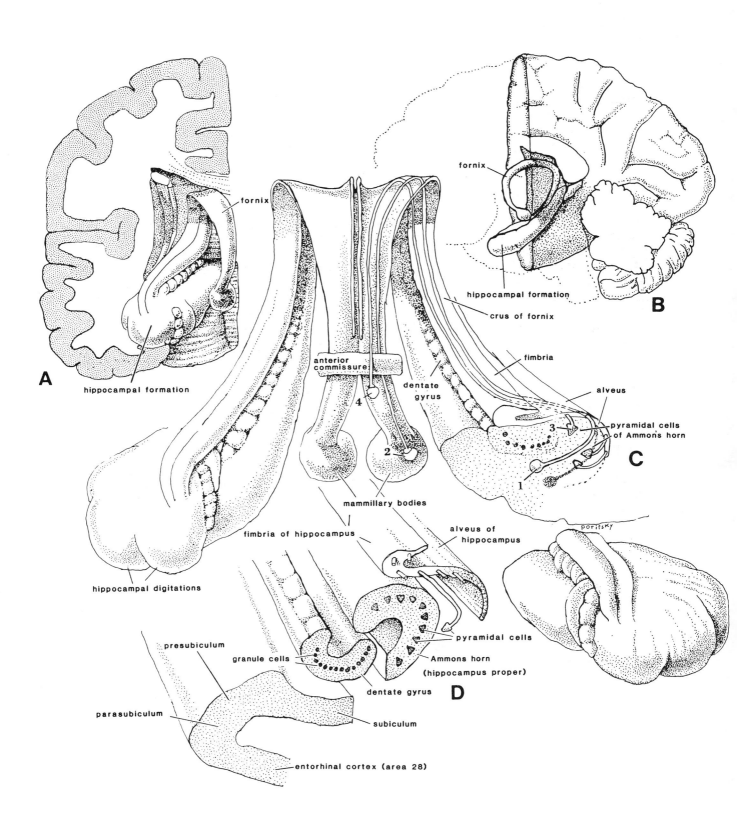

A

fornix

hippocampal formation

B

fornix

hippocampal formation

crus of fornix

fimbria

alveus

pyramidal cells of Ammon's horn

anterior commissure

dentate gyrus

mammillary bodies

4

2

3

1

C

hippocampal digitations

fimbria of hippocampus

alveus of hippocampus

poritsky

presubiculum

parasubiculum

granule cells

pyramidal cells

Ammons horn (hippocampus proper)

dentate gyrus

subiculum

entorhinal cortex (area 28)

D

The figure on the opposite page shows some of the internal connections within the hippocampal formation. The major source of afferent fibers to the hippocampus is the entorhinal cortex.

Trace and color neuron 1 in the medial entorhinal cortex and **neuron 2** in the lateral entorhinal cortex, both of which send their axons into the dentate gyrus where they synapse upon the dendrites of granule cells. Granule cells, which are the most conspicuous feature of the dentate gyrus, give rise to mossy fibers that enter the hippocampus proper and end as giant boutons upon the proximal portion of the apical dendrites of the pyramidal neurons. Only granule cells 3 and 4 are shown with their axons.

Color and trace the course of granule cell fibers 3 and 4 as they synapse upon pyramidal cells 5, 6, 7, and 8.

Color hippocampal pyramidal cells 5, 6, 7, and 8. Note that the axons of the pyramidal cells course toward the ventricular surface where they form the alveus. The fibers of the alveus group together into the fimbria, which then becomes the fornix. Pyramidal cell 8 gives off a recurrent collateral axon that synapses upon both the proximal axons and apical dendrites of other pyramidal cells.

Trace and color basket cell 9 (in the lower right) as its axon courses in the pyramidal cell layer of the Ammon's horn, where its terminal fibers make synaptic baskets around the cell bodies of several pyramidal neurons.

Fibers 10, 11, and 12 represent afferent fibers that arrive by way of the cingulum. Fiber 10 ends in the parasubiculum, fiber 11 in the subiculum, and fiber 12 in the hippocampus proper.

Color fibers 10, 11, and 12.

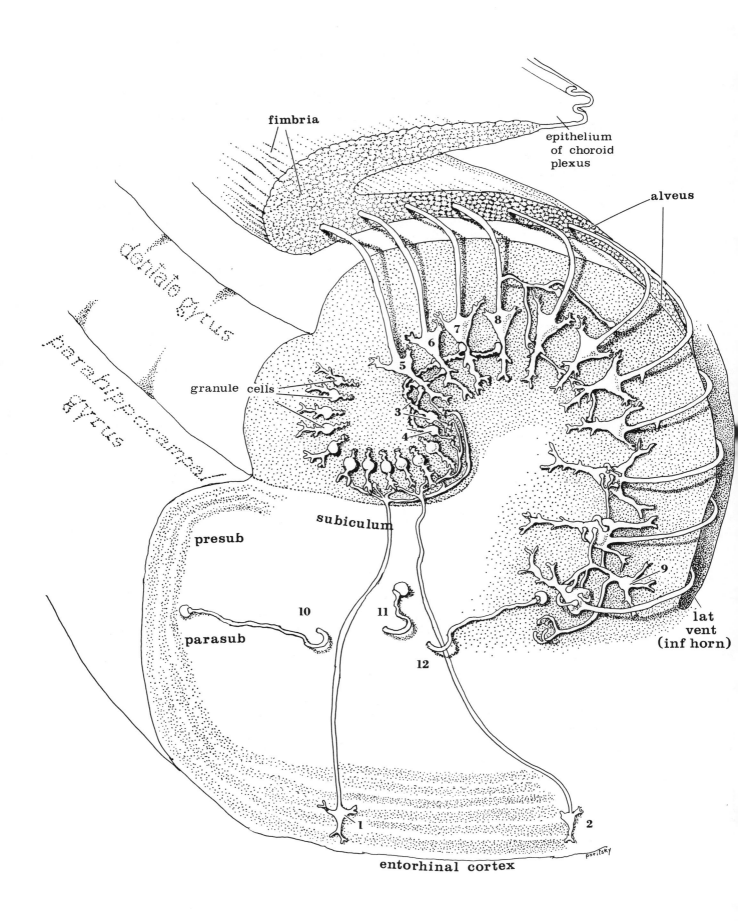

fimbria

epithelium
of choroid
plexus

alveus

dentate gyrus

parahippocampal gyrus

granule cells

6

7

8

5

3

4

9

subiculum

presub

parasub

10

11

12

lat
vent
(inf horn)

1

2

entorhinal cortex

poritsky

The autonomic nervous system (ANS) oversees our fundamental visceral processes such as digestion, assimilation, the flow of blood, and the rate and amplitude of the heartbeat. It regulates the secretion of glands, the contraction of smooth muscle, the caliber of blood vessels, and cardiac output. The ANS works as an involuntary system, reflex in nature, essentially at the subconscious level.

General plan (Figure A): The ANS consists of two antagonistic secretomotor systems, the **parasympathetic** and **sympathetic**, which have opposing actions on the organs innervated. Some organs, however, such as the sweat glands, arrector muscles of hair, and blood vessels, receive only sympathetic fibers.

The autonomic outflow, in contrast to the somatic efferents, consists of a two-neuron chain. The first neuron's cell body is either in the brain stem or spinal cord. The second neuron's soma is in a ganglion somewhere outside the CNS. The first neuron is the **preganglionic** neuron and the second the **postganglionic** neuron. The axon of the first (preganglionic) neuron synapses upon the soma and dendrites of the second (postganglionic) inside a ganglion.

Preganglionic parasympathetic somata reside in four nuclei in the brain stem, the Edinger-Westphal nucleus (EW nucleus), the superior salivatory nucleus (sup sal nucleus), the inferior salivatory nucleus (inf sal nucleus), and the dorsal vagal nucleus (dorsal nucleus X). The preganglionic parasympathetic fibers arising from neurons in these ganglia leave the brain stem with cranial nerves III, VII, IX, and X, respectively. **Color preganglionic parasympathetic neurons 1–5.**

Postganglionic parasympathetic somata reside in four ganglia in the head and receive the terminal synapses of preganglionic fibers in the following manner: Preganglionic fibers in nerve III synapse upon postganglionic neurons in the ciliary ganglion; preganglionic fibers in nerve VII end upon postganglionic neurons in two ganglia, the pterygopalatine and submandibular; preganglionic fibers in nerve IX synapse upon postganglionic neurons in the otic ganglion, and preganglionic fibers in nerve X make synaptic contact with postganglionic neurons in numerous ganglia spread throughout the thorax and abdomen. **Color postganglionic parasympathetic neurons 7–12.**

Additional parasympathetic preganglionic fibers arise from somata in the sacral spinal cord and emerge with spinal nerves S2-S4 (6). **Color** preganglionic parasympathetic neuron 6 in the lower spinal cord and postganglionic parasympathetic neuron 13 near the bladder. The **preganglionic sympathetic** somata 14–17 lie in the gray matter of the spinal cord at levels T1-L2. They emerge with ventral roots of the corresponding spinal nerves. They then turn off in short, white communicating rami and enter the sympathetic trunk and ganglia. The preganglionic fibers may synapse upon postganglionic neurons in these ganglia; or they may ascend or descend in the trunk to end at a ganglion higher or lower; or they may continue into the thorax and abdomen without synapsing as **splanchnic nerves.** Color preganglionic sympathetic neurons 14–17.

Postganglionic sympathetic somata 18, 19, and 20 are found in the ganglia of the sympathetic chain. Additional postganglionic sympathetic somata reside in **prevertebral** ganglia, such as the celiac ganglia. Postganglionic fibers arising from somata in the ganglia of the sympathetic chain may either join spinal nerves via gray communicating rami or pass into the arms and legs with blood vessels. **Color** postganglionic sympathetic neurons 18, 19, and 20.

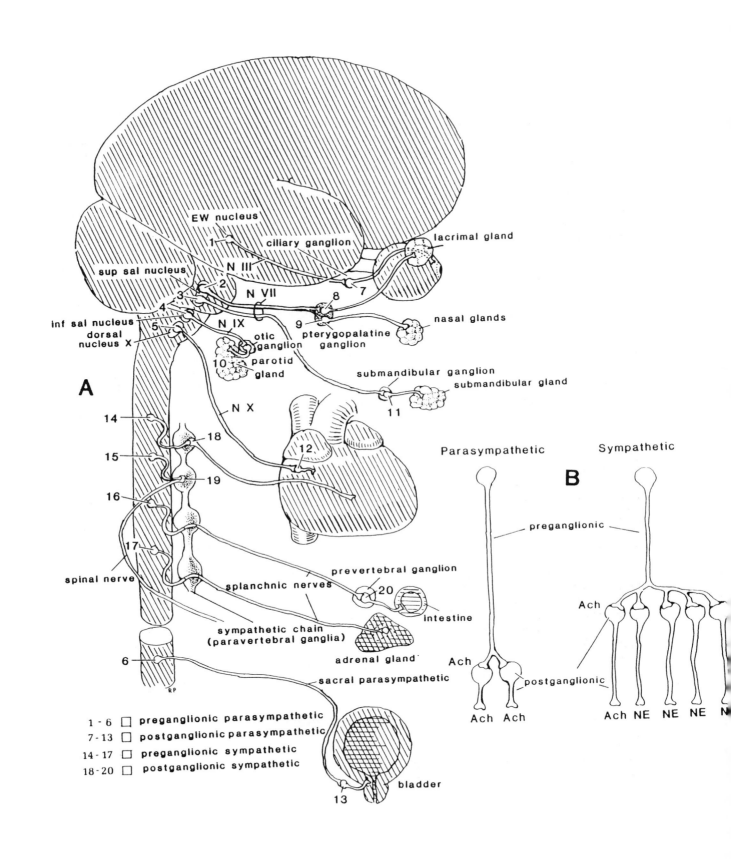

EW nucleus

1

ciliary ganglion

N III

lacrimal gland

sup sal nucleus

2

N VII

3

4

inf sal nucleus

5

dorsal nucleus X

N IX

otic ganglion

8

7

9

pterygopalatine ganglion

nasal glands

10

parotid gland

A

submandibular ganglion

submandibular gland

11

14

N X

18

12

15

19

16

17

spinal nerve

prevertebral ganglion

splanchnic nerves

20

intestine

sympathetic chain (paravertebral ganglia)

adrenal gland

6

sacral parasympathetic

RP

13

bladder

1 - 6 □ preganglionic parasympathetic
7 - 13 □ postganglionic parasympathetic
14 - 17 □ preganglionic sympathetic
18 - 20 □ postganglionic sympathetic

Parasympathetic

Sympathetic

B

preganglionic

Ach

Ach

postganglionic

Ach   Ach

Ach   NE   NE   NE   N

Cholinergic versus adrenergic (Figure B):   These terms refer to the mode of action of the two systems, specifically, the neurotransmitter released at the terminals of the postganglionic fibers. The postganglionic parasympathetic fibers release **acetylcholine** (Ach); thus, it is a **cholinergic** system. The postganglionic sympathetics release **norepinephrine** (NE); thus, it is an **adrenergic** system. Exceptions to this are the postganglionic sympathetic fibers to sweat glands (sudomotor), which are cholinergic.

The **parasympathetic** (cholinergic) **system** is concerned with the vegetative aspects of day-to-day living. It promotes the digestion and absorption of food, gastric secretion, the motility of the intestinal tract (peristalsis), the relaxation of the pyloric and urinary sphincters, and slowing of the heart. Its action tends to be limited and discrete. This is due to each parasympathetic preganglionic neuron synapsing on relatively few postganglionic neurons (the reverse is true of the sympathetic system), and acetylcholine being rapidly broken down by the enzyme cholinesterase. The parasympathetic system promotes the acquisition and storing of free energy within the organism.

The **sympathetic** (adrenergic) **system** accelerates the heart (tachycardia) and raises the blood pressure by constricting blood vessels in the viscera and skin (which also limits heat loss from the skin). It dilates the bronchioles by relaxing the smooth muscles in their walls and inhibits peristalsis of the intestines. It causes the breakdown of glycogen into glucose and the liberation of free fatty acids, both of which supply more energy. When needed, the adrenergic action may be significantly augmented by the liberation of epinephrine from the adrenal medulla into the bloodstream. The cells of the adrenal medulla receive preganglionic sympathetic fibers in the splanchnic nerves. In time of stress the adrenergic effect is massive due to the widespread action of epinephrine in the blood stream, plus norepinephrine's not being broken down as readily as acetylcholine, plus each preganglionic fiber exciting a large number of postganglionic fibers.

Figure B shows some of the differences between the two divisions: Parasympathetic preganglionic fibers are longer and tend to synapse with fewer postganglionic neurons, which tend to lie near or inside the target organ. Sympathetic preganglionic fibers are not as long and each fiber synapses upon many postganglionic neurons. All preganglionic neurons, parasympathetic and sympathetic, release acetylcholine (Ach); all postganglionic parasympathetic fibers release acetylcholine (Ach). Most postganglionic sympathetic neurons release norepinephrine (NE), but those to sweat glands (sudomotor) release acetylcholine (Ach).

It is usually stated that there are no sympathetic cell bodies in the head and that sympathetic fibers in the head arise from cell bodies in the superior cervical ganglion. However, some postganglionic sympathetic cell bodies are found in small groups along the internal carotid artery. These have apparently migrated cephalically from the superior cervical ganglion. Parasympathetic fibers do not extend into the arms or legs, nor do they run along with or innervate blood vessels. The apparently contradictory action of norepinephrine (both excitatory on some organs and inhibitory on others) is believed to be due to the existence of two types of receptors to norepinephrine; one type of receptor will respond with an excitatory action; the other, with an inhibitory action.

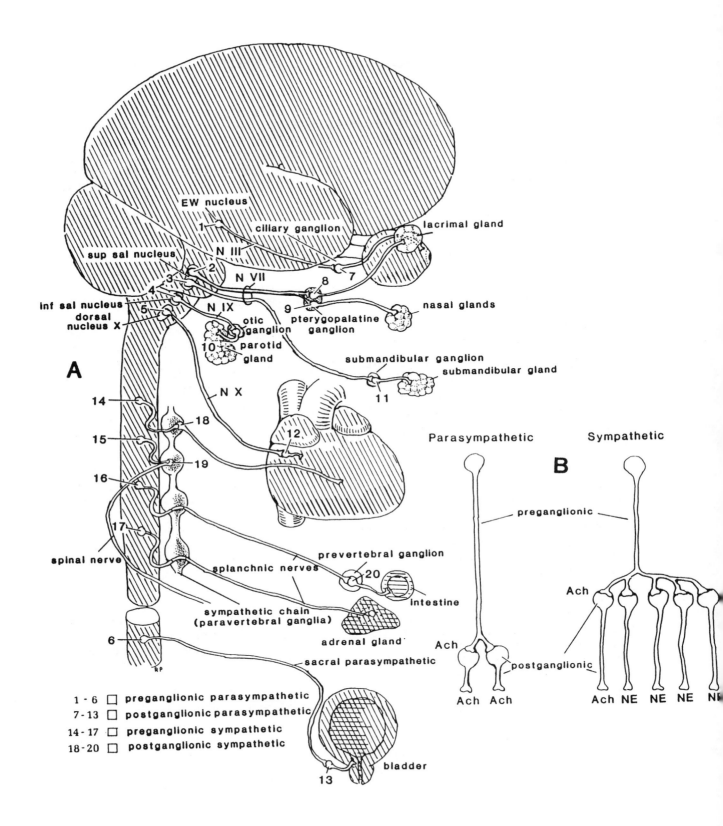

EW nucleus

ciliary ganglion

lacrimal gland

sup sal nucleus

N III

inf sal nucleus
dorsal nucleus X

N VII

nasal glands

N IX

otic ganglion

pterygopalatine ganglion

parotid gland

submandibular ganglion
submandibular gland

A

N X

spinal nerve

splanchnic nerves

sympathetic chain
(paravertebral ganglia)

prevertebral ganglion

intestine

adrenal gland

sacral parasympathetic

1 - 6 ☐ preganglionic parasympathetic
7 - 13 ☐ postganglionic parasympathetic
14 - 17 ☐ preganglionic sympathetic
18 - 20 ☐ postganglionic sympathetic

bladder

Parasympathetic

Sympathetic

B

preganglionic

Ach

Ach

postganglionic

Ach   Ach

Ach   NE   NE   NE   N

The drawing shows a small portion of the thoracic spinal cord and related autonomic neurons. All preganglionic sympathetic perikarya are located in the **intermediolateral column** of the spinal cord gray matter. The intermediolateral column extends from the first thoracic level (T1) to the second lumbar level (L2) of the spinal cord. The axons of these preganglionic sympathetic neurons leave the spinal cord within the ventral roots of spinal nerves T1 through L2. Thus the sympathetic division leaves the CNS within the 12 thoracic nerves and upper two lumbar nerves. The parasympathetic division, on the other hand, leaves the CNS within four cranial nerves and sacral nerves S2, S3, and S4.

Directions: Starting with neuron 1a, a preganglionic sympathetic neuron lying in the intermediolateral column of the spinal cord, **color the neuron 1a cell body** and its axon as it passes out the ventral root into the spinal nerve and then via a white communicating ramus into a ganglion of the sympathetic trunk, where it ends by synapsing upon **postganglionic sympathetic neuron 2c**. Using another color for postganglionic sympathetic neurons, **color neuron 2c** and its fiber as it runs via a gray communicating ramus back into the spinal nerve. **Color neuron 1b** and follow its axon, which ascends in the sympathetic trunk to the superior cervical ganglion, where it synapses upon postganglionic sympathetic neurons 2a and 2b. **Color neurons 2a and 2b** and notice that the axons of 2a form a plexus around the internal carotid artery. These postganglionic sympathetic axons ascend into the head as the internal carotid plexus, eventually reaching organs such as the eye and salivary glands. Postganglionic sympathetic neurons 2b have axons that innervate the heart via the cardiac plexus.

Follow and color the course of preganglionic fiber 1c. Notice that 1c passes through the sympathetic ganglion without synapsing, travels in a splanchnic nerve, and does not end until it reaches a ganglion such as the celiac ganglion. The **thoracic splanchnic nerves** contain preganglionic axons such as 1c. In the celiac ganglion, preganglionic fibers synapse upon postganglionic neurons 2h and 2i. Postganglionic neuron 2h directs its axon to a blood vessel on the intestine. Postganglionic neuron 2i sends its axon into the smooth muscle of the intestine. **Color** and follow the course of **postganglionic sympathetic neurons 2d, 2e, and 2f,** whose cell bodies lie in another ganglion of the sympathetic trunk. Their axons either run into spinal nerves or run as a plexus around blood vessels and eventually end on such structures as sweat glands, arrector muscles of hair, and blood vessels of the skin.

Locate preganglionic sympathetic neuron 1e in the opposite intermediolateral column and trace its axon. Note that the axon 1e does not synapse in the sympathetic chain ganglia but continues into the abdomen within a splanchnic nerve. It synapses upon cells in the adrenal medulla (2g) that secrete epinephrine (adrenalin) and lesser amounts of norepinephrine (noradrenalin) into blood vessels passing through the gland.

Neuron 3 represents a **preganglionic parasympathetic neuronal cell body** lying in the dorsal nucleus of the vagus nerve. Axons from somata such as 3 travel within the vagus nerve and supply a very wide range of viscera in both the thorax and abdomen. The preganglionic parasympathetic fibers in the vagus nerve tend to be much longer than the postganglionic parasympathetic fibers. Neurons labelled 4 are **postganglionic parasympathetic neurons.** Note that they lie entirely within the structure innervated. Postganglionic parasympathetic somata found in this position are therefore termed **intramural** (Latin, within the walls). Neuron 5 represents a **visceral afferent neuron.** Its cell body lies in the dorsal root ganglion and has the typical unipolar shape of all the perikarya found in the dorsal root ganglion.

Directions: Use the boxes as color keys for each category.

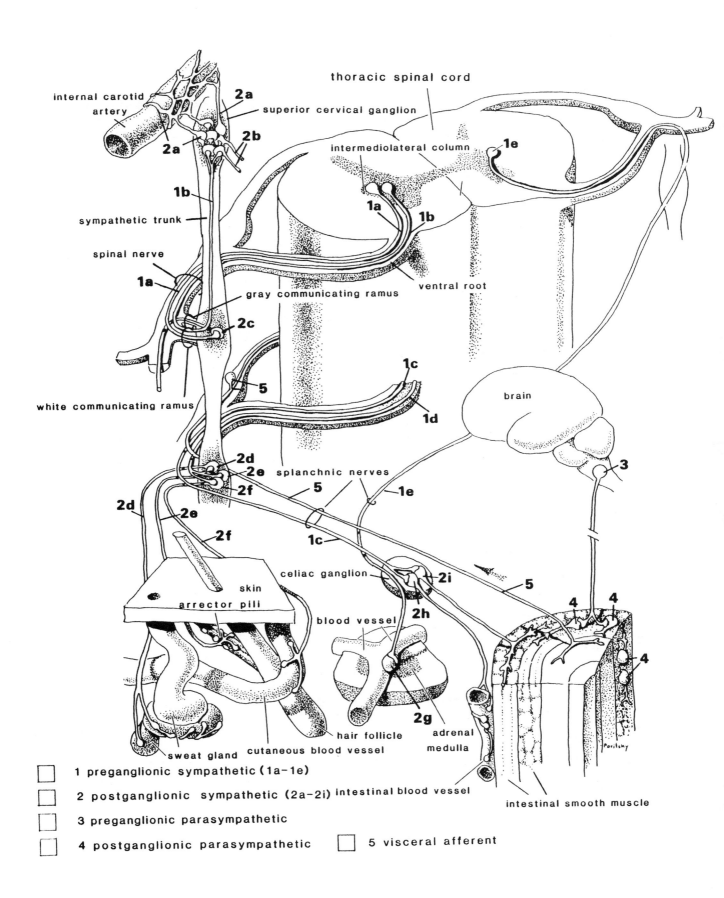

internal carotid artery

2a

superior cervical ganglion

2a   **2b**

2a

thoracic spinal cord

intermediolateral column   **1e**

1b

1a

1b

sympathetic trunk

spinal nerve

1a

gray communicating ramus

ventral root

2c

5   **1c**

white communicating ramus   **1d**

brain

2d

2e   splanchnic nerves

2f   **5**   **3**

2d   **1e**

2e

1c

2f

5

skin   celiac ganglion   **2i**

arrector pili   **2h**   **4**   **4**

blood vessel   **4**

2g

hair follicle   adrenal medulla

sweat gland   cutaneous blood vessel   **4**

intestinal smooth muscle

□ 1 preganglionic sympathetic (1a-1e)

□ 2 postganglionic sympathetic (2a-2i) intestinal blood vessel

□ 3 preganglionic parasympathetic

□ 4 postganglionic parasympathetic   □ 5 visceral afferent

Pain fibers from the heart (1, 2) have their cell bodies (1p and 2p) in the dorsal root ganglia of thoracic spinal nerves T1–T5. Starting with the terminals of pain fibers 1 and 2 on the heart, **trace and color fibers 1 and 2** as they extend into the central nervous system. Note that fiber 1 ascends to the **inferior cervical ganglion** where it turns down within the sympathetic trunk until it reaches one of the upper four or five thoracic ganglia. It then leaves the sympathetic trunk via a white ramus communicans, enters the spinal nerve at that level, proceeds centrally by way of dorsal root, and finally enters the spinal cord where it synapses upon a second-order pain neuron (11). **Trace** pain fiber 2 as it leaves the heart and ascends to the **middle cervical ganglion** where, like fiber 1, it passes through with no interruption and descends to the level of thoracic nerve T2. It also leaves the sympathetic chain and enters the spinal cord by the dorsal root of the corresponding spinal nerve.

Each of the three cervical sympathetic ganglia in the neck give off **cardiac branches** to the heart. The cardiac branch from the superior cervical ganglion is believed to carry no pain fibers, only efferents. The efferent sympathetic fibers arise from the three cervical sympathetic ganglia plus the upper five thoracic sympathetic ganglia (the first thoracic ganglion is often missing, having fused with the inferior cervical ganglion to form the stellate ganglion). The sympathetic fibers from these ganglia converge on the heart, where they form the **cardiac plexus** (the smaller top figure shows an exaggerated cardiac plexus; in reality it is found at the back of the heart).

As mentioned previously, the outflow (efferents) of the sympathetic nervous system occurs only at thoracic nerves T1–L2. **Locate** the perikaryon of preganglionic sympathetic neuron 3p and note that it lies in the intermediolateral column of the spinal cord gray matter. All preganglionic sympathetic perikarya are located in the intermediolateral column. **Color and follow the axon of 3** out the ventral root, through the white ramus communicans, and into the sympathetic chain, where it synapses upon postganglionic neuron 7, which sends its axon (cut) to the cardiac plexus. Fiber 3 continues to ascend up into the neck where it makes synaptic contact upon postganglionic neurons 6 (cut), 5 (cut), and 4 in the inferior, middle, and superior cervical ganglia, respectively. **Color and trace the fiber of postganglionic neuron 4** in the superior cervical ganglion. **Color postganglionic neuron 8** in thoracic sympathetic ganglion T2, which also sends its axon to the cardiac plexus. The postganglionic sympathetic fibers release norepinephrine, which increases the force and rate of the heart beat and dilates the coronary arteries.

Color preganglionic sympathetic neuron 9p, which lies in level T6 of the spinal cord. Its axon will become a thoracic splanchnic nerve. The greater splanchnic nerve receives fibers from thoracic ganglia T5–T9, most of which are preganglionic. Additional postganglionic sympathetic cell bodies (10) are located in ganglia such as the celiac, which are collectively called **prevertebral** ganglia. The preganglionic parasympathetic fibers travel within the vagus nerve (not shown). The postganglionic parasympathetic fibers (not shown) are within the walls of the heart. Afferent fibers from the heart that mediate cardiac reflexes travel with the vagus. Unlike the sympathetic pain fibers, these vagal cardiac afferents function at the subconscious level. Removal of the upper four or five thoracic sympathetic ganglia bilaterally interrupts the path of the cardiac pain fibers and abolishes pain from the heart (plus removing direct sympathetic influence on the heart).

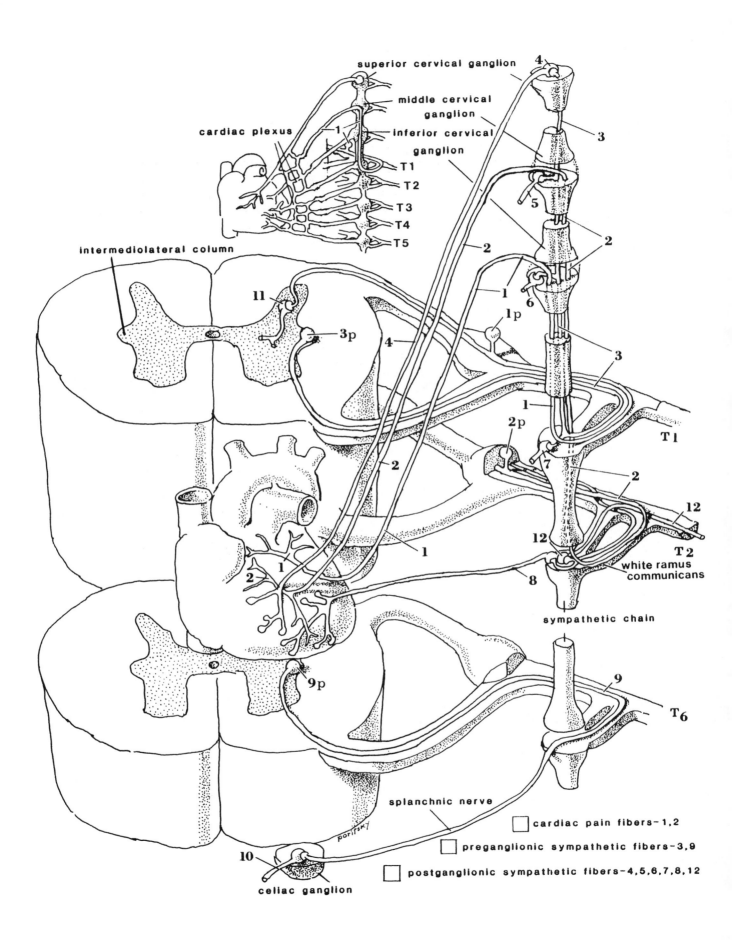

superior cervical ganglion

middle cervical ganglion

cardiac plexus

inferior cervical ganglion

T1
T2
T3
T4
T5

intermediolateral column

T1

T2

white ramus communicans

sympathetic chain

T6

splanchnic nerve

celiac ganglion

cardiac pain fibers-1,2

preganglionic sympathetic fibers-3,9

postganglionic sympathetic fibers-4,5,6,7,8,12

117 Thalamus: Internal medullary lamina

The thalamus is divided into three nuclear masses by the internal medullary lamina, which is a sheet of myelinated fibers. The lower figure shows the right thalamus and left thalamus seen from the left, from behind, and slightly superior. The **internal medullary lamina** (1) is seen inside the two transparent thalami. The upper figure shows the right thalamus disassembled into its three nuclear groups: **medial** (Med), **anterior** (Ant), and **lateral** (Lat). Note that the internal medullary lamina internally expands to encompass the so-called **intralaminar nuclei** (2), the most prominent of which is the centromedian nucleus. Altogether each thalamus contains close to 50 nuclei.* Only a few of the best known nuclei are pictured here, and these are not broken down into their numerous subsidiary nuclei. For example, the anterior nuclear group contains three subsidiary nuclei, and the pulvinar contains four nuclei, but these smaller nuclei are not shown.

Color and label

1	Internal medullary lamina
2	Intralaminar nuclei (simplified and schematic)
3	Interthalamic adhesion
4	Medial geniculate body
5	Lateral geniculate body
Med	Medial nuclear group
Ant	Anterior nuclear group
Lat	Lateral nuclear group

---

*Jones lists 48 nuclei in the cat thalamus.

Jones EG: Organization of the thalamocortical complex and its relation to sensory processes. In Brookhart JM, Mountcastle VB, Darian-Smith I, Geiger SR (eds): The Handbook of Physiology. Section 1: The Nervous System. Volume III: Sensory Processes. Bethesda, MD, American Physiological Society, 1984.

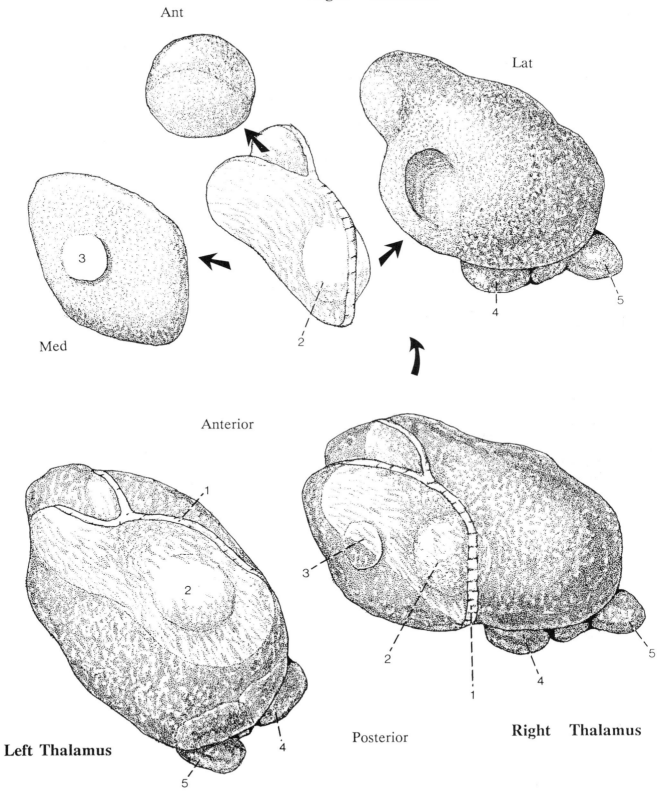

Right Thalamus

Ant

Lat

3

Med

2

4

5

Anterior

1

2

3

2

1

4

5

Left Thalamus

4

5

Posterior

Right Thalamus

Bottom Figure: Superior view of the two thalami cut into six coronal sections: A, B, C, D, E, and F. Sections A and B are shown above. The remainder (C, D, E, and F) are on the following pages.

The thalamus is divided into three nuclear masses by a thin sheet of myelinated fibers called the internal medullary lamina (1). These three nuclear masses are the lateral, medial, and anterior. They are indicated in the lower left figure by the large Lat, Med, and Ant. The lateral surface of the thalamus is covered by a curved sheet of myelinated fibers called the external medullary lamina (4). Lateral to the external medullary lamina is a thin, curved nucleus, the thalamic recticular nucleus (5). The external medullary lamina and thalamic reticular nucleus are shown in sections B, C, D, and E but not in section A or in the bottom figure.

Color and label

1	Internal medullary lamina
2	Stria medullaris thalami
3	Interthalamic adhesion (formerly, massa intermedia)
4	External medullary lamina
5	Thalamic reticular nucleus
Pin	Pineal body
Hab	Habenular nucleus
Pul	Pulvinar
LGB	Lateral geniculate body
MGB	Medial geniculate body
Vent III	Third ventricle
Ant	Anterior nuclear group
Lat	Lateral nuclear mass
Med	Medial nuclear mass
VA	Ventral anterior nucleus
VL	Ventral lateral nucleus
VP	Ventral posterior nucleus (this contains nuclei ventral posterolateral, or VPL, and ventral posteromedial, or VPM)
LD	Lateral dorsal nucleus
LP	Lateral posterior nucleus
MD	Mediodorsal nucleus
CM	Centromedian nucleus

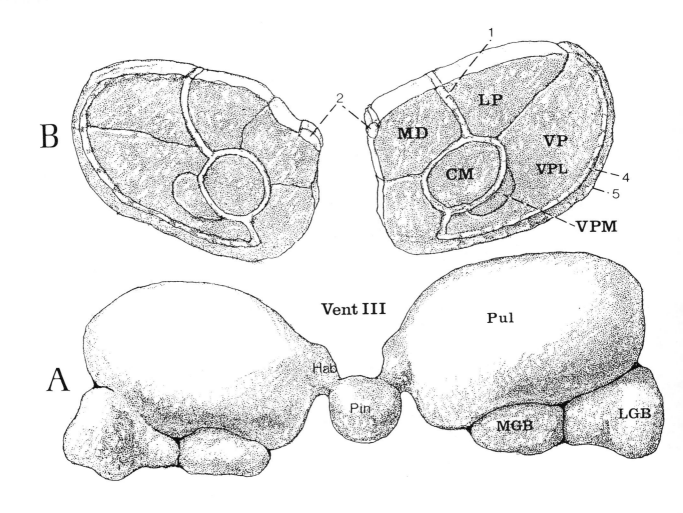

B

LP

MD

VP

VPL

CM

4

5

VPM

1

2

Vent III

Pul

Hab

A

Pin

MGB

LGB

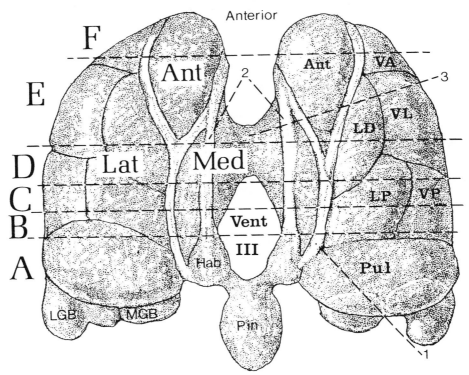

Thalami. Superior Aspect

Anterior

F

Ant

Ant

VA

2

3

E

VL

LD

D

Lat

Med

C

LP

VP

B

Vent

III

A

Hab

Pul

LGB

MGB

Pin

1

Color and label

1	Internal medullary lamina
2	Stria medullaris thalami (medullary stria of thalamus)
3	Interthalamic adhesion (formerly, massa intermedia)
4	External medullary lamina
5	Thalamic reticular nucleus
Ant	Anterior nuclear group
VA	Ventral anterior nucleus
VL	Ventral lateral nucleus
VP	Ventral posterior nucleus
VPM	Ventral posteromedial nucleus
LD	Lateral dorsal nucleus
LP	Lateral posterior nucleus
MD	Mediodorsal nucleus
CM	Centromedian nucleus

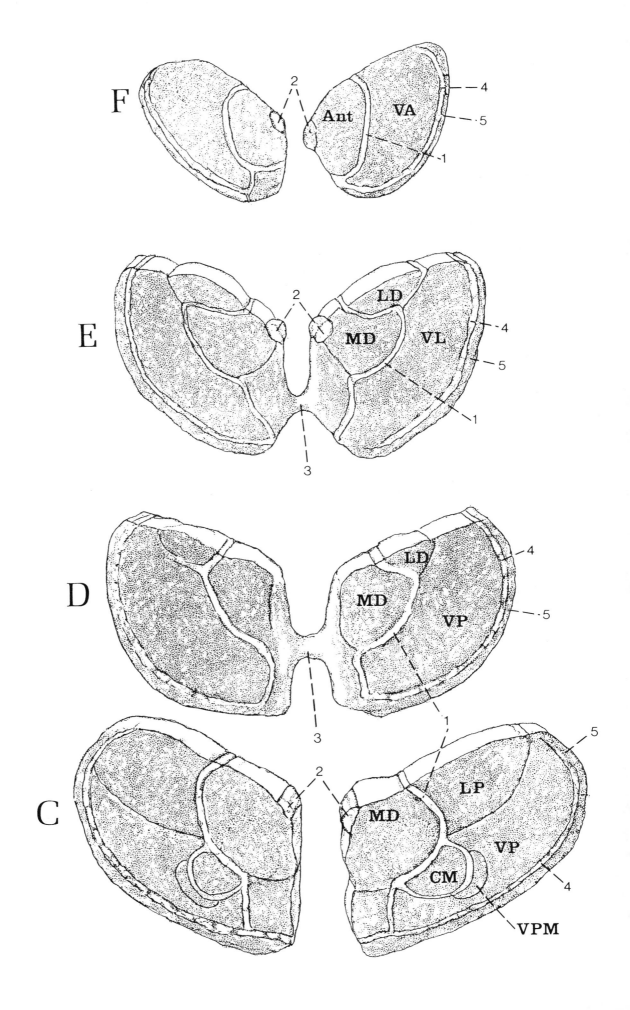

The reticular nucleus of the thalamus is a thin sheet of neurons only two or three neurons thick that overlies the anterior, lateral, and ventral surfaces of the thalamus. All the thalamocortical fibers and corticothalamic fibers pass through the reticular nucleus, which appears to monitor the activity between the thalamus and cerebral cortex. Thalamocortical fibers, corticothalamic fibers, and thalamostriate fibers give off synaptic terminals to neurons in the reticular nucleus as they pass through it.

At one time it was believed that the reticular nucleus was the upward extension of the brain stem reticular formation and that its discharge would bring about a widespread activation of the cerebral cortex. However, it has now been shown that the reticular nucleus does not project to the cortex at all; rather, the reticular nucleus projects only to the thalamus and it projects in a very orderly pattern so that each group of reticular neurons sends inhibitory fibers back to the same thalamic neurons whose fibers passed through and excited those reticular neurons. Thus the reticular nucleus may ". . . provide an inhibitory effected on the dorsal thalamic* neurons, tending to reduce their levels of excitability immediately after the firing of a thalamocortical volley and immediately after their activation by corticothalamic fibers."†

Top Figure. The left thalamus seen from behind, above, and slightly lateral. Note the thin sheet-like reticular nucleus (Ret N) lateral to the external medullary lamina (EML).

Bottom Figure. The left thalamus cut horizontally. **Follow and color fiber 1**, which carries touch, vibratory sense, or proprioception from the opposite side of the body to thalamic nucleus **VPL**, where it synapses upon VPL neuron 2.

Follow and color fiber 3 carrying similar sensation from the opposite side of the face to thalamic nucleus **VPM** where it synapses upon VPM nucleus 4.

Color neuron 2, which sends **thalamocortical fiber 5** to the trunk region of the somatosensory cortex. Note that thalamocortical fiber 5 gives off a **collateral** fiber to reticular nucleus neuron 6, which sends back a fiber to neuron 2 in the VPL nucleus.

Trace and color reticular neuron 6. VPM nucleus neuron 4 sends **thalamocortical fiber 7** to the face region of the somatosensory cortex. Note that fiber 7 also gives off a **collateral** to reticular neuron 8, which sends back its axon to neuron 4 in the VPM.

Trace and color reticular neuron 8. Cortical neuron 9 sends a corticothalamic fiber 10 back to VPM neuron 4 and in so doing gives a collateral to reticular nucleus neuron 8.

Color cortical neuron 9. Likewise cortical neuron 11 sends its corticothalamic fiber 12 back to VPL neuron 2 and also gives a collateral to reticular nucleus neuron 6.

Color cortical neuron 11.

---

*Many researchers now refer to the thalamus as the dorsal thalamus and use the term ventral thalamus for the reticular nucleus, zona incerta, fields of Forel, and ventral lateral geniculate nucleus.

†Jones EG: Organization of the thalamocortical complex and its relation to sensory processes. In Brookhart JM, Mountcastle VB, Darian-Smith I, Geiger SR (eds): The Handbook of Physiology. Section 1: The Nervous System. Volume III: Sensory Processes. Bethesda, MD, American Physiological Society, 1984.

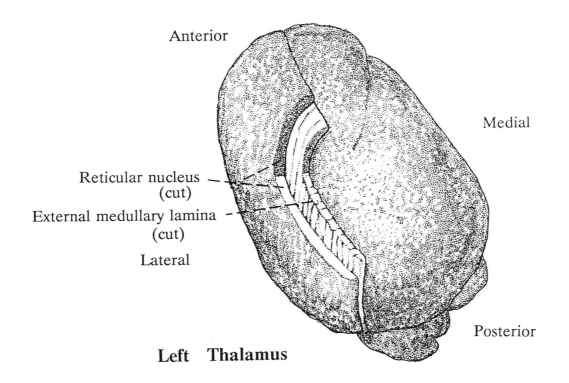

Anterior

Medial

Reticular nucleus
(cut)

External medullary lamina
(cut)

Lateral

Posterior

Left Thalamus

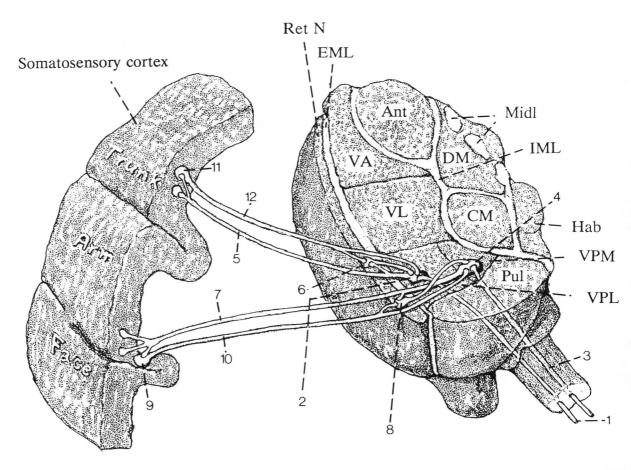

Somatosensory cortex

Ret N

EML

Ant

Midl

VA

DM

IML

VL

CM

4

Hab

Trunk

11

VPM

12

Arm

Pul

VPL

5

7

6

3

Face

10

9

2

8

1

Left Thalamus cut horizontally

121 Etymological cartoon: Somesthesia (Greek, body feeling)

If an animal such as the rabbit pictured here could draw his own image, he might create something like this disproportionate self-portrait. This is because the snout in a rabbit has the largest representation in both the thalamus and the cerebral cortex. The ventral posterior nucleus* in the thalamus receives the terminations of the medial lemniscus and the spinothalamic tract. The opposite surface of the body is projected into the VP nucleus, as diagrammed on the opposite page. The most caudal body parts, such as the tail, lie anterior and lateral in the VPL nucleus, and the rostral parts, such as the face, lie posterior and medial in the VPM nucleus. Parts of the body that have the densest aggregations of cutaneous receptors and play predominant roles in somesthetic sensation have the largest thalamic and cortical representation.

The lower figure shows a section through the ventrobasal complex in the thalamus of an animal such as a rabbit. Note the relatively large representation in the thalamus of the snout, which receives the trigeminothalamic tract.

The orderly projection of sense pathways and motor pathways up and down the neural axis is a common feature of the CNS. For example, the lateral geniculate nucleus of the thalamus, which is the visual relay center, is organized in a retinotopic pattern. The medial geniculate nucleus, which is the auditory relay center, is organized in a tonotopic manner, with the high tones at one place and the low tones at another.

All types of sensation except olfaction are sent to the thalamus, where they are integrated in some fashion and then relayed on the cerebral cortex. Olfactory stimuli reach the olfactory cortex without first passing through the thalamus.

---

*Because the ventral posterior nucleus also includes smaller nuclei that have no somesthetic function, the term **ventrobasal complex** is now used to describe only those nuclei that receive and relay somesthesia (touch, pressure, and proprioception).

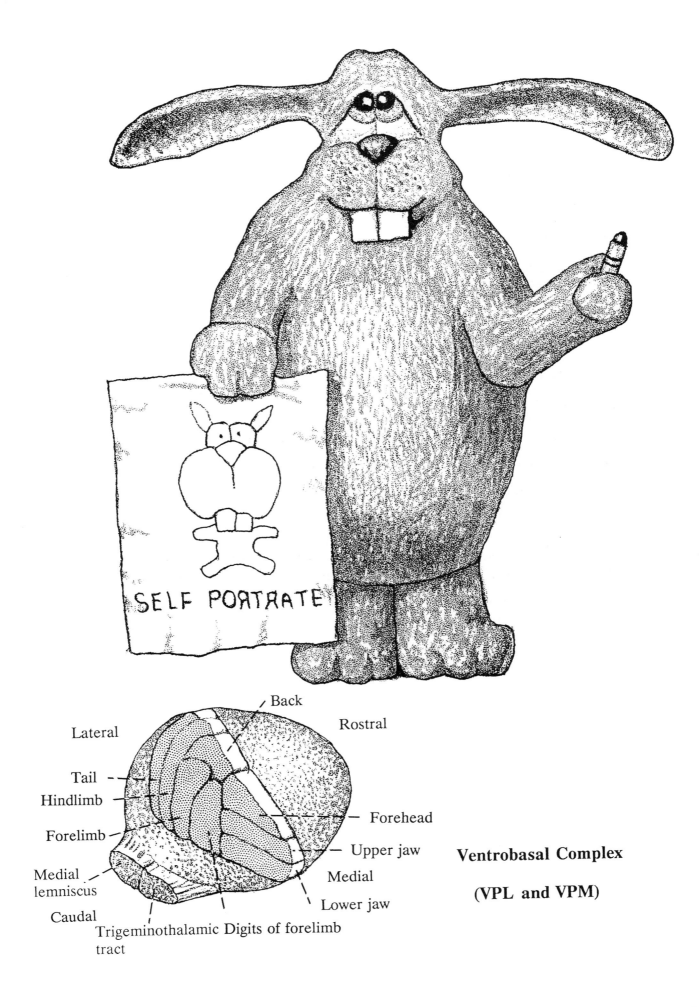

SELF PORTRATE

Back

Rostral

Lateral

Tail

Hindlimb

Forelimb

Forehead

Medial
lemniscus

Upper jaw

Medial

Lower jaw

Caudal

Trigeminothalamic Digits of forelimb
tract

Ventrobasal Complex

(VPL and VPM)

Color and label

1   Interthalamic adhesion. This joins the two thalami together (old name, massa intermedia).

2   Thalamus

3   Hypothalamus. The thalamus and hypothalamus form the lateral walls of the third ventricle.

4   Pituitary gland

5   Optic chiasm

6   Anterior commissure

7   Fornix (column)

8   Septum pellucidum

9   Corpus callosum (genu)

10   Corpus callosum (body)

11   Corpus callosum (splenium)

12   Pineal gland

13   Tectum (that part of the midbrain dorsal to the cerebral aqueduct)

14   Midbrain tegmentum (that part of the midbrain or mesencephalon ventral to the tectum and dorsal to the cerebral peduncle; it contains the red nucleus and the decussation of the superior cerebellar peduncle)

15   Oculomotor nerve

16   Mamillary body (part of the hypothalamus). The mamillary body is the only clearly identifiable hypothalamic nucleus in brain sections.

17   Mesencephalic aqueduct

18   Medullary stria of thalamus. This is a bundle of fibers visible on the medial dorsal border of the thalamus that arises from several sources, including the amygdala, the hippocampal formation and other structures. It ends in the forebrain habenular nuclei.

19   Cingulate gyrus

20   Lamina terminalis. This non-nervous membrane forms the anterior wall of the third ventricle. In the embryo this formed the most rostral wall of the prosencephalon.

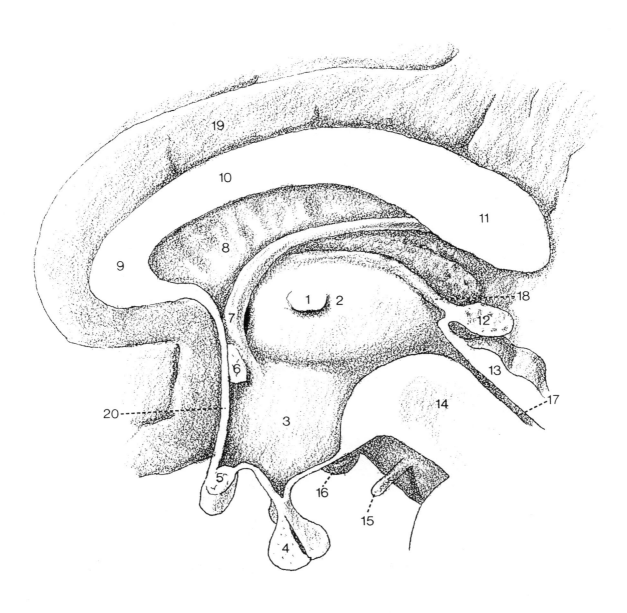

123 Some connections of the limbic system: The circuit of Papez

In 1937 James Wenceslas Papez, a U.S. anatomist (1883–1958), proposed a "mechanism" of neural circuitry to explain how intellectual function, which is presumed to involve the cerebral cortex, is connected to certain diencephalic nuclei that appear to be responsible for feeling and for producing emotion, and to hypothalamic centers that produce visceral responses. This "circuit" involves the cingulate gyrus, which is part of the neocortex (the evolutionarily recent, six-layered cerebral cortex), the anterior thalamus, the hypothalamus, and the hippocampal formation. These structures are all connected reciprocally by fibers that carry impulses both ways. While Papez's proposal is an interesting concept, exactly how this circuit relates to emotions remains unclear.

Color and label

1 Anterior thalamic nuclei. These project to the cingulate gyrus.
2 Thalamocortical fibers. Also present are reciprocal corticothalamic fibers (not shown).
3 Cingulate gyrus. Part of the neocortex (six-layered cortex).
4 Cingulum. This is a bundle of fibers that arises from neurons in the cingulate gyrus, encircles the corpus callosum, travels into the parahippocampal gyrus, and ends in the entorhinal cortex on the temporal lobe.
5 Entorhinal cortex (area 28). Entorhinal neurons project into the hippocampal formation.
6 Hippocampal formation. This is the phylogenetically ancient, three-layered cortex, the archicortex. It consists of the hippocampus proper (or Ammon's horn) and the dentate gyrus.
7 Pes hippocampi or the paw of the hippocampus
8 Fornix. This arched bundle of 1,200,000 fibers is the main outflow of the hippocampal formation and the underlying part of the parahippocampal gyrus. It ends mainly in the mamillary body, but also ends in other hypothalamic nuclei and in the septal nuclei that lie in front of the column of the fornix
9 Fornix (body)
10 Fornix (column). Here it passes through the hypothalamus, which is shown as if it were transparent.
11 Mamillary body. Part of hypothalamus.
12 Mamillothalamic tract. This easily identifiable bundle of fibers begins in the mamillary body and ends in the anterior thalamic nuclei.

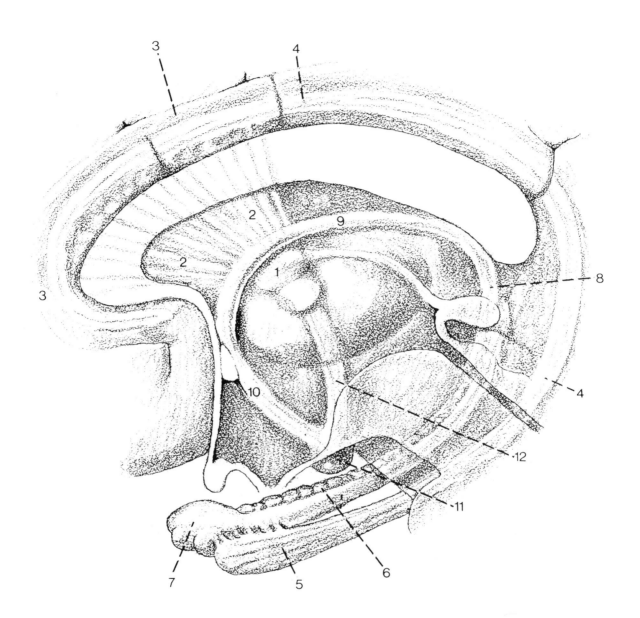

Color and label

1	Adenohypophysis (anterior lobe)	10	Superior hypophyseal artery
2	Neurohypophysis (posterior lobe)	11	Inferior hypophyseal artery
3	Median eminence	12	Capillary network in median eminence
4	Pars tuberalis	13	Long portal vessel
5	Mamillary body	14	Capillary network in adenohypophysis
6	Optic chiasm	15	Hormone-secreting cells in
7	Supraoptic nucleus in hypothalamus		adenohypophysis
8	Paraventricular nucleus in hypothalamus	16	Short portal vein
9	Pituitary stalk (infundibulum)	17	Capillary network in neurohypophysis

18   Peptidergic* neuron in paraventricular nucleus. These neurons synthesize the peptide hormones vasopressin and oxytocin, which travel down their axons into the neuro-hypophysis where they are released into the general circulation. The discovery of neurosecretion by hypothalamic neurons into the posterior lobe of the pituitary gland was made by Sharrer and Sharrer in 1954.

19   Peptidergic neuron in supraoptic nucleus. These neurons also secrete vasopressin and oxytocin, which are likewise released at their axon terminals into capillaries in the neurohypophysis (17).

20   Hypothalmo-hypophyseal tract. This is formed by the axons of the supraoptic and paraventricular neurons and is the pathway taken by the neurosecretory hormones oxytocin and vasopressin. Oxytocin, which means swift labor, causes uterine contraction and milk ejection. Vasopressin causes vasoconstriction and water reabsorption by the kidneys.

21   Hypothalamic neuron that produces hormone-regulating hormones. These are also peptide hormones, which may be as small as four amino acids, e.g., the thyrotropin-releasing hormone. The hormone-regulating hormones, which have either an inhibitory or stimulating effect, are released into capillaries in the median eminence that carry them by the long hypophyseal portal system to the adenohypophysis, where they bring about hormone release or inhibition.

22   Hypothalamic neuron making axoaxonic synapses on endings of hormone-regulating neuron.

23   Hypothalamic neuron that produces hormone-regulating peptide hormone that reaches the adenohyphysis via the short portal vessels.

24   Hypothalamic neuron with synapses on the cell body of the hormone-regulating neuron.

25   Hormone-regulating hormone. These blood-borne messages cause the cells of the anterior pituitary either to release their hormones or to inhibit their release.

26   Anterior pituitary hormones. The adenohypophysis has been shown to secrete 14 hormones. These include growth hormone, thyrotropin, adrenocorticotropin, prolactin, and follicle-stimulating hormone. Each hormone that is synthesized and released in the adenohypophysis has a releasing hormone made by cells in the hypothalamus. These releasing hormones are carried into the adenohypophysis by the hypophyseal portal system. To date four hormone-inhibiting hormones have been discovered.

Kupfermann I: Hypothalamus and limbic systems 1: Peptidergic Neurons, homeostasis, and emotional behavior. In Kandel ER, Schwartz JH (eds): Principals of Neural Science, 2nd ed. New York, Elsevier, 1985 pp. 611-625.

*A peptid is a compound that consists of two or more amino acids. Peptidergic means the neuron employs small peptid molecules as its neurotransmitter.

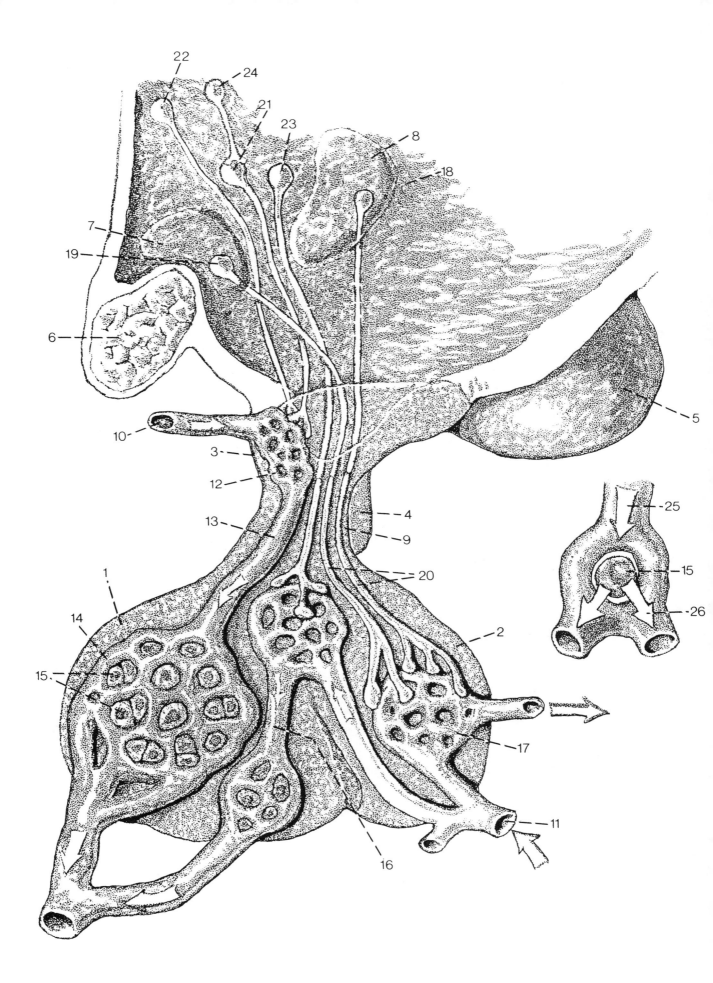

Olfaction (the sense of smell) begins with receptors at the top of the nasal cavities (Figure A). The olfactory receptor is a bipolar **neuroepithelial cell** with **chemosensitive cilia** (1) projecting from its free surface. These cilia are bathed in a serous fluid that covers the olfactory mucosa. The cilia are stimulated by the various odor-causing molecules that become dissolved in the serous fluid.

The axons of the olfactory receptors (5) group together into small bundles that collectively form the **olfactory nerve** (cranial nerve I). These bundles of axons penetrate the cribriform plate of the ethmoid bone, enter the **olfactory bulb,** branch extensively, and form whorl-like synaptic formations called **olfactory glomeruli** with the apical dendrites of **mitral cells** (6).

The axons of the mitral cells (8) carry the stimuli backward in the olfactory tract until they reach the olfactory trigone. The mitral cell axons turn laterally into the lateral olfactory stria (lat olf st). Some mitral cell axons synapse upon scattered neurons in the olfactory tract. These scattered neurons, which together comprise the anterior olfactory nucleus, send axons into either the medial olfactory stria (med olf st) (9), or into the lateral olfactory stria. Some fibers in the medial olfactory stria enter the anterior commissure, cross to the opposite side, enter the opposite olfactory tract, proceed forward as efferent fibers, and finally end in the opposite olfactory bulb.

In addition to axons of mitral cells, the olfactory tract contains the axons of tufted cells (not shown) and the above-mentioned efferent fibers (not shown). Fibers within the lateral olfactory stria encircle the limen (Latin, threshold) of the insula and travel from the base of the frontal lobe to the temporal lobe (Figure E). These fibers end either in the olfactory cortex (olf cortex, upper right figure) or in the cortical nucleus of the amygdala (12). The olfactory cortex, which is quite small in humans, consists of two gyri, the gyrus semilunaris (gyr semil) (10) and the gyrus ambiens (11). Indeed, humans are small smellers or **microsmatic** (Greek, *micros*, small; *osme*, smell or odor) and rely mainly upon vision and hearing rather than smell. Most mammals are big smellers or **macrosmatic.** Olfaction is the only sense that reaches the cerebral cortex without first passing through the thalamus.

Color the olfactory pathways:

1 Chemosensitive cilia
2 Olfactory vesicle
3 Dendrite of olfactory receptor
4 Cell body of olfactory receptor
5 Axon of olfactory receptor (= olfactory nerve, N I)
6 Olfactory glomerulus (in olfactory bulb)
7 Mitral cell
8 Mitral cell axon
9 Olfactory trigone
10 Gyrus semilunaris
11 Gyrus ambiens
12 Cortical nucleus of amygdala

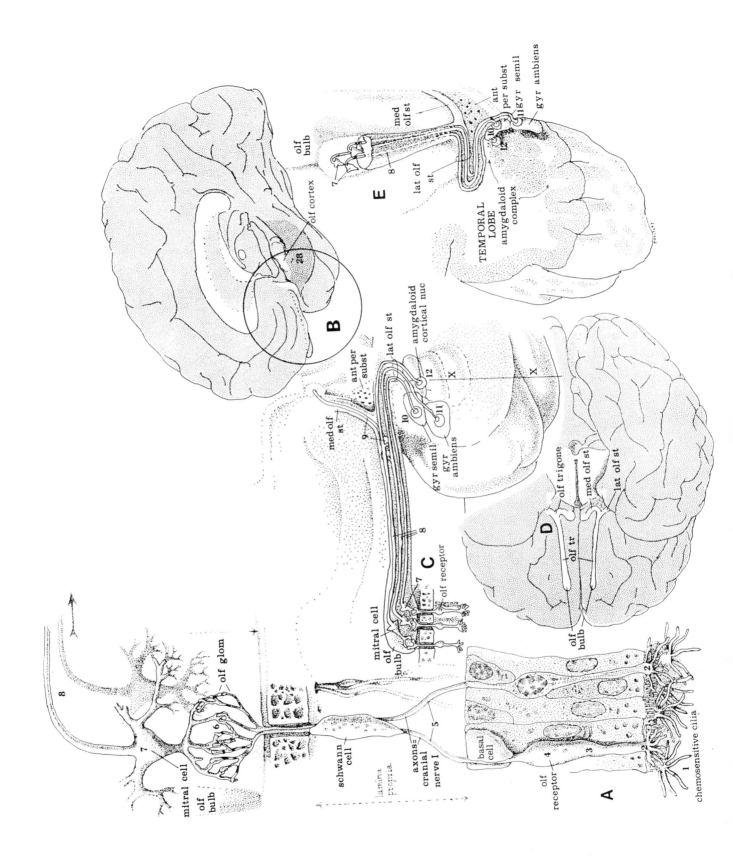

A

chemosensitive cilia

olf receptor

basal cell

olf receptor

axons= cranial nerve I

schwann cell

lamina propria

1
2
3
4
5

C

olf bulb
mitral cell
olf receptor

7
8

med olf st

ant per subst

lat olf st

9
10
11
12

gyr semil
gyr ambiens

amygdaloid cortical nuc

X
X

D

olf tr
olf bulb

olf trigone
med olf st
lat olf st

B

28

olf cortex

E

olf bulb

7
8

med olf st

lat olf st

ant per subst
gyr semil
gyr ambiens

TEMPORAL LOBE
amygdaloid complex

10
12

mitral cell
olf bulb
olf glom

6
7
8

Principal Types of Neurons and Some of Their Connections

Color the labelled neurons, their processes, and the afferent (corticopetal) fibers

P **Pyramidal cell.** These cells have a single thin axon directed downward (centripetally). Its pyramidal-shaped body sprouts several basal dendrites, and a single apical dendrite that extends to the superficial level I where it ramifies and runs tangentially. The dendrite spines are sites of axodendritic synapses. The pyramidal cell axon gives off a collateral that remains in the cortex and excites other cortical cells. The arrowheads in the axons are, of course, artifactual and indicate the direction of impulse.

S **Stellate cells.** These are present in all lamina except lamina I, with the greatest concentrations in lamina II and IV. Their axons, which are rather short, divide and end upon other cortical cells without leaving the cortex.

B **Basket cell.** These cells have axons that run horizontally and form basket-like endings about the pyramidal cell body. Basket cell endings are believed to have an inhibitory effect on the pyramidal cells by releasing the inhibitory neurotransmitter GABA.

F **Fusiform cell.** These cells sprout processes at either end, one bunch projecting centripetally and the other projecting centrifugally. The latter processes, which look like dendrites, are actually axons that contact cells in all layers of the cortex.

N **Neurogliaform cell.** These are small cells with dense localized dendritic fields within which the short axon ramifies and ends.

H **Horizontal cells (of Cajal).** These are found only in lamina I, the molecular layer. They are small cells with short dendrites that sprout in opposite directions and remain in the molecular layer. Their axons which often arise from one of the dendrites, divide into two branches, which run for considerable distances in the molecular layer.

M **Cells of Martinotti.** These small multipolar cells are found in levels II to VI. They have localized dendritic fields and long ascending axons that run to the molecular layer, where they divide and spread out.

Label the six lamina of the cerebral cortex

I **Molecular (plexiform) layer.** This layer contains scattered horizontal cells (of Cajal), tangentially oriented fibers arising from cells of Martinotti, axons of stellate cells, and the endings of cortical association fibers and callosal fibers from the opposite hemisphere.

II **External granular layer.** This layer contains densely-packed stellate cells and small pyramidal cells.

III **External pyramidal layer.** This layer contains medium-sized pyramidal cells, stellate cells, basket cells and fusiform cells.

IV **Internal granular layer.** This layer contains densely arranged stellate cells. Horizontally-coursing axons form the outer band of Baillarger in this layer (IV).

V **Internal pyramidal (ganglionic) layer.** The largest pyramidal cell somata are in this layer, along with stellate cells and cells of Martinotti. Horizontal fibers form the inner band of Baillarger in this layer (V).

VI **Multiform layer.** Various small neurons are found here, with fusiform cells predominating.

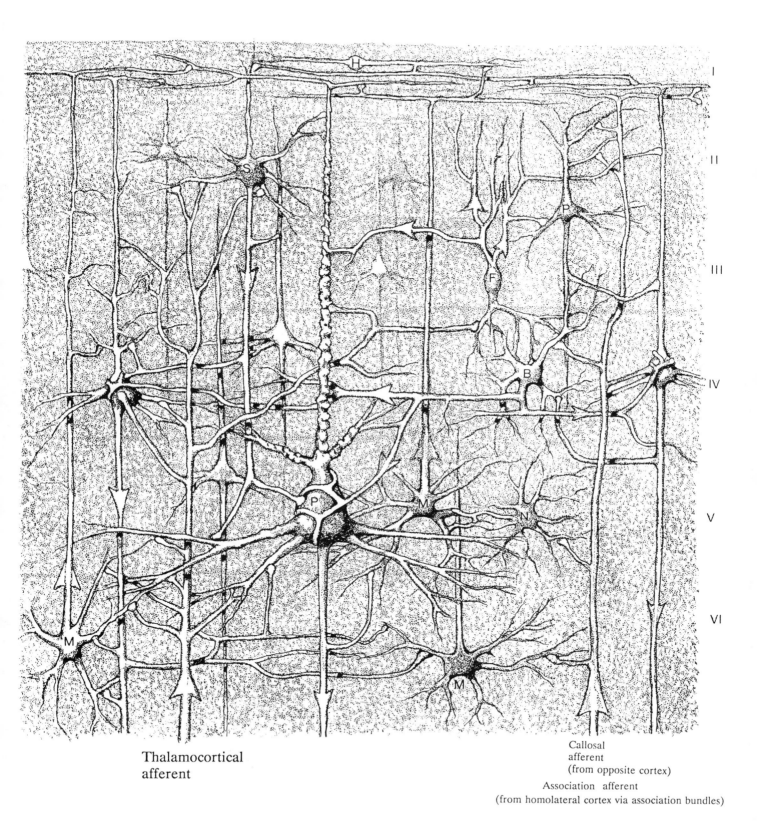

I

II

III

IV

V

VI

Thalamocortical
afferent

Callosal
afferent
(from opposite cortex)

Association afferent
(from homolateral cortex via association bundles)

Directions: Color and label each of the numbered cortical areas

Figure 127 shows a few of the cortical areas in which certain functions habe veen localized. Each cerebral hemisphere is divided into four lobes: **occipital lobe, parietal lobe, temporal lobe** and **frontal lobe**. These roughly correspond to the bones of the skull that overlie them. The folds or convolutions of cortex are called **gyri** (singular, gyrus), and the fissures between them are **sulci** (singular, sulcus).

Some authors divide the cerebral hemispheres into five lobes by the addition of the limbic lobe as the fifth lobe (Figure 21). The limbic cortical areas, which lie on the medial surface of the hemispheres and surround the corpus callosum and brain stem (Latin, *limbus*, border), include the cingulate gyrus and parahippocampal gyrus. The numbers on the cortex are those of Korbinian Brodmann, a German neurologist (1868–1918), who categorized some 50 areas of the cerebral cortex on the basis of different cell formations. Note that the central sulcus (fissure of Rolando) separates the frontal lobe from the parietal lobe. The lateral fissure (fissure of Sylvius) partially separates the temporal lobe from the frontal lobe and parietal lobe. Within the lateral fissure there is additional hidden cortex, the insula. The **central sulcus** is a very important landmark because it lies between the primary motor cortex (area 4) and the primary somatosensory cortex (areas 3, 1, and 2). Note that in the lower figure, area 4 and areas 3, 1, and 2 overlap onto the medial surface of the cortex.

Language (motor aphasia). Area 44 on the posterior end of the inferior frontal gyrus in the left cerebral hemisphere is Broca's area and is responsible for muscular control in normal speech. Damage to area 44 on the left hemisphere results in motor aphasia (or expressive aphasia), of which the individual is unable to speak because of lack of control of the muscles that produce speech. He is, however, able to comprehend what he hears and reads. In complete motor aphasia the individual may be mute. Interestingly, the patient may be capable of swearing.

Receptive aphasia (Wernicke's aphasia). A patient with receptive aphasia cannot understand what he hears or what is being spoken to him. He is able to speak but his speech tends to be meaningless. He frequently uses the wrong word so that what he utters is a confused unintelligible jargon. This occurs when there is damage to Wernicke's area in the left hemisphere. Wernicke's area encompasses a large surface of the parietal and temporal lobes of the left cerebral hemisphere, corresponding approximately to Brodmann's areas 40, 39, and 22. Area 41, which is the primary auditory cortex, lies on the superior temporal gyrus, hidden from view in the lateral fissure. Area 41 receives the auditory projection from the medial geniculate body of the thalamus. Areas 42 and 22, which surround area 41, are the auditory association areas and are necessary for language and sound to be understood. In general, the cortical areas in the left cerebral hemisphere around the lateral fissure (the perisylvian region) are essential for the normal expression, reading, writing, and understanding of language, both spoken and written.

OCCIPITAL LOBE AND VISION. Brodmann divided the occipital cortex into three areas, 17, 18, and 19. Area 17 is the primary **visual cortex** and receives the optic radiation from the lateral geniculate body. Note that in the lower figure, most of area 17 is on the medial surface of the occipital lobe. Area 17 is also called the **striate cortex** because of the prominent white line, the line of Gennari, in its fourth layer. Area 17 is the neural substrate for vision at the conscious level. It is responsible for the visual localization of objects in space, for color perception, and for the three-dimensional appearance of the world about us. Complete destruction of area 17 on one side of the brain will result in a loss of vision in the opposite half of both visual fields, which would be either a right or left hemianopsia. The retinal field loss will be on the same side as the lesion, but the visual field damage, that is, what the patient sees or does not see, is always on the side opposite to where the damage is.

Stimulation of area 17 either electrically by a wire applied directly to the cortex, or by a focal epileptic seizure that begins in area 17, causes the patient to see flashes of light, stars, and color, and geometric forms such as circles, squares, and hexagons. These false perceptions are called **simple visual hallucinations**.

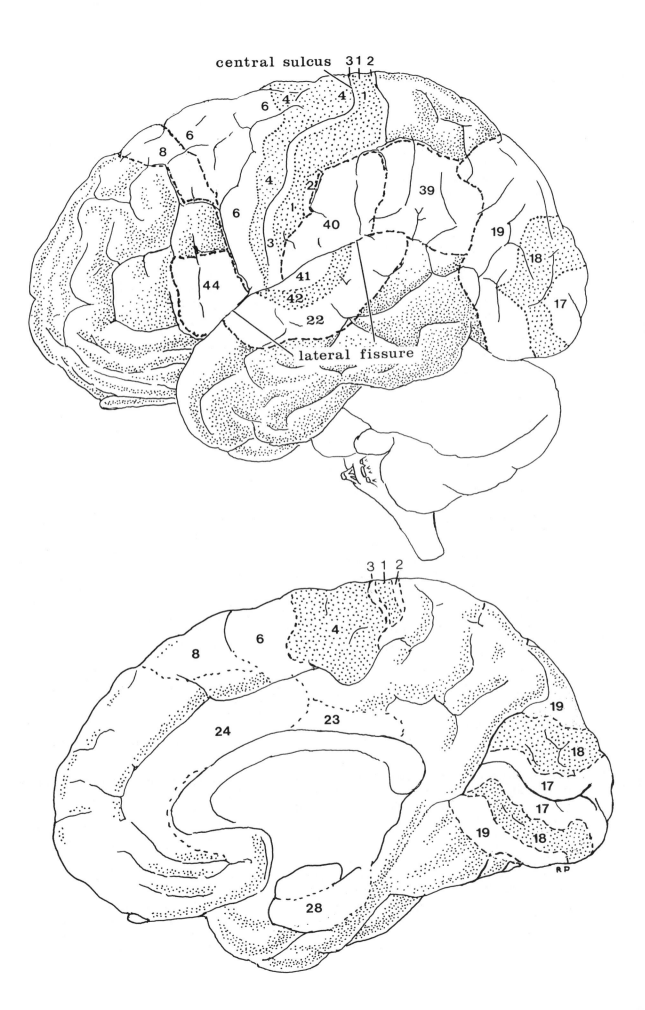

central sulcus 3 1 2

6 4 4 1

6

8

4 2

6 39

4 3 40 19

44 41 18

42 17

22

lateral fissure

3 1 2

4

8 6

19

24 23 18

17

17

19 18

28

RP

Areas 18 and 19 are the visual association areas and are essential for interpreting and understanding what one sees. They integrate the present visual perception with one's past experience and in doing so impart a significance and meaning to the visible world about us. In the simple terms, they inform us and remind us what is good for us and what is bad for us, based on our own past experience. We quickly learn that a lighted match will cause pain if we touch it and that the next time we see one we must avoid touching it. Damage in the visual association areas will resut in **visual agnosia**, in which the person does not understand what he sees. A lighted match to such an individual will merely be something bright, and he may well reach out and touch it. He can see in the sense that the visual perception, a lighted match in this case, reaches the conscious level, but he is not able to tie it in with his memories of lighted matches, fire, and pain. A gold watch held in front of the patient is merely "something shiny." But if the watch is held close enough for him to hear its ticking, he will instantly recognize it as a watch. He may not even be able to recognize his own relatives when he sees them. They are just "people" or "someone" until they speak and he recognizes them by their voices. Looking at an orange will mean nothing, but upon smelling it, recognition is immediate.

THE PARIETAL LOBE. This extends from the central sulcus backward to the occipital lobe. Its most anterior gyrus, the postcentral gyrus (or post-Rolandic gyrus), which lies immediately posterior to the central sulcus, contains Brodmann's areas 3, 1, and 2 and constitutes the primary somatosensory cortex. It is here that sensation from the opposite side of the body is projected in an orderly manner from thalamic nuclei VPL and VPM, so that a topographical cortical representation or a crude image of the contralateral body is formed. Thus the somatosensory cortex contains the sensory homunculus (Latin, little man). The sensory homunculus is the cortical representation of the opposite side of the body in a disproportionate form.

Immediately in front of the central sulcus on the precentral gyrus (pre-Rolandic gyrus) lies the motor homunculus. Because these two critical cortical areas occupy both banks of the central sulcus, one can appreciate the importance of correctly identifying the central sulcus and not injuring it in brain surgery. The somatosensory cortical image (or sensory homunculus) is disproportionate, in that the parts of the body with the greatest sensitivity, such as the fingers, toes, lips, and tongue, have the largest cortical representation; whereas parts of the body such as the back, which is considerably less sensitive, have relatively small cortical areas. The contralateral body is projected in an upside-down fashion, so that the cortical representation of sensation from the pharynx is most inferior and nearest the lateral fissure. Proceeding up the convexity of the postcentral gyrus, the body is projected in the following order: pharynx, tongue, jaws, face, hand, arm, trunk, and thigh. The knee area is at the highest point, and the lower leg and foot are projected onto the paracentral lobule on the vertical medial surface of the hemisphere. Fibers carrying sensation from the skin (cutaneous sensation) end mainly in the anterior lip (area 3) of the somatosensory cortex, whereas fibers carrying sensation from deep receptors end mainly in the posterior part (area 2).

Electrical stimulation of points within the primary somatosensory cortex by neurosurgeons evokes feelings such as itching, tingling, numbness, and a desire to move. These sensations are experienced at the opposite body surface and tend to be sharply localized. Similar feelings are brought on by focal epileptic seizures, which have their irritative source or focus in or near the postcentral gyrus. Following damage to the primary somatosensory cortex, the patient would not be able to precisely feel or discern the nature of a wound to that part of the body, although he would still feel diffuse and burning pain.

Proprioception and the parietal lobe. The parietal lobe as a whole maintains a mental image of the body in terms of where each part of the body is in relation to the rest of the body (position sense or proprioception) as well as where the individual is in relation to his surroundings. The word proprioception is derived from Latin, *proprius* (one's own) and *captus* (comprehension), hence, knowledge of one's own body. Proprioception is a complex mental phenomenon that results from the parietal lobe somehow combining information from multiple sources such as joint receptors, tendon organs, touch receptors, and pressure receptors, and building a mental picture of the opposite side of the body. Following World War I, Holmes and Head examined British soldiers who had suffered parietal lobe damage. They found that these patients could only detect gross movement in their limbs. If the examiner moved a leg or arm while the patient's eyes were closed, the patient could not tell which direction the foot or hand was being moved. He could only feel that the hand or foot was being moved. When given weights to hold, such patients were not able to detect small differences in weights. Two points touching the skin were felt to be one point unless the two points

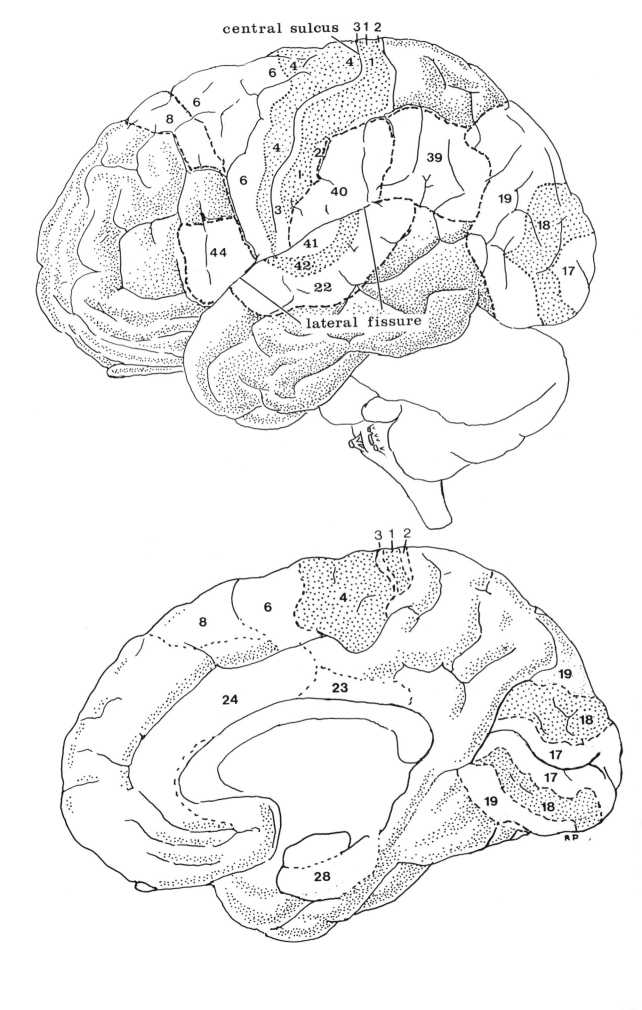

central sulcus

lateral fissure

Touch and the parietal lobe. The sense of touch (or tactile sensation) depends upon an intact parietal lobe. Parietal lobe damage seriously impairs the sense of touch, particularly the ability to use the fingers to identify objects by their shape and texture. This ability is called **stereognosis** (Greek, solid knowledge), and, like proprioception, it depends upon the several sensory modalities such as joint sense, tactile sense, and pressure sense. Loss of this ability, which often occurs in parietal lobe injury, is called **astereognosis.**

Amorphosynthesis. Extensive parietal lobe damage may result in the patient's completely ignoring the opposite side of the body, even to the extent of not dressing that side, or washing it, or shaving it. He may even deny the existence of the affected side and claim that it does not belong to him. This loss of awareness of a part or half of the body is called amorphosynthesis.

THE TEMPORAL LOBE. As mentioned earlier, the temporal lobe contains the primary auditory cortex, area 41 of Brodmann, and the auditory association areas 42 and 22. Focal epileptic seizures that originate in area 41 will begin with an auditory aura that may sound like birds flapping their wings, or wind blowing through the trees, or water cascading over a waterfall.

Experiential hallucinations. Certain types of epilepsy that have their focus in the temporal lobe begin with a strange aura in which the patient feels he is reliving an event from his past. These may take the form of complex visual hallucinations or complex auditory hallucinations or they may be a combination of both. The Canadian neurosurgeon Wilder Penfield was able to induce these hallucinations by electrically stimulating the temporal cortex of epileptics during brain surgery. Under local anesthesia these patients described themselves as being participants in vivid recall of their past. These evoked memories, which Penfield called experiential hallucinations and J. Hughlings Jackson called **dreamy states,** were sometimes frightening childhood experiences.

The dreamy states of J.V. Penfield wrote about one of his patients (J.V.), a 14-year-old girl who had developed seizures at 11. Penfield believed that her seizures were triggered by a terrifying event from her past in which she was accosted by a man with a bag of snakes who threatened to put her in the bag with the snakes.* The hallucination consisted of seeing herself as a little girl of 7 years walking through a field of grass. Suddenly she felt as though someone from behind was going to smother her or hit her on the head and she became terrified. The scene was almost exactly the same in each epileptic attack. At operation the right hemisphere was exposed and a meningo-cerebral cicatrix was found involving the temporal lobe."†

Illusions and altered feelings. In addition to seizure-induced hallucinations, epileptic discharge in the temporal lobe can bring on a variety of seizures in which there is an impairment or alteration of consciousness, but without any motor convulsions. These include distorted perceptions or **illusions,** and **altered feelings.** Illusions may be **visual** in which objects appear larger than they actually are (macropsia), or smaller (micropsia), or appear to move away from the viewer or towards the viewer. There may be a loss of three-dimensional vision, in which everything looks flat. Or the the visual image may persist even with the eyes closed (palinopsia). Objects may even appear to be disproportionately elongated (imagine what this would be like if the patient had a dachshund). The illusions may be **auditory** in which sounds seem abnormally loud, or unreal, or certain words may sound unpleasant.

---

*Epilepsy is due to malfunctioning neurons that fire off uncontrollably. Whether a frightening experience by itself could induce seizures is not clear.
†Penfield W, Perot P: The Brain's Record of Auditory and Visual Experience. Brain 86:595-696, 1963.

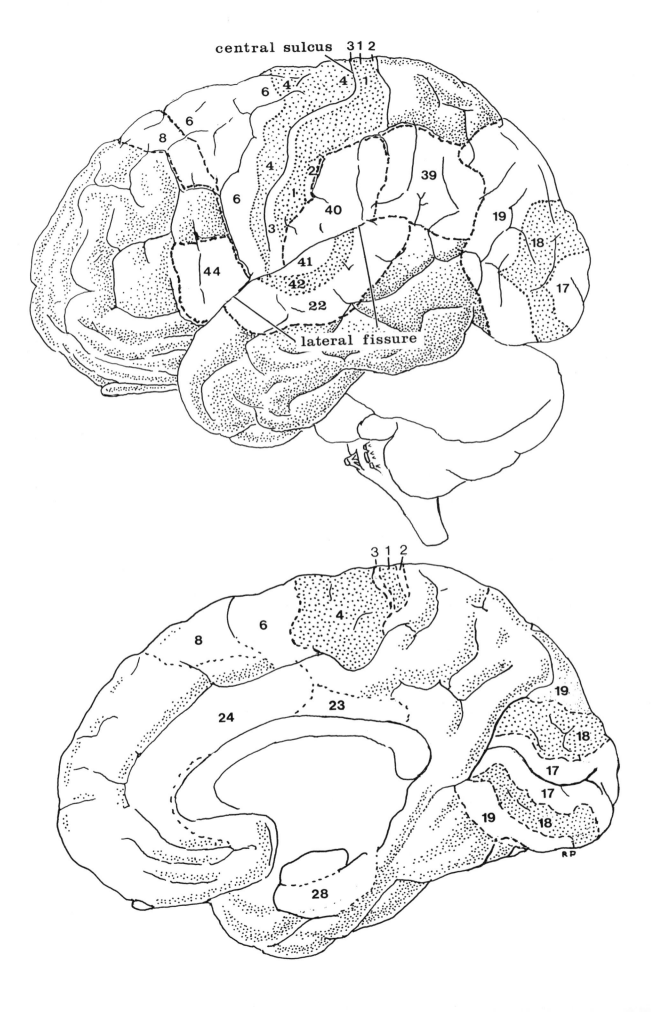

central sulcus 3 1 2

6 4 4 1
6
8
6 4 2
39
6 40
3 19
44 41 18
42
22 17

lateral fissure

3 1 2

8 6 4
24 23 19
18
17
17
28 19 18

R.P.

Altered feelings are sudden feelings such as fear, familiarity (*deja vu*), strangeness (*jamais vu*), and even euphoria (see Figure 130, Dostoyevsky's Epilepsy). An epileptic discharge causing a sudden feeling of dread or fear most likely involves the amygdala, which lies directly beneath the uncinate gyrus on the medial surface of the temporal lobe. Because one part of the amygdala functions in olfaction and the other part in defensive reactions and self preservation, **uncinate seizures** usually consist of an olfactory hallucinations along with an impairment of consciousness, and they frequently have an accompanying feeling of fear. A powerful and inexplicable sense of familiarity (in an unfamiliar situation) or *deja vu* (French, already seen) would appear to be the result of the misfiring of certain temporal lobe neurons that normally are activated only when something familiar is encountered. *Jamais vu* (French, never seen), on the other hand, is a strong sense of unreality or strangeness (even in the company of old acquaintances or in familiar circumstances) that occurs in temporal lobe epilepsy. Most of us have probably experienced fleeting episodes of deja vu at some time in our lives.

THE FRONTAL LOBE reaches its greatest elaboration in the human where it is the largest of the four lobes. The most posterior part of the frontal lobe is the precentral gyrus immediately in front of the central sulcus. It corresponds to area 4 of Brodmann and contains the primary motor cortex, in which the opposite side of the body is represented in the form of a motor homunculus similar in proportion to the sensory homunculus, which lies immediately behind it on the postcentral gyrus. Within the primary motor cortex parts of the body capable of the most complicated movements such as the fingers, toes, lips, and tongue have the largest cortical areas. Stimulation of points within the primary motor cortex causes twitching of small groups of muscles in the opposite side of the body. A seizure that has its focus (starting point) within the primary motor cortex is a **jacksonian fit.** It is triggered by malfunctioning neurons in the primary motor cortex abnormally firing off (all forms of epilepsy are caused by abnormal neurons firing off somewhere in the brain), and exciting a small area of the precentral gyrus. These abnormally excited cortical neurons send a volley of impulses down the brainstem, across the midline, to the opposite side, where they trigger the firing off of alpha motor neurons, which in turn cause a limited group of muscles to twitch.

A more serious affliction is a **jacksonian march,** which also has its focus in the primary motor cortex. However, in this case the wave of excitation spreads across the motor cortex. Seizures such as these often begin with convulsions in the muscles of the thumb, and then spread to the hand and other fingers, and then march up the arm to the shoulder. The convulsions may spread until the entire half of the body is affected. By carefully observing epileptic patients in the latter half of the 1800s, the British neurologist J. Hughlings Jackson, regarded as the founder of modern neurology, was able to arrive at a number of conclusions about the motor cortex that are still valid today. He recorded where each of the seizures began and, after the patients' deaths, examined their brains for any scar or malformation, particularly in the precentral gyrus. By doing this he was able to link where the convulsions began (thumb, lips, etc.) with its representation in the precentral gyrus and was thus able to map out the motor homunculus within the precentral gyrus.

Jacksonian Principles
1. The motor part of the mind resides in the precentral gyrus.
2. Within the precentral gyrus there is an orderly topographical representation of the body.
3. Regions of the body capable of the most complex movements have the largest cortical representation.
4. The motor cortex is connected to the anterior horn cell (alpha motor neuron) by direct and indirect pathways.
5. The major projection of the motor cortex to the anterior horn cell is contralateral.
6. Certain parts of the body receive projections from both cortices.
7. Cortical representation is predominate but not absolute. For example, the thumb region may also have a bit of index finger in it.
8. Areas of the cortex are not exclusively motor or sensory, but rather predominantly motor with some sensory, or predominantly sensory with some motor.

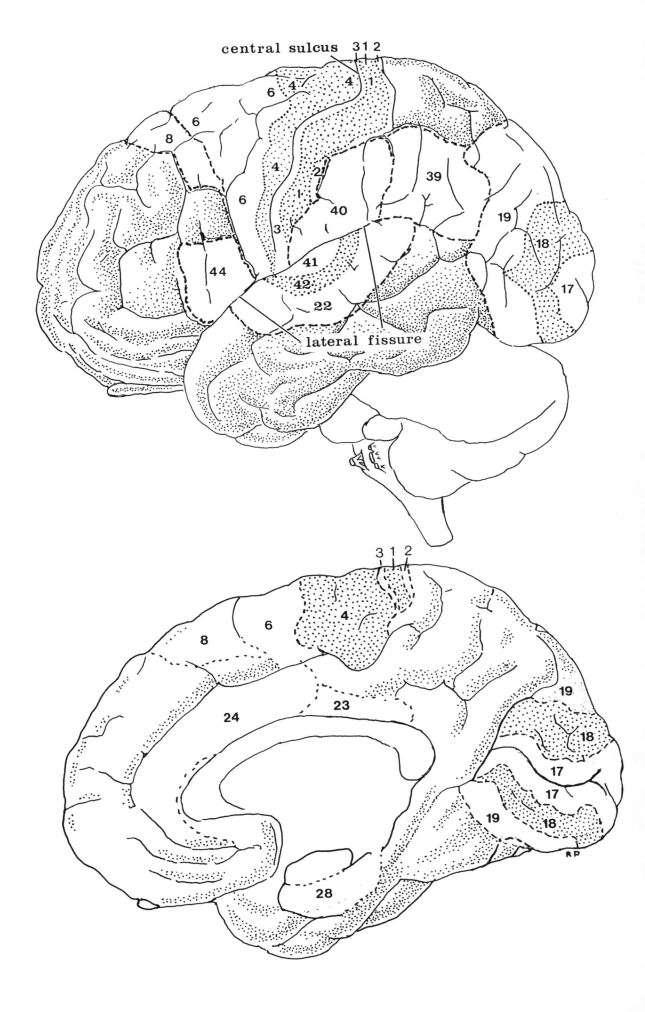

central sulcus 3 1 2

6 4 4 1

6

8 6

4 2

6 I 39

3 40

19

44 41 17

42 18

22 17

lateral fissure

3 1 2

4

8 6

19

24 23 18

17

17

19

28 18

RP

Premotor areas 6 and 8. Movements can also be elicited by stimulating premotor area 6, but these movements are likely to involve more muscles and require stronger stimulation. Area 8 in front of 6 is another premotor area and contains the frontal eye fields. Stimulation in area 8 causes both eyes to turn to the side opposite that of the stimulation.

Prefrontal cortex. An intact prefrontal lobe and prefrontal cortex are essential for certain higher human functions, such as the ability to plan ahead and contemplate the consequences of one's actions, particularly in terms of how they will affect other people. Extensive damage to the prefrontal lobe usually results in the following symptoms: a profound change in one's personality so that one becomes socially indifferent or tactless; an inability to follow an extended course of action; an emotional lability, such as flying into sudden rages or breaking into tears over trifles; and inability to think abstractly. For example, if asked what a proverb means, such as "The pitcher which goes oft to the well gets broken at last," the individual with prefrontal lobe damage would likely say, "But a pitcher can't walk."*

Psychosurgery and prefrontal lobotomy. During the 1950s operations called prefrontal lobotomies were performed on patients in mental hospitals, with the aim of alleviating their incapacitating mental states (the basis for the movie "One Flew Over the Cuckoo's Nest" with Jack Nicholson). These operations consisted mainly of severing the connections between the orbital cortex and the thalamus. With the advent of tranquilizers and other mind-altering drugs, these lobotomies (or leukotomies) are now rarely performed. The most recently performed psychosurgery, although it, too, is no longer done, was the cingulotomy to relieve intractable pain. In this operation the fibers running in the cingulum were cut. This seemed to greatly reduce the overwhelming intensity of the pain. After the operation the patient was still conscious of the pain, but it no longer seemed to bother him. When asked about the pain, he might reply "Oh yea, it's still there. Say, Doc, how did the Red Sox do last night?"

Cerebral dominance. An increasing amount of evidence indicates that the two cerebral hemispheres perform different functions. The comprehension and production of language are located, in the great majority of cases, in the left cerebral hemisphere. The left cerebral hemisphere is regarded as the dominant hemisphere and the right hemisphere as the nondominant hemisphere. More than 95% of right-handed individuals have language dominance in the left hemisphere, and even about 70% of left-handed people have language dominance in the left hemisphere. About 15% of left-handers have language in both hemispheres and 15% have language dominance in the right hemisphere. There are actual anatomical differences between the two hemispheres, especially in the area around the sylvian fissure, which has considerably more cortical tissue than does the right side. In addition to controlling language, the left hemisphere possesses mathematical ability and the ability to solve problems in a logical sequential manner. The right hemisphere appears to be superior in the tasks involving spatial relations, drawing, recognition of human faces, and musical skills. The right hemisphere solves problems in a comphrehensive holistic manner and not in a logical step-by-step manner as the left hemisphere appears to do.

The corpus callosum is the great cerebral commissure of about 300,000,000 fibers that connects the two cerebral hemispheres and informs one hemisphere about what is happening in the other hemisphere. Studies of epileptic patients who have had the corpus callosum and anterior commissure cut (commissurotomized, split-brain procedure) have demonstrated that each half of the brain is capable of some independent function, although the right hemisphere is usually mute and cannot communicate verbally.

---

*Rylander G: Quoted in Gray GW: The great ravelled knot. Scientific American 13:26-39, 1948.

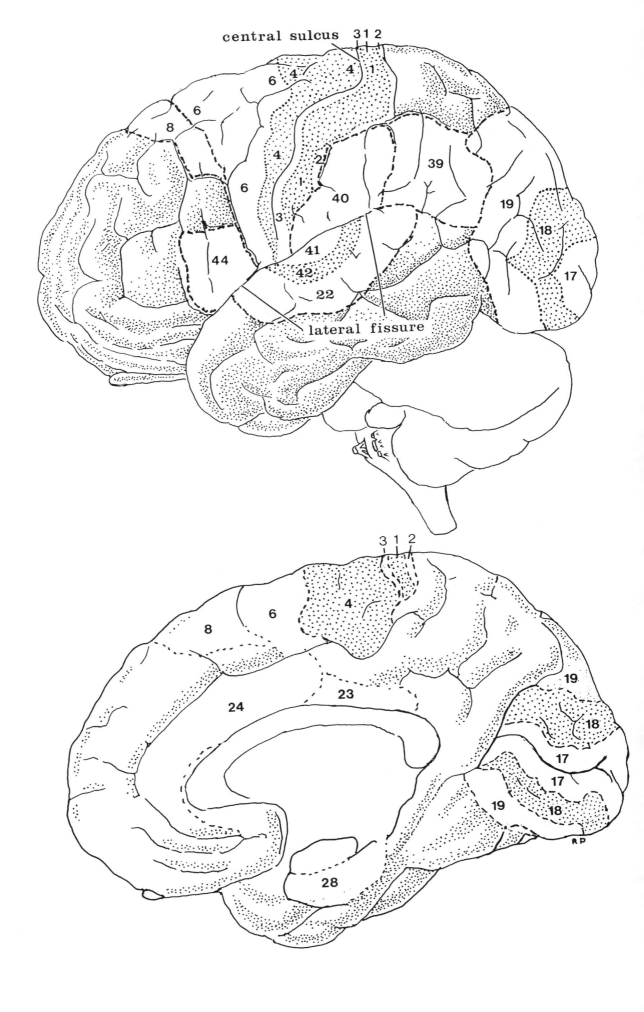

Thalamus meant bedroom or inner chamber in both Latin and Greek. Why the thalamus, which is a solid mass of neurons, should be named a room or chamber is something of a mystery. It probably goes back to the ancients' belief that hollow chambers in the brain stored particles of sensation conveyed to the brain by hollow nerves. The optic nerve supposedly carried particles of vision to its chamber, the optic thalamus. A careful examination of the brain would have revealed to the ancients that the lateral geniculate body, which is that part of the thalamus where the optic nerve ends, is not hollow but rather solid; nor is any other part of the thalamus hollow. Unfortunately the ancients' knowledge of brain anatomy was founded more on doctrine than on actual dissection and examination. For a long time the term **optic thalamus** was used for the thalamus, even after it was shown that it was solid, not hollow. Eventually the "optic" was discarded and the name was shortened to simply thalamus.

Pituitary gland. At one time the pituitary gland was believed to secrete phlegm. Its name is derived from the Latin **pituita**, which meant phlegm. Pituita itself is an onomatope, which means it is imitative of the sound associated with it, which in this case is the sound of spitting, much like our expression "ptooey." The ancients thought that the brain extracted phlegm from the blood. The phlegm was then funneled into the pituitary gland. In fact, the name of the pituitary stalk **infundibulum** means funnel in Latin. From the pituitary gland the phlegm was supposedly conveyed to the roof of the nose, where it migrated through tiny holes in the cribriform plate into the nose.

Ostium (Latin) meant door. It is now used in anatomy for a small opening of a vessel. It is derived from **os** (mouth).

Tectum (Latin) was either a ceiling or a roof. The tectum is that part of the midbrain dorsal to the cerebral aqueduct. The former name for the tectum was **lamina quadrigemina**, the "plate with the quadruplets," that is, the four colliculi.

Colliculus (Latin) meant little hill from collis, hill. **Folia** (Latin) meant leaves. One leaf was a **folium.** The transverse folds of the cerebellar cortex are called folia. **Ramus** (Latin) meant branch. **Arbor** (Latin) meant tree. The **arbor vitae,** "tree of life," was the old name for the white matter in the cerebellum.

Dendrite is derived from the Greek **dendron** (tree) and means little tree or tree-like.

Radix (Latin) meant root. **Radicular** relates to a root. **Radiculitis** means inflammation of a nerve root. A **radical** change is a change so drastic that it gets down to the roots, and may even pull out the roots!

Funiculus (Latin) is derived from **funis** (rope) and meant little rope or string. The white matter of the spinal cord is divided into three funiculi.

Pulivinar (Latin) meant a cushion. **Pulivinar** meant couch. The pulivinar of the thalamus resembles a cushion.

Kline was a bed in ancient Greece. Words such as **clinic, recline, incline** all come from this root. A **clinician** was originally one who visited and treated at the bedside.

Murus (Latin) was a wall. **Intramural** ganglia are groups of nerve cells within the walls of the heart, the intestines, and other viscera. **Intramural** sports are held within the walls of the school or college.

Clinoid process means bed post, being derived from **kline** (bed). The four **clinoid processes** are found in the skull, where they make up part of the **sella turcica** or "Turkish saddle," which holds the pituitary gland.

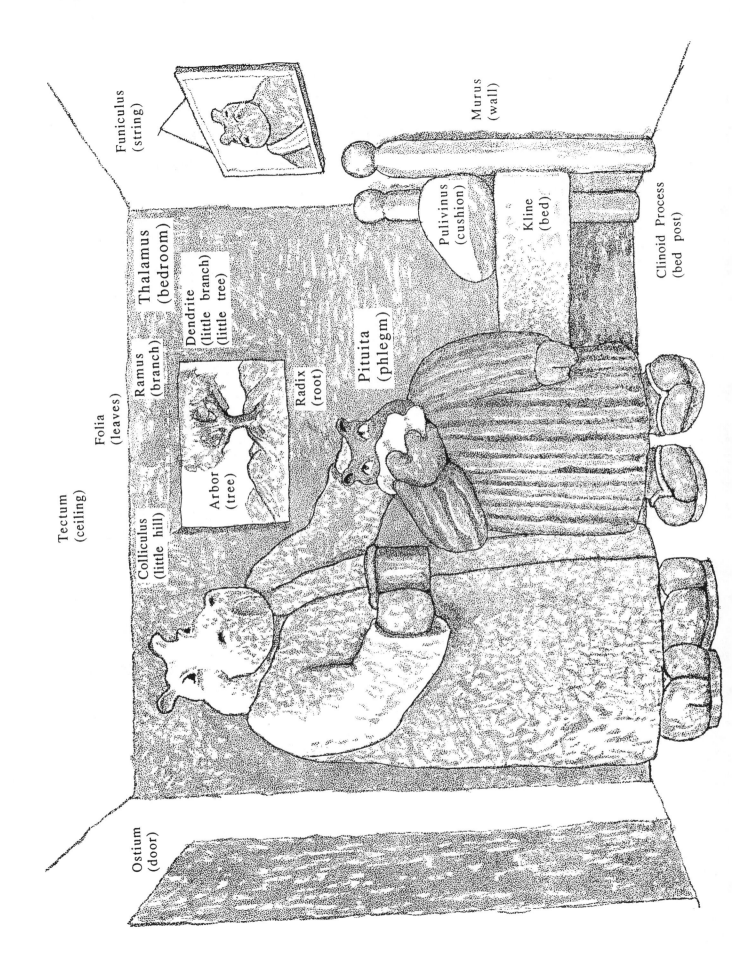

Phineas P. Gage was a railroad worker who, in 1848, miraculously survived an accidental explosion in which a 3 1/2 foot iron bar was blown through his head. A considerable part of his forebrain was destroyed. The profound personality and behavioral changes that Gage displayed following the accident were recorded by Dr. John M. Harlow who treated Gage after his injury. Up to the time of his accident, Gage was a normal, well-liked young man who had never been sick a day in his life. Following this tragic mishap, Harlow noted that Gage had changed drastically, and unlike his previous self he had become stubborn, lacking in sound judgment, inconsistent in his plans, and inconsiderate towards others. In those days practically no one could survive an injury this serious. Gage, however, did not die. He recovered, lived for 12 1/2 more years, and passed away in San Fransico in 1861. Eventually Harlow obtained the skull of Gage along with the iron tamping bar. From Harlow's article and published pictures, it appears that the metal bar passed through the left frontal lobe and that the right frontal lobe may have been spared.

This is a brief summary of Harlow's article

Phineas P. Gage was a foreman of a gang of railroad workers constructing a railroad track near Cavendish, Vermont. On September 13, 1848, while in the act of tamping down an explosive charge of gun powder, his attention was diverted to his men who were working in a pit behind him. He turned his head and at the same time dropped his tamping iron, which "struck fire upon a rock causing the gun powder to explode and shooting the iron bar completely through his head." The iron bar was later found by his men "smeared with blood and brain. The patient was thrown upon his back by the explosion and gave a few convulsive motions of the extremities, but spoke in a few minutes. His men (with whom he was a great favorite) took him in their arms and carried him to his hotel where Gage was attended by Dr. Harlow and another physician.

Harlow found Gage to be "perfectly conscious" and "bearing his suffering with firmness." Gage pointed to the hole in his cheek and said "the iron bar entered here and passed through my head." The tamping iron had apparently entered the left side of his face immediately in front of the angle of the mandible, passed through the back of the left orbit (Gage lost the use of his left eye), then through the left frontal lobe of the brain, and emerged from the top of the skull in the midline at the junction of the frontal bone and the two parietal bones.

In the days immediately following the accident, Harlow held no hope for Gage's recovery. He wrote that "friends and attendants are in hourly expectancy of his death, and have his coffin and clothes in readiness to remove his remains to his native place in Lebanon, New Hampshire. . . . One of his attendants implored me not to do anything more for him as it would only prolong his suffering. . .that if I would only keep away and let him alone, he would die." Harlow, however, continued to treat Gage, dressing and cleaning his wounds three times a day and bathing his face and head with ice water. "With a pair of curved scissors, I cut off the fungi which were sprouting out from the top of the brain and filling the opening, and made free application of caustic to them." On the 32nd day Harlow recorded, "progressing favorably. . . remembers passing and past events correctly, as well before as since the injury. Intellectual manifestations feeble, being exceedingly capricious and childish, but with a will as indomitable as ever; is particularly obstinate, will not yield to restraint when it conflicts with his desires." A month later Harlow noted that Gage continued to improve but "is impatient of restraint, and could not be controlled by his friends." By April of the following year, Harlow is convinced that Gage has recovered his physical health.

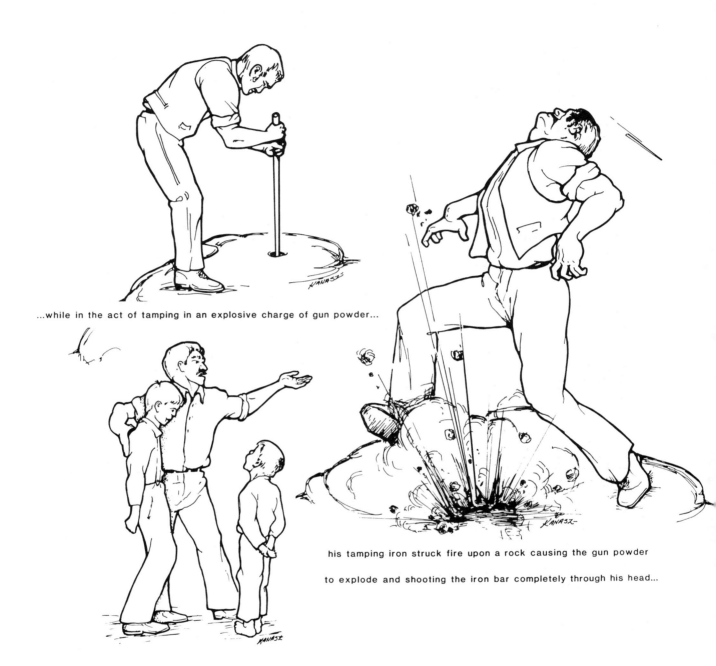

...while in the act of tamping in an explosive charge of gun powder...

his tamping iron struck fire upon a rock causing the gun powder

to explode and shooting the iron bar completely through his head...

...wonderful feats and hairbreadth escapes

without any foundation except in his fancy...

He has no pain in the head, but says he has a queer feeling (in his head) which he is not able to describe. His contractors, who regarded him as the most efficient and capable foreman in their employ previous to his injury, considered the change in his mind so marked that they could not give him his place again. The equilibrium or balance, so to speak, between his intellectual faculties and animal propensities, seems to have been destroyed. He is fitful, irreverent, indulging at times in the grossest profanity (which was not previously his custom), manifesting but little deference for his fellows, impatient of restraint or advice when it conflicts with his desires, at times pertinaciously obstinate, yet capricious and vacillating, devising many plans for future operation, which are no sooner arranged than they are abandoned in turn for others appearing more feasible. A child in his intellectual capacity and manifestation, he has the animal passions of a strong man. Previous to his injury, though untrained in the schools, he possessed a well-balanced mind....In this regard, his mind was radically changed, so that his friends and acquaintances said he was no longer Gage.

After his accident Gage displayed peculiar child-like quirks, such as regaling his nephews and nieces with "the most fabulous recitals of his wonderful feats and hair-breadth escapes without any foundation except in his fancy. He conceived a great fondness for pets and souvenirs, especially for children, horses, and dogs, only exceeded by his attachment for his tamping iron, which was his constant companion during the remainder of his life."

In spite of the profound behavioral and personality changes, Gage lived an independent and productive life in his remaining 12 1/2 years. He worked with horses in New Hampshire and then spent 8 years in Chile running a stage coach line. In 1859, his health began to fail and he left Chile for San Francisco, where his mother and sister were then living. After arriving in San Francisco, his health improved and he worked there as a farm laborer. However, his health once again began to fail and he died on May 21, 1861 after a series of epileptic convulsions. As for Gage's survival and Harlow's account of it, many physicians of the day refused to believe the story when they first heard it. On June 3, 1866 Harlow gave a lecture to the Massachusetts Medical Society in which he demonstrated the skull and the tamping iron to his audience. He concluded his lecture with these words, "I can only say in conclusion, with good old Ambrose Pare, 'I dressed him, God healed him' ". Harlow donated both the skull and tamping iron to the medical museum at Harvard.

Harlow JM: Recovery from the passage of an iron bar through the head. Publications of the Massachusetts Medical Society 2:320-347, 1868.

Figure drawn by Joseph Kanasz.

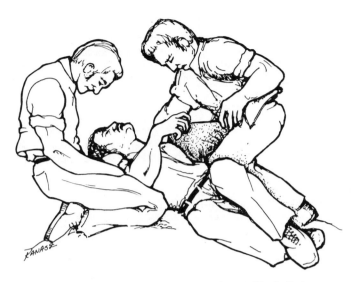

his men (with whom he was a great favorite) took him in their arms......

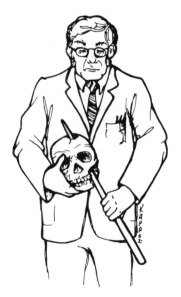

...his mind was radically changed so

decidedly that his friends and acquaintances said

he was "no longer Gage"......I dressed him, God healed him.

One of the most moving and personal accounts of epilepsy was written by the Russian author Feodor Mikhailovich Dostoyevsky (1821–1881), who was an epileptic. In his novels and his letters he describes an intensely beautiful feeling he experienced at the onset of his seizures. This peculiar sensation, which signals the beginning of a seizure, is called the aura (Latin, breeze) and may be auditory, visual, or olfactory, depending on where in the brain the malfunctionong neurons are firing off. In Dostoyevsky's case, his seizures were preceded by an overwhelming euphoria.

In *The Idiot* the principal character, Prince Muichine, suffers from epileptic attacks very similar to those of the author. In the following passage from *The Idiots,* the prince reflects on his seizures and gives the reader an insight into Dostoyevsky's own experience.

> He remembered among other things that he always had one minute just before the epileptic fit (if it came on while he was awake), when suddenly in the midst of sadness and oppression, there seemed a sudden flash of light in his brain and with extraordinary impetus all his vital forces seemed to swell to their greatest powers. The sense of life, the awareness of self, were increased ten fold at these moments which passed like a flash of lightning. His mind and his heart were flooded with extraordinary light; all his worries, all his doubts, all his anxieties were relieved at once; they were all merged into a lofty calm, full of serene, harmonious joy and hope. But these moments, these flashes were only the prelude of that final second (it was never more than a second) with which the fit began. That second was, of course, unendurable.

The prince further reflects. "What if it is disease? What does it matter that it is an abnormal intensity, if the result, if the moment of sensation, remembered and analysed afterwards in health, turns out to be the summation of harmony and beauty, and gives a feeling, unknown and unperceived 'til then, of completeness, of harmony, of reconciliation, and of rapturous ardent love merging into the highest synthesis of life?"

Dostoyevsky described a particular seizure he experienced while serving a prison term in Siberia after being arrested and convicted for illegal reformist activities. One day he had the unexpected joy of receiving a visit from one of his best friends. It was Easter Eve, and the two friends, though it was late, continued to talk and, like the true Russians they were (Russians of that time), the subject was God. Suddenly Dostoyevsky exclaimed: "God exists, He exists." At the same time from a nearby church a bell began to toll for the midnight mass. Dostoyevsky recalled: "The air was filled with a big noise and I couldn't move. I felt that heaven had come down upon the earth and engulfed me. I felt I had touched God. He seemed to come into my body. 'Yes, God exists,' I cried, and I don't remember anything else. You all, healthy people, can't imagine the happiness which we epileptics feel during the second before our fit. . . . I would not exchange it for all the joys that life may bring."

Alajounine T: Dostoyevsky's epilepsy. Brain 86(Part 2):14, 1963.

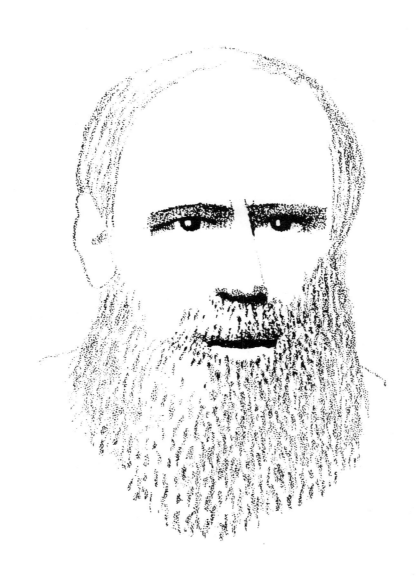

FEODOR MIKHAILOVICH DOSTOYEVSKY

INDEX

Entries are indexed to figure numbers. See figures for anatomical detail.